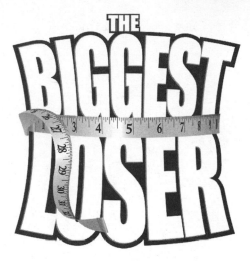

# Complete Calorie Counter

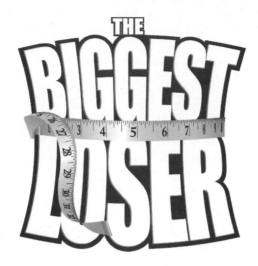

# Complete Calorie Counter

**The Quick and Easy Guide to Thousands of Foods
from Grocery Stores and Popular Restaurants
—As Seen on NBC's Hit Show!**

**Cheryl Forberg, RD,
and *The Biggest Loser* Experts and Cast
Foreword by Michael Dansinger, MD**

RODALE

© 2006 by Universal Studios Licensing LLLP. *The Biggest Loser*tm and NBC Studios, Inc., and Reveille LLC. All rights reserved.

Rodale books may be purchased for business or promotional use or for special sales. For information, please write to:
Special Markets Department,
Rodale Inc., 733 Third Avenue, New York, NY 10017

Printed in the United States of America

Rodale Inc. makes every effort to use acid-free ∞, recycled paper ♲.

Interior design by Christina Gaugler
Cover design by Christopher Rhoads

ISBN-13 978–1–59486–595–4 paperback
ISBN-10 1–59486–595–7 paperback

Distributed to the trade by Holtzbrinck Publishers

2    4    6    8    10    9    7    5    3    1    paperback

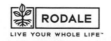

We inspire and enable people to improve their lives and the world around them

For more of our products visit **rodalestore.com** or call 800-848-4735

Product Development & Direction: Chad Bennett, Dave Broome, Cindy Chang, Mark Koops, Kim Niemi
Project Coordinator: Neysa Gordon

NBCU, Reveille, and 25/7 Productions would like to thank the many people who gave their time and energy to this project:

3 Ball Productions, Stephen Andrade, Sean Bangert, Keith Biery, *The Biggest Loser* Contestants, Scot Chastain, Elayne Cilic, Hope Clarke, Tami Booth Corwin, Dr. Michael Dansinger, Lisa Dolin, Milissa Douponce, Kat Elmore, John Farrell, Dawn Fiore, Cheryl Forberg, Kurt B. Ford, Jeff Gaspin, Chris Gaugler, Linda Gilbert, Beth Goss, Marc Graboff, Erica Gruen, Bob Harper, Heather Halloway, Kim Hedland, Dr. Robert Huizenga, Frederick Huntsberry, Helen Jorda, Allison Kaz, Jessica Kirby, Laura Kuhn, Beth Lamb, Roni Lubliner, Kim Lyons, Vince Manze, Rebecca Marks, John Miller, Kam Naderi, Todd Nelson, Jennifer O'Connell, Carole Panick, Joanne Park, Trae Patton, Liz Perl, Jerry Petry, Craig Plestis, Kevin Reilly, Chris Rhoads, Lindsay Rickel, Beth Roberts, J. D. Roth, Lauren Santiago, Leslie Schneider, Ben Silverman, Charles Steenveld, Lee Straus, Amy Super, Deborah Thomas, Matt Vassallo, Brian Wendel, Bob Wright, Yong Yam, Jeff Zucker

# Contents

# Preface

Calories, calories everywhere! The world around us often seems to be overflowing with high-calorie foods. Over the past several decades, the food in our grocery stores, local restaurants, shopping malls, and even our homes has changed dramatically, and often for the worse. If we don't know what we're doing—if we fail to master a practical eating strategy for good health—most of us will succumb to the temptations of unhealthy, high-calorie, appetite-stimulating food. If we let our guard down for too long, most of us will eat far too many calories, pile on excess body fat, and develop medical problems caused by obesity.

Let this calorie-counting guide help you take and keep control! Let it serve as one of your greatest tools for beating obesity and eating healthily! Any eating strategy that produces weight and fat loss ultimately reduces daily caloric intake—the greater the caloric reduction, the greater the weight and body fat loss. Combined with the state-of-the-art eating and exercise advice in *The Biggest Loser: The Weight-Loss Program to Transform Your Body, Health, and Life*, this calorie counter can be used to develop and fine-tune a personal eating strategy that leaves you both satisfied and healthy.

Set a daily calorie budget and then record your daily food and beverage intake. The Biggest Loser Diet calls for 7 calories per pound of current body weight until you reach your target weight. (If you weigh over 300 pounds, count 300 pounds as your starting "weight" for this formula. Likewise, count 150 pounds as your starting "weight" if you currently weigh less than 150 pounds.) Twelve calories per pound will usually maintain your target body weight. Faithfully keeping a calorie budget or limit will teach you to work toward discovering the most favorable foods for your eating strategy—those that leave you most satisfied without breaking the caloric bank. Exploring new food and recipe possibilities is one key toward mastering this approach. Another key is recognizing and avoiding appetite-stimulating foods (usually processed foods with high starch, sugar, and/or fat content) and trigger foods that lead to excessively large portions.

Change your food environment! As you learn which foods work best for you, make sure they are around when you need them. Eat these foods at home, and whenever possible, bring them with you when you work or travel. Similarly, keep your trigger foods out of your home environment whenever possible.

Become a role model! I have such great respect and admiration for everybody out there who has taken the plunge and given it their all—they are role models for all of us. Talk to everyone and anyone you can find who has learned how to keep the weight off. Listen to their stories, learn from their experiences, and let *The Biggest Loser Complete Calorie Counter* help you follow their lead. Success comes once you decide you'll never give up trying. I wish you great success and excellent health for many years to come.

Sincerely,
Michael Dansinger, MD
Weight-Loss, Nutrition, and Fitness Team, *The Biggest Loser*
Director, Tufts Popular Diet Trial
Tufts-New England Medical Center
Boston, Massachusetts

# Acknowledgments

I have many colleagues and friends to thank for helping me write this book. Susan Bowerman, MS, RD, of the UCLA Center for Human Nutrition, and Dr. Rob Huizenga, of Robertson Diagnostic in Beverly Hills, were not only supportive but also instrumental by introducing me to the weight loss phenomena and the NBC program called *The Biggest Loser*. Dr. Huizenga's endless flow of brilliant ideas is a constant source of inspiration to me—thank you, Rob!

Dr. Michael Dansinger, director of Clinical Studies and Obesity Research at Tufts-New England Medical Center, has been steadfast with his guidance and support—thank you, Michael!

I am eternally grateful to Chad Bennett and Mark Koops, of Reveille, for all of the incomparable opportunities they afford me—thank you, my friends. I cannot say enough.

Many kind thanks to Dave Broome of 25/7 Productions, JD Roth, and many colleagues at 3 Ball Productions who have provided generous support to my work with *The Biggest Loser* program.

My heartfelt gratitude to my good friend Marie Chrabaszewski, RD, of Los Angeles, who has been generous with insightful suggestions and in helping me analyze the thousands of foods in this book.

Thanks to our trainers, Bob Harper and Kim Lyons, who dedicate themselves tirelessly to the contestants and to the show. My special thanks to Bob for his creative food suggestions to include in this book.

Amy Super at Rodale lives up to her name. Thank you for your sage advice, your brilliant ideas, and mostly for believing in me. I am so proud to be working with you.

Biggest thanks to *The Biggest Loser* contestants—past and present, onscreen and offscreen. You all have such amazing stories; it has been a gift to know you and to work with each of you. Without you, this book wouldn't have been written. With you, a nation is inspired—thank you!

# The Biggest Loser Calorie Counter

If you've ever wondered why some people are able to shed those pounds and keep them off, it's probably because they know the five secrets to lasting weight loss.

1. They eat breakfast.
2. They eat fruit and/or vegetables with each meal.
3. They have protein with each meal and snack.
4. They're physically active.
5. They plan their meals, their snacks, and their exercise.

Counting calories alone isn't the answer, but it is an important factor in this winning equation. *The Biggest Loser Complete Calorie Counter* is an indispensable part of your successful weight loss plan.

Carry *The Biggest Loser Complete Calorie Counter* wherever you go. You may even want an extra copy to keep at work or in your car. Is every food in this book a part of the Biggest Loser Weight Loss Plan? No. The numbers will jump off the page for the foods you shouldn't be having. But we all have weak moments now and then. When you do, you'll still be able to record everything you eat by looking it up in this book (and make up for any indulgences by overcompensating at your next workout or undercompensating at your next meal).

# THE BIGGEST LOSER DIET IN A NUTSHELL

Before explaining how to use this guide, here's a brief review of the Biggest Loser Weight Loss Plan. It's based on two principles.

- With a regular exercise program in place, you must burn off more calories than you take in each day.
- Your recommended daily caloric intake for weight loss is made up of about 45 percent carbohydrate calories, 30 percent lean protein calories, and 25 percent healthy fat calories.

These guidelines are not meant to replace the advice of your personal health care provider. Please consult with him or her for specific guidelines tailored to your situation and medical condition.

## Carbohydrates

Carbohydrates include vegetables, fruits, and whole grains. Each gram of carbohydrate contains 4 calories. Aim for a minimum of 4 cups of a variety of nondried fruits and nonstarchy vegetables daily. Favor fruits and vegetables over grain products, choose whole grain foods in moderation, and select whole grain foods with a high fiber content.

## Vegetables

Vegetables should make up the majority of your carbohydrate intake.

- Cook your vegetables for the minimal amount of time possible to preserve nutrients.
- Avoid added fat; steam, grill, or stir-fry veggies in a nonstick pan.
- Try to eat at least one raw vegetable each day.

- Eat a vegetable salad most days of the week.
- Plan ahead. Keep cut-up vegetables such as bell peppers, broccoli, and jicama in your fridge for easy snacking at home or to take to work or school.
- Starchier vegetables such as pumpkin, winter squash, and sweet potatoes are higher in calories and carbs, so you should limit them to a serving or two per week.
- Fresh vegetables are best, but it's okay to choose frozen. If you opt for canned, watch the sodium content; you'll need to rinse the veggies before cooking them.

### Fruit

Fruit is naturally sweet, refreshing, and delicious. Be sure to enjoy at least one raw fruit each day and try a new fruit each week to add variety to your menu.

- Savor fruits from different color groups—dark green, light green, orange, purple, red, and yellow. This ensures you're getting a variety of nutrients each day.
- Avoid dried fruits, such as dried berries and raisins. They're more concentrated in calories and sugar, and they're not as filling as their raw counterparts.
- Choose whole fruit over fruit juices. Fruit juice contains less fiber so it's not as filling as whole fruit, and it's more concentrated in sugars. When you do choose juice, a serving size is 4 ounces (½ cup).
- Fresh fruits are preferable, but frozen is fine if it is not packaged with sugar or syrup. If you choose canned, be sure it is packed in water, not syrup.

## Whole Grains

Whole grains have undergone minimal processing and thus are more nutritious. When whole grains are refined, important nutrients are removed. All that's usually left is starch, which is loaded with carbohydrate calories and little else.

- When choosing bread products, check out the label first. If the label says "enriched," it probably contains white flour, meaning it's low in fiber and nutrition.
- Choose breads with at least 2 grams of fiber per serving.
- The first ingredient listed should be "whole wheat" or "whole grain." If the label says "wheat flour," you may want to make a different choice. Wheat flour is enriched flour with some whole wheat added.
- Most packaged breakfast cereals are highly processed and loaded with sugar. Try to choose packaged cereals with less than 5 grams of sugar and at least 5 grams of fiber per serving.

## Protein

On the Biggest Loser Diet, approximately 30 percent of your daily calorie intake will come from lean proteins. Each gram of protein contains around 4 calories. Remember to include protein with each meal and each snack so your body can use it throughout the day. There's plenty to choose from in three different protein groups: animal protein, low-fat (or fat-free) dairy protein, and vegetarian protein.

- Choose a variety of proteins each day in order to meet your calorie goal.

- Limit your servings of lean red meat to twice a week. Red meat tends to be higher in saturated fat.
- Fish is an excellent source of protein, omega-3 fatty acids, vitamin E, and selenium. Cold-water fish (such as salmon, mackerel, and herring) contain more hearty-healthy fats—though they also have more calories.
- Avoid processed meats, such as bologna, hot dogs, and sausage; they're generally high in fat and calories. If you do indulge in these meats, try to find products that are nitrate-free. Nitrates can react with foods in your stomach to form potentially cancer-causing compounds.

## Protein Sources

**Meat:** Choose lean cuts of meat, such as pork tenderloin and lean cuts of beef including round, chuck, sirloin, and tenderloin. USDA choice or USDA select grades of beef usually have lower fat content. Avoid meat that is heavily marbled, and remove any visible fat. Try to find ground meat that is at least 95 percent lean.

**Poultry:** The leanest poultry is the skinless white meat from the breast of chicken or turkey. When choosing ground chicken or turkey, ask for the white meat and try to avoid dark meat from the thigh and wing. Egg whites are an excellent source of protein and are fat free.

**Seafood:** Try to choose fish rich in omega-3 fatty acids. These fish include salmon, sardines (water-packed), herring, mackerel, trout, and tuna. Indulge in shark and swordfish sparingly, as these fish have been shown to have high levels of mercury.

## THE BIGGEST LOSER TIPS FOR SUCCESS

- Plan meals in advance.
- Schedule your three small meals plus two or three small snacks every day. Skipping meals leads to excess hunger, extreme eating, and extra calories.
- Pay attention to your portion sizes.
- Minimize saturated fats, trans fats, added sugars, processed foods, and excess salt.
- Record all meals in a food journal.
- Drink at least eight 8-ounce glasses of water a day.
- Exercise daily according to the recommendations of your personal trainer and/or physician.

**Dairy:** Top choices include skim (fat-free) milk, low-fat (1%) milk, buttermilk, plain fat-free (or low-fat) yogurt, fat-free (or low-fat) yogurt with fruit (no sugar added), fat-free (or low-fat) cottage cheese, and fat-free or low-fat ricotta cheese. Light soy milks and soy yogurts are also good choices. Avoid full-fat dairy products, such as whole milk and sauces made with heavy cream.

**Vegetarian Protein:** Excellent sources of vegetarian protein include beans, legumes, and a variety of soy foods. Many of these healthy proteins are also loaded with fiber, which aids your digestion and helps you feel full after eating.

### Healthy Fats

On the Biggest Loser Diet, approximately 25 percent of your calories should come from fat. Each gram of fat contains 9 calories. Many of these fat calories will be hidden in your carbohydrate and protein food choices. You will have a small budget of leftover calories to spend on healthy fat and "extras." Healthy fats include an occasional spray or splash of olive oil or canola oil for your salads or cooked dishes. It also includes healthy fats from small servings of nuts and seeds.

## Extras

Many of the Biggest Losers like to allocate a small number (100 to 150) of calories each day for "extras." Try to spend these on healthy food choices instead of candy or sweets. Your meals should mostly be made of whole foods, with less emphasis on "diet-food" substitutes.

## HOW TO USE *THE BIGGEST LOSER COMPLETE CALORIE COUNTER*

The first thing you'll need to know is, how big is a serving size? Weighing and measuring food is extremely important to calculate an accurate number of your daily calories. For this, you will need:

- A liquid measuring cup (2-cup capacity)
- A set of dry measuring cups (1 cup, ½ cup, ⅓ cup, and ¼ cup)
- Measuring spoons (1 tablespoon, 1 teaspoon, ½ teaspoon, and ¼ teaspoon)
- Food scale
- Calculator

Be sure that your food scale measures grams. (A gram is very small, about ⅟₂₈ ounce.) Most of your weight measurements will be in ounces, but certain foods, such as nuts, are very concentrated in calories, so a portion size will be much smaller. Food scales range in price from a few dollars to $30 or more. Digital scales are often more accurate, but they tend to be a little more expensive. In the end, any scale that measures grams will do.

## Getting Started

If you like having your cereal in your favorite bowl each morning, measure ½ cup (or your designated serving size) into the bowl. Then measure the milk in the liquid measuring cup and pour it on your cereal. Take a mental picture and remember how this looks. That way, you won't have to measure every single time. No more quart-size bowls of cereal; your food portions are now smaller, and soon, your clothes will be, too.

For consistency, weigh and measure your food *after* cooking. A food's weight can change dramatically when cooked. For example, 4 ounces of boneless skinless chicken breast has around 130 calories when raw. When it's cooked, it'll weigh closer to 3 ounces but will have nearly the same caloric content. The same holds true for vegetables and other cooked foods. Dry cereals or grains, on the other hand, can double or even triple in volume after being cooked with water.

After measuring all of your foods for a week or so, you'll be able to make fairly accurate estimates without having to measure everything each time you eat. Of course you'll always need to weigh and measure when trying a new food for the first time, so keep your measuring tools in a handy location. Over time, you'll know what's just right for you, whether you're cooking a meal in your own kitchen or deciding how much of your entrée to eat in a restaurant—and how much of it to wrap up and take home! But in the beginning, you'll need a few tools so that you can get it just right.

If you're not accustomed to spending time in the kitchen, the following conversion table may be helpful for you.

## CONVERSION TABLE FOR MEASURING PORTION SIZES

| TEASPOON | TABLESPOON | CUPS | PINTS/QUARTS/ GALLONS | FLUID OUNCE | MILLILITER |
|---|---|---|---|---|---|
| ¼ teaspoon | | | | | 1 ml |
| ½ teaspoon | | | | | 2 ml |
| 1 teaspoon | ⅓ tablespoon | | | | 5 ml |
| 3 teaspoons | 1 tablespoon | ¹⁄₁₆ cup | | 0.5 oz | 15 ml |
| 6 teaspoons | 2 tablespoons | ⅛ cup | | 1 oz | 30 ml |
| 12 teaspoons | 4 tablespoons | ¼ cup | | 2 oz | 60 ml |
| 16 teaspoons | 5 ⅓ tablespoons | ⅓ cup | | 2.5 oz | 75 ml |
| 24 teaspoons | 8 tablespoons | ½ cup | | 4 oz | 125 ml |
| 32 teaspoons | 10 ⅔ tablespoons | ⅔ cup | | 5 oz | 150 ml |
| 36 teaspoons | 12 tablespoons | ¾ cup | | 6 oz | 175 ml |
| 48 teaspoons | 16 tablespoons | 1 cup | ½ pint | 8 oz | 237 ml |
| | | 2 cups | 1 pint | 16 oz | 473 ml |
| | | 3 cups | | 24 oz | 710 ml |
| | | 4 cups | 1 quart | 32 oz | 946 ml |
| | | 8 cups | ½ gallon | 64 oz | |
| | | 16 cups | 1 gallon | 128 oz | |

Remember that an ounce of *weight* is not the same as a *fluid* ounce. You cannot convert the two without knowing the density of the ingredient you are measuring.

Some of the foods in the lists in this book will provide calories based on a measured or cup amount. Others will provide calories based on weight, such as an ounce or more.

Your calculator will be indispensable for adding your daily calories in a hurry. But sometimes the portion size you desire may be different than the portion size provided in the food list. You may have to do a little multiplication or division to find the perfect fit. This is great practice for the real world because you will rarely find your ideal portion sizes when you dine out.

## Food Journal

Keeping a food journal is paramount to a successful weight loss plan. It will help you identify the times that you eat certain things, allowing you to learn from your eating patterns. It is imperative to keep track of the number of calories you take in (and burn off through exercise) each day, especially when you're just getting started.

Buy a notebook and a pen just for this purpose. Keep them in your desk, your handbag, your backpack, or wherever is handy or most convenient for you. Take notes throughout the day, because it's easy to forget an unplanned snack or tasting. Find a routine, a favorite place, and a time to record in your journal. This is one of the biggest keys to your success. On the opposite page, we've included a sample format for a food journal. If you're feeling a bit more high-tech, go ahead and record your food intake on your computer. Just pick a method that's easy and convenient for you.

# THE BIGGEST LOSER SAMPLE FOOD JOURNAL PAGE

|  | CALORIES | CARB (45%) | PRO (30%) | FAT (25%) |
|---|---|---|---|---|
| Sample Goal | 1200 | 540 | 360 | 300 |

| MEAL/TIME | FOOD | CALORIES | CARB | PRO | FAT |
|---|---|---|---|---|---|
|  |  |  |  |  |  |
|  |  |  |  |  |  |
|  |  |  |  |  |  |
|  |  |  |  |  |  |
|  |  |  |  |  |  |
|  | Totals |  |  |  |  |
|  | Goal Totals |  |  |  |  |
|  | + /− |  |  |  |  |

## How to Read Labels

As you page through *The Biggest Loser Complete Calorie Counter*, you'll notice that some of your favorite packaged foods are missing from the food lists. That's because labels on packaged foods will provide all of the information you need.

Manufacturers are required to provide information on nutrients under a food label's "Nutrition Facts" panel. When you're shopping for healthy foods, labels can help you choose between similar products based on calories and certain nutrients (such as fat or protein).

**Serving size:** Serving size is the most important piece of information. Everything else on the label is based on the serving size. Some products (especially bottled sodas and beverages) may appear to be single-serving, but they can hold two or more servings; be sure to check carefully. Also, if a food label gives a serving size as 1 cup, that doesn't necessarily mean that it's the right serving size for your weight loss goals. Look at the calories and fat before you decide. If you need to, cut the serving size in half (or double it).

# Nutrition Facts
Serving Size
Servings Per Container

**Amount Per Serving**

**Calories** 0        Calories from Fat 0

**% Daily Value***

| | |
|---|---|
| **Total Fat** 0g | **0%** |
| Saturated Fat 0g | **0%** |
| Polyunsaturated Fat 0g | |
| Monounsaturated Fat 0g | |
| **Cholesterol** 0mg | **0%** |
| **Sodium** 0mg | **0%** |
| **Total Carbohydrate** 0g | **0%** |
| Dietary Fiber 0g | **0%** |
| Sugars 0g | |
| **Protein** 0g | |

Vitamin A 0%    •    Vitamin C 0%

Calcium 0%    •    Iron 0%

* Percent Daily Values are based on a 2,000 calorie diet. Your daily values may be higher or lower depending on your calorie needs:

| | | Calories: | 2,000 | 2,500 |
|---|---|---|---|---|
| Total Fat | Less than | | 0g | 0g |
| Sat Fat | Less than | | 0g | 0g |
| Cholesterol | Less than | | 0mg | 0mg |
| Sodium | Less than | | 0mg | 0mg |
| Total Carbohydrate | | | 0g | 0g |
| Dietary Fiber | | | 0g | 0g |

**Calories:** Before you record the number of calories on the label into your food journal, be sure it corresponds with your actual serving size. If the label says a serving is 1 cup and you're having 2 cups, double the calories you record in your food journal.

*Reduced-calorie* means the food contains at least 25 percent fewer calories than the regular version. *Low-calorie* means it has no more than 40 calories per serving (except sugar substitutes). *Calorie-free* means that a food has less than 5 calories per serving.

**Fat:** This number is determined by totaling the grams of saturated fat, polyunsaturated fat, and monounsaturated fat. *Reduced-fat* products have 25 percent less fat than the regular counterpart, *light* means a product has 50 percent less fat, *low-fat* means there are no more than 3 grams of fat per serving, and *fat-free* means that a product contains no more than a half gram of fat per serving. Pay special attention to the calories on lighter, reduced, low-fat, and fat-free products. When the fat is removed from many recipes, salt or sugar are sometimes added back to make sure there's still plenty of flavor. This can result in a fat-free or low-fat product that actually has *more* calories than the regular version. Be careful!

**Saturated fat:** Saturated fat is fat that is solid at room temperature. Most saturated fats are derived from animal products, though a few plant oils such as coconut and palm oil are also saturated. Examples of saturated fat include butter, chicken skin, visible fat on meats, lard, and shortening. Less than one-third of your daily fat grams should be from saturated fats, as the saturated fat from animal foods is the primary source of cholesterol in American diets.

**Sodium:** For most people, the daily recommendation for sodium is 2,400 milligrams. *Light in sodium* means this product has half the sodium of its counterparts.

**Total carbohydrate:** This number is calculated by totaling the grams of complex carbohydrates, fiber, and sugar. If the total carbohydrate is more than double the amount of sugars, that means there are more "good carbs," which help tame your hunger.

**Dietary fiber:** Fiber is found in plant foods but not in animal foods. *High-fiber* means that one serving has at least 5 grams of dietary fiber. *Good source of fiber* means the food product has 2.5 to 4.9 grams of fiber per serving. *More fiber* or *added fiber* on the label means the product has at least 2.5 grams of fiber per serving. Unless you're on a fiber-restricted diet, aim for at least 25 to 35 grams of fiber per day.

**Sugar:** The grams of sugar in a food can be naturally occurring, added, or both. Check the ingredient list to find out. The total grams of carbohydrate in a food serving should be more than twice the amount of sugar grams. *Reduced-sugar* means that a food contains at least 25 percent less sugar per serving than the regular version. Be careful with this because some products, such as cereals, sport this label because some of the sugar has been replaced with other carbs. The caloric content may be the same, so there isn't necessarily a huge improvement. *Sugar-free* means there's less than half a gram of sugar per serving.

**Protein:** If a food has more than 9 grams of protein per serving, it's considered a high-protein food, and protein is key to your weight loss. Foods high in protein include cheese, dried beans and legumes, eggs, fish, meat, milk, nuts, poultry, soybeans, and yogurt.

**Ingredient list:** The ingredients are listed in order of decreasing weight in the food product. If the list begins with sugar (such as white sugar, corn syrup, or sucrose) or fats and oils, it's probably not a good product choice for the Biggest Loser Diet. Also, a shorter ingredient list often means the product is more natural. A long list of ingredients with a plethora of chemicals and preservatives is probably a good product to leave on the store's shelf.

## TOP TWENTY LISTS

In order to give you a jump-start on your food choices, we've asked the Biggest Losers to share their favorite foods in various categories. Read on for some of their hard-earned advice!

### Top 20 Low-Calorie Foods

1. **Mark Yesitis**—I always keep extra lean ground beef hamburger patties in the freezer to barbecue on the grill. There are only 33 calories per ounce (raw weight) with 6 grams of protein and 1 gram of fat.
2. **Suzy Preston**—My cupboards always have sugar-free, fat-free pudding snack cups and sugar-free gelatin snack cups—my favorite snack foods! Sometimes I stir in a little fat-free whipped topping.
3. **Lisa Andreone**—I keep whole wheat pita bread on hand so that I can bake my own chips to serve with hummus. I also love to spread frozen fat-free whipped topping on graham cracker squares! Yummy!

4. **Ryan Kelly**—I never get bored with snacking on grilled chicken or asparagus.
5. **Drea Baptiste**—String cheese sticks have only 50 calories, and they're great with a piece of fruit or a few veggie sticks for a last-minute or on-the-go snack.
6. **Ken Coleman**—I like to roll thinly sliced lean ham in lettuce leaves with a little mustard and onions.
7. **Dana DeSilvio**—Four ounces of fat-free vanilla yogurt with a few berries and a sprinkle of ground flax seed is my favorite low-cal snack, especially after a workout.
8. **Melony Samuel**—I love fat-free ricotta cheese; it doesn't taste low-cal. I like to put a couple spoonfuls on apple or pear slices and sprinkle it with sliced almonds and cinnamon.
9. **Scott Senti**—Salsa adds flavor to everything, and it has only 40 calories in ½ cup. I like to mix it half and half with fat-free cottage cheese, and sometimes I add extra Tabasco.
10. **Robert Lovane**—I keep a low-cal spinach dip in the fridge made from frozen chopped spinach, low-fat or fat-free cottage cheese, and lots of garlic and onion. It's great with veggies or whole wheat pita chips.
11. **Jennifer Eisenbarth**—Lean deli meat wrapped around blanched asparagus is fast, easy, and low-cal.
12. **Brian Starkey**—This would be my favorite even if it weren't low-cal—grilled chicken breast drizzled with balsamic vinegar.
13. **Heather Hansen**—Fat-free sour cream tastes rich and has a fraction of the calories of the real thing (and no fat). Just a spoonful here and there adds a lot to a dessert or to top cooked beans.

14. **Tiffany Flores Hernandez**—I love beans. Pinto beans with chopped onions and a little salsa or ketchup is my favorite low-cal snack.

15. **Amber Gross**—I love to wrap pickles with a thin slice of smoked turkey or lean deli ham for a quick snack.

16. **Rasha Spindel**—I usually have a few nuts and a small piece of fruit. Almonds and a pear is my favorite combination.

17. **Kelly McFarland**—I sometimes grab ¼ cup fat-free dressing and a couple cups of fresh veggies to dip: cauliflower, jicama, bell pepper strips—whatever's on hand.

18. **Emily Senti**—I like the small single-serving cans of tuna. I mix it with salsa and fat-free cottage cheese for a quick snack.

19. **Nelson Potter**—Edamame (immature green soybeans) is my latest favorite snack. It takes a little longer to eat because you have to remove them from the pod. But ¼ cup of the shelled edamame has 50 calories, 4 grams of protein, and only 5 grams of carbs.

20. **Dave Fioravanti**—I like to bake corn chips from wedges of small corn tortillas. I usually have them with salsa and fat-free refried black beans.

## Top 20 Evening Snacks

1. **Mark Yesitis**—I have given up so many of my favorite foods, but I just can't live without chocolate. Hands down, my favorite snack is fat-free frozen fudge bars.

2. **Lisa Andreone**—Sugar-free hot chocolate (the 25-calorie kind) made with water and a dollop of fat-free whipped topping (5 calorie kind) or carrot sticks with hummus.

3. **Al Stephens**—I love sandwiches. I make a wrap with a small low-carb tortilla. Sometimes I just use lettuce, tomato, and hummus. Other times I have a little leftover grilled chicken with spicy mustard.

4. **Ruben Hernandez**—I have finally learned to satisfy my sweet tooth with fruit instead of rich desserts and pastries. Apple slices with low-fat peanut butter or fresh berries with fat-free whipped topping are my favorite satisfying snacks.

5. **Suzy Preston**—If you know the evening is when you usually binge, save your calories for that time. Make them work for you and don't fight it all day. I save up for the evening and have air-popped popcorn with low-cal butter spray. I always have precut veggies ready for my "snacky" moments.

6. **Ryan Kelly**—Low-fat popcorn is my favorite anytime snack.

7. **Ruben Hernandez**—I never thought nuts could be part of a weight loss plan. My favorite guilt-free snacks are low-fat or fat-free yogurt with just a few unsalted cashews or almonds, or a piece of fresh fruit and unsalted nuts.

8. **Lisa Andreone**—For my snacks, I always combine a carbohydrate and a protein, such as peanuts, almonds, or cashews and a piece of fruit or turkey slices and low-fat yogurt.

9. **Ryan Kelly**—The only time I really have cravings is at night. I have to have something sweet. I love fresh fruit, but I can't live without sugar-free chocolate Popsicles.

10. **Shannon Mullen**—Frozen fruit is a refreshing snack (and easy to prepare if you think ahead). Frozen grapes and bananas are my favorites. They're great to have on hand when that sweet tooth strikes.

11. **Stacie Farr**—My favorite nighttime snack is Parmesan popcorn—2 cups air-popped popcorn sprinkled with ¼ teaspoon garlic salt and 2 teaspoons Parmesan cheese—only 80 calories.

12. **Amy Hildreth**—I make a mini-sandwich with a high-fiber cracker and a wedge of light cheese—only 60 calories.

13. **Marty Wolf**—I like to make a smoothie with ¼ cup vanilla soy milk, fresh strawberries or blueberries, and a spoonful of fat-free vanilla yogurt.

14. **Tiffany Flores Hernandez**—I have a weakness for peanut butter. I spread a tablespoon on celery sticks for a filling evening snack.

15. **Jessica Lanham**—Sometimes I have grilled veggies left over from dinner. I like to wrap sliced turkey or a little smoked salmon around a piece of grilled asparagus or roasted bell pepper.

16. **Matt Kamont**—When it's cold out, I like to make a small bowl of oatmeal. I usually have vanilla yogurt and a few chopped pecans with it.

17. **Kai Hibbard Martin**—I like to make a mini quesadilla with a small high-fiber tortilla and low-fat mozzarella or Cheddar.

18. **Amy Tofanelli**—I try to have a cup of herbal tea at night when I get hungry. My nighttime snack is usually fat-free or low-fat yogurt of some sort, topped with a few fresh berries.

19. **Jeff Levine**—I like to have a little smoked salmon on a whole grain rye cracker. Sometimes I add mustard or horseradish.

20. **Tami Bastian**—I like to have a cup of miso soup. If I'm extra hungry, I add a little bit of diced tofu.

## Top 20 Low-Cal Desserts to Die For

1. **Steve Tofanelli**—I fill a wine glass with mostly berries, a little fat-free ricotta cheese, and a crumbled amaretto cookie on top.

2. **Ryan Benson**—Skinny Cow brand ice-cream sandwiches are delicious and only 130 calories.

3. **Mark Yesitis**—Sugar-free pudding snack cups are only 60 calories. Mmm!

4. **Lisa Andreone**—A really great dessert is sugar-free hot chocolate (the 25-calorie kind) with a dollop of fat-free whipped topping (the 5-calorie kind).

5. **Ryan Kelly**—I love a sandwich of fat-free chocolate graham crackers with sugar-free whipped topping in the middle. Put your sandwich in the freezer for about 1 hour, and it will taste just like an ice-cream sandwich with hardly any calories!

6. **Heather Hansen**—I call it my apple treat: I core half of an unpeeled apple and put it into a small microwaveable bowl. I cover it with plastic wrap and microwave it for a couple minutes and then drizzle it with sugar-free maple syrup and a sprinkling of cinnamon. Sometimes I also add a dollop of fat-free vanilla yogurt.

7. **Kathyrn Murphy**—I like to stir a teaspoon or two of peanut butter into a sugar-free, fat-free chocolate pudding cup. It tastes just like a peanut butter cup!

8. **Kai Hibbard Martin**—I love a bowl of sliced fresh strawberries with vanilla soymilk. Sometimes I add a little Splenda for extra sweetness.

9. **Susan Tofanelli**—When I have extra ripe bananas on hand, I peel them, cut them into 1-inch pieces, and freeze them. I

blend the frozen chunks in a food processor or blender, sometimes adding a little water and maybe a drop of vanilla extract. It's really creamy and tastes rich like ice cream. I figure ½ cup probably has about 50 calories and no fat.

10. **Tina Meyers**—I like having melon because I can have a bigger serving size than some other fruits. Frozen yogurt goes well with it, but sometimes I just have plain melon with a little fresh mint and a few sliced almonds sprinkled on top.

11. **Suzanne Mendonca**—I like to spread a graham cracker square with fat-free cream cheese. I usually put fruit spread or fresh berries on top of it.

12. **Tammy Senti**—If there's extra coffee in the kitchen, I'll ice a glass of decaf with a little scoop of fat-free vanilla frozen yogurt, with nutmeg or cocoa powder on top. It's more like a dessert than a drink.

13. **Edwin Chapman**—I like to make homemade rocky road by topping sugar-free chocolate ice cream with a couple of miniature marshmallows and a few chopped pecans.

14. **Gary Deckman**—I make "croutons" of toasted angel food cake. I put a few in a glass with diced fruit and a spoonful of fat-free frozen yogurt or sugar-free ice cream and a drizzle of chocolate sauce.

15. **Nick Keeler**—My weakness is sugar-free raspberry sorbet. I like it with tangerine or orange slices and top it with a few almonds.

16. **Lael Dandan**—I like fat-free vanilla or strawberry frozen yogurt with fresh blueberries.

17. **Toniann "Toni" Sapienza**—I buy the super jumbo fresh strawberries and dip them into a few tablespoons of fat-free chocolate sauce.

18. **Steve Rothermel**—I like to grill fruit on kebabs; sometimes cantaloupe, honeydew, or a little pineapple in chunks on skewers. If it's a special occasion, I have a little sugar-free ice cream with it.

19. **Ruben Hernandez**—A pudding parfait is one of my favorite dessert recipes. I layer sugar-free, fat-free chocolate pudding with fresh blueberries, raspberries, unsalted pistachios, and fat-free whipped cream . . . yum!

20. **Kelly Minner**—I like poached pears with a little honey and chopped pecans.

## Top 20 Dining Out Tips

1. **Ruben Hernandez**—Request all sauces and dressings on the side, and then use them sparingly. Order nothing fried; food should be steamed or grilled only. Avoid restaurants that are "all you can eat" or are known for their large portions.

2. **Ryan Benson**—Know the restaurant you're going to so you can plan what you will eat. Don't let what other people are ordering sway you or change your plans.

3. **Suzy Preston**—I stick with the salads, always with dressing on the side. Don't feel bad about being picky. Ask the restaurant to leave off things you don't want and pick off all the other foods you know aren't good for you. Have it made your way!

4. **Lisa Andreone**—Tell the server, "no bread." If you are with friends who want bread, ask the server to bring you a salad (with the dressing on the side) when he brings the bread, so you have something to munch on. If you *have* to eat a piece of lasagna (and it seems to be calling your name) just order it. When it arrives, cut it in half, and put the other half in a to-go box. If they have a kid-size lasagna, order that and you can eat the whole thing!

5. **Mark Yesitis**—Be a pain and have it your way; count your calories. Use Splenda or low-calorie sweetener.

6. **Ryan Kelly**—Plan ahead. Pick out what you'll eat prior to arrival and then stay focused. If you waver on your choices, you'll be more likely to pick things that are tempting and fattening. Don't pick your food on a whim!

7. **Rosalinda Guadarrama**—When going out for your favorite coffee drink, be sure to request fat-free milk and no whipped cream. This will drastically cut fat and calories. Also, some coffee bars make hot beverages in smaller sizes than what's listed on the menu. Ask for an 8-ounce size, which is sometimes called "short."

8. **Maurice "Mo" Walker**—Have a low-fat, high-fiber snack (such as fruit and yogurt or raw veggies) before you go out, to avoid feeling too hungry and to prevent the temptation of overeating once you get there.

9. **Nelson Potter**—Don't be afraid to ask your server questions about the food. How is it prepared? What are the ingredients used? Are there substitutions available?

10. **Andrea Overstreet**—Avoid added fat and ask for skin to be removed on chicken or turkey. Also ask for steamed, baked, broiled, boiled, or poached food instead of creamed, fried, sautéed, or breaded. Always ask for no added fat or oil.

11. **Jen Kersey**—Carry packets of fat-free or low-fat salad dressing with you in case you wind up somewhere that only has regular (full-fat) choices.

12. **Lizzeth Davalos**—Whether it's dinner or lunch, try to be sure that your plate is half veggies (and fruit).

13. **Shaun Muha**—I eat my calories (instead of drinking them). I usually order water or unsweetened iced tea to drink—no calories there!

14. **Sarah Eberwein**—If I have soup, it's always brothy and much lower in calories than the creamy ones. (Plus vegetable soup counts as a vegetable!) I've learned to love mustards, and I never use mayonnaise anymore.

15. **Pete Thomas**—I know it's not always an option, but when I have the choice, I try to choose a restaurant within walking distance from work or home. Sneaking in a miniworkout before and after dinner can only be good.

16. **Jennifer Eisenbarth**—I drink a full glass of water before ordering. It's kind of like grocery shopping on a full stomach. You'll wind up ordering something your body needs instead of what your mouth wants.

17. **Bobby Moore**—When I go out for Mexican food, I order a small portion of fajitas without tortillas. I pass on the sour cream and guacamole and have chicken, lots of veggies, and fresh salsa.

18. **Dave Fioravanti**—If the main course doesn't come with veggies, I order a side of steamed veggies, but no starch.
19. **Melinda Suttle**—If I know in advance that I'm going out for dinner, it really makes me stick to my planned meal and snack schedule for the rest of the day.
20. **Ken Coleman**—Stay home and cook! You don't have to worry about hidden calories and fat, you can put just the right amount on your plate and have it your way every time.

# The Calorie Counter

In order to compile this book, we used a number of sources, including the ESHA Research Food Processor program, manufacturers' Web sites, restaurant submissions and Web sites, and the USDA National Nutrient Database for Standard Reference—Release 18. In some cases, analyses for specific nutrients were not available. We've marked those columns "n/a."

## BEANS AND LEGUMES

| FOOD ITEM | SERVING SIZE | CALORIES | PRO (g) | CARB (g) | FIBER (g) | SUGAR (g) | FAT (g) | SAT FAT (g) | SOD (mg) |
|---|---|---|---|---|---|---|---|---|---|
| adzuki beans, cooked with salt | ½ cup | 147 | 9 | 28 | 8 | 0 | 0 | 0 | 281 |
| adzuki beans, cooked without salt | ½ cup | 147 | 9 | 28 | 8 | 0 | 0 | 0 | 9 |
| adzuki beans, dry | ¼ cup | 130 | 8 | 26 | 5 | 1 | 0 | 0 | 0 |
| baked beans | ⅓ cup | 113 | 4 | 21 | 4 | 4 | 1 | 0 | 293 |
| baked beans, vegetarian | ⅓ cup | 113 | 5 | 21 | 5 | 5 | 1 | 0 | 147 |
| bean sprouts (mung beans) | ½ cup | 13 | 1 | 3 | 1 | 2 | 0 | 0 | 6 |
| black beans, cooked with salt | ½ cup | 114 | 8 | 20 | 7 | 0 | 1 | 0 | 204 |
| black beans, dry | ¼ cup | 160 | 9 | 29 | 4 | 4 | 0 | 0 | 0 |
| black turtle beans, cooked without salt | ½ cup | 120 | 8 | 23 | 5 | 0 | 0 | 0 | 221 |
| black-eyed peas (cowpeas), cooked with salt | ½ cup | 80 | 3 | 17 | 4 | 3 | 0 | 0 | 198 |
| black-eyed peas (cowpeas), cooked without salt | ½ cup | 90 | 6 | 16 | 4 | 1 | 1 | 0 | 25 |
| black-eyed peas (cowpeas), dry | ¼ cup | 135 | 9 | 24 | 8 | 4 | 1 | 0 | 5 |

| FOOD ITEM | SERVING SIZE | CALORIES | PRO (g) | CARB (g) | FIBER (g) | SUGAR (g) | FAT (g) | SAT FAT (g) | SOD (mg) |
|---|---|---|---|---|---|---|---|---|---|
| black-eyed peas, fresh | ¼ cup | 33 | 1 | 7 | 2 | 1 | 0 | 0 | 1 |
| broad beans (fava beans), cooked with salt | ½ cup | 53 | 4 | 9 | 3 | 2 | 0 | 0 | 235 |
| broad beans (fava beans), cooked without salt | ½ cup | 62 | 5 | 10 | 4 | 0 | 0 | 0 | 41 |
| broad beans (fava), raw | 1 cup | 78 | 6 | 13 | 5 | 6 | 1 | 0 | 110 |
| butter beans (lima), canned | ½ cup | 70 | 6 | 18 | 5 | 1 | 0 | 0 | 440 |
| butter beans (lima), cooked with brine | ½ cup | 90 | 6 | 16 | 4 | 1 | 0 | 0 | 450 |
| butter beans (lima), cooked with salt | ½ cup | 105 | 6 | 20 | 5 | 1 | 0 | 0 | 215 |
| butter beans (lima), cooked without salt | ½ cup | 105 | 6 | 20 | 5 | 1 | 0 | 0 | 14 |
| butter beans (lima), raw | ½ cup | 88 | 5 | 16 | 4 | 1 | 1 | 0 | 6 |
| cannellini beans, cooked without salt | ½ cup | 100 | 6 | 17 | 5 | 1 | 1 | 0 | 40 |
| cannellini beans, dry | ¼ cup | 153 | 11 | 28 | 11 | 1 | 0 | 0 | 11 |
| chickpea flour | ¼ cup | 89 | 5 | 13 | 2 | 3 | 2 | 0 | 15 |
| chickpeas (garbanzo beans), cooked with salt | ½ cup | 134 | 7 | 22 | 6 | 4 | 2 | 0 | 199 |
| chickpeas (garbanzo beans), cooked without salt | ½ cup | 134 | 7 | 22 | 6 | 4 | 2 | 0 | 6 |
| cranberry beans, cooked with salt | ½ cup | 120 | 8 | 22 | 9 | 0 | 0 | 0 | 210 |
| cranberry beans, cooked without salt | ½ cup | 120 | 8 | 22 | 9 | 0 | 0 | 0 | 1 |
| cranberry beans, raw | ¼ cup | 163 | 11 | 29 | 12 | 0 | 0 | 0 | 3 |
| edamame (immature green soybeans), out of shell, cooked with salt | ½ cup | 100 | 8 | 9 | 4 | 1 | 3 | 1 | 225 |
| edamame (immature green soybeans), out of shell, cooked without salt | ½ cup | 100 | 8 | 9 | 4 | 1 | 3 | 0 | 30 |
| falafel, cooked | 2.25" patty | 57 | 2 | 5 | 0 | 0 | 3 | 0 | 50 |
| falafel, dry | ¼ cup | 120 | 7 | 21 | 6 | 3 | 2 | 0 | 370 |
| fava beans | ½ cup | 94 | 6 | 17 | 5 | 2 | 0 | 0 | 4 |
| French beans, cooked with salt | ½ cup | 114 | 6 | 21 | 8 | 0 | 1 | 0 | 214 |
| French beans, cooked without salt | ½ cup | 114 | 6 | 21 | 8 | 0 | 1 | 0 | 5 |
| French beans, raw | 3 oz | 30 | 1 | 6 | 2 | 2 | 0 | 0 | 0 |
| great Northern beans, cooked with salt | ½ cup | 104 | 7 | 19 | 6 | 0 | 0 | 0 | 210 |

| FOOD ITEM | SERVING SIZE | CALORIES | PRO (g) | CARB (g) | FIBER (g) | SUGAR (g) | FAT (g) | SAT FAT (g) | SOD (mg) |
|---|---|---|---|---|---|---|---|---|---|
| great Northern beans, cooked without salt | ½ cup | 104 | 7 | 19 | 6 | 0 | 0 | 0 | 2 |
| great Northern beans, dry | ½ cup | 134 | 9 | 24 | 8 | 0 | 1 | 0 | 2 |
| hummus | ⅛ cup | 56 | 3 | 6 | 1 | 0 | 3 | 0 | 76 |
| hummus, dry | ⅛ cup | 80 | 3 | 11 | 1 | 0 | 3 | 1 | 280 |
| hummus, low-fat | ⅛ cup | 59 | 5 | 6 | 2 | 0 | 2.5 | 0 | 111 |
| hummus, low-fat, dry | ⅛ cup | 75 | 3 | 8 | 2 | 0 | 3 | 0 | 240 |
| kidney beans, red, cooked with salt | ½ cup | 110 | 8 | 20 | 8 | 0 | 0 | 0 | 212 |
| kidney beans, red, cooked without salt | ½ cup | 110 | 8 | 20 | 8 | 0 | 0 | 0 | 4 |
| kidney beans, red, dry | ¼ cup | 136 | 10 | 25 | 10 | 0 | 0 | 0 | 5 |
| lentils, brown, cooked with salt | ½ cup | 115 | 9 | 20 | 8 | 2 | 0 | 0 | 236 |
| lentils, brown, cooked without salt | ½ cup | 115 | 9 | 20 | 8 | 2 | 0 | 0 | 2 |
| lentils, brown, dry | ¼ cup | 161 | 13 | 28 | 11 | 3 | 1 | 0 | 3 |
| lentils, green, dry | ¼ cup | 150 | 10 | 27 | 7 | 1 | 1 | 0 | 5 |
| lentils, pink, dry | ¼ cup | 165 | 12 | 28 | 5 | 0 | 1 | 0 | 3 |
| lentils, red, dry | ¼ cup | 160 | 12 | 27 | 3 | 3 | 0 | 0 | 5 |
| mung beans, cooked with salt | ½ cup | 106 | 7 | 19 | 8 | 2 | 0 | 0 | 240 |
| mung beans, cooked without salt | ½ cup | 106 | 7 | 19 | 8 | 2 | 0 | 0 | 2 |
| mung beans, dry | ¼ cup | 133 | 9 | 24 | 10 | 3 | 0 | 0 | 3 |
| navy beans, cooked with salt | ½ cup | 127 | 7 | 24 | 10 | 0 | 1 | 0 | 216 |
| navy beans, cooked without salt | ½ cup | 127 | 7 | 10 | 0 | 0 | 1 | 0 | 0 |
| navy beans, dry | ¼ cup | 167 | 10 | 31 | 13 | 0 | 1 | 0 | 0 |
| pinto beans, cooked with salt | ½ cup | 122 | 8 | 22 | 8 | 0 | 1 | 0 | 203 |
| pinto beans, cooked without salt | ½ cup | 122 | 8 | 22 | 8 | 0 | 1 | 0 | 1 |
| pinto beans, dry | ¼ cup | 162 | 10 | 30 | 10 | 0 | 1 | 0 | 1 |
| refried beans | ½ cup | 119 | 7 | 20 | 7 | 0 | 2 | 1 | 378 |
| refried beans, fat-free | ½ cup | 130 | 9 | 24 | 7 | 0 | 0 | 0 | 490 |
| refried beans, vegetarian | ½ cup | 140 | 5 | 23 | 7 | 1 | 3 | 1 | 530 |
| soybean sprouts, raw | ½ cup | 24 | 3 | 2 | 0 | 0 | 1 | 0 | 3 |

## BEANS AND LEGUMES (cont.)

| FOOD ITEM | SERVING SIZE | CALORIES | PRO (g) | CARB (g) | FIBER (g) | SUGAR (g) | FAT (g) | SAT FAT (g) | SOD (mg) |
|---|---|---|---|---|---|---|---|---|---|
| soybean sprouts, steamed with salt | ½ cup | 38 | 4 | 3 | 0 | 0 | 2 | 0 | 116 |
| soybean sprouts, steamed without salt | ½ cup | 38 | 4 | 3 | 0 | 0 | 2 | 0 | 5 |
| soybeans, black, organic, cooked without salt | ½ cup | 120 | 11 | 8 | 7 | 1 | 6 | 1 | 30 |
| soybeans, cooked | ½ cup | 148 | 14 | 8 | 5 | 3 | 7 | 1 | 1 |
| soybeans, dry roasted, salted | ¼ cup | 202 | 15 | 14 | 8 | 0 | 11 | 2 | 70 |
| soybeans, dry roasted, unsalted | ¼ cup | 202 | 15 | 14 | 8 | 0 | 11 | 2 | 2 |
| soybeans, green, boiled | ½ cup | 127 | 11 | 10 | 4 | 0 | 6 | 1 | 13 |
| split peas, cooked with salt | ½ cup | 116 | 8 | 21 | 8 | 3 | 0 | 0 | 233 |
| split peas, cooked without salt | ½ cup | 115 | 8 | 20 | 8 | 3 | 0 | 0 | 2 |
| split peas, yellow or green, dry | ¼ cup | 165 | 10 | 30 | 14 | 1 | 1 | 0 | 1 |
| white beans, small, cooked with salt | ½ cup | 80 | 7 | 19 | 6 | 1 | 1 | 0 | 440 |

## BEVERAGES

| FOOD ITEM | SERVING SIZE | CALORIES | PRO (g) | CARB (g) | FIBER (g) | SUGAR (g) | FAT (g) | SAT FAT (g) | SOD (mg) |
|---|---|---|---|---|---|---|---|---|---|
| **Alcohol** | | | | | | | | | |
| aquavit, 80 proof | 1.5 fl oz | 96 | 0 | 0 | 0 | 0 | 0 | 0 | 0 |
| aquavit, 86 proof | 1.5 fl oz | 104 | 0 | 0 | 0 | 0 | 0 | 0 | 0 |
| aquavit, 90 proof | 1.5 fl oz | 110 | 0 | 0 | 0 | 0 | 0 | 0 | 0 |
| aquavit, 94 proof | 1.5 fl oz | 115 | 0 | 0 | 0 | 0 | 0 | 0 | 0 |
| aquavit, 100 proof | 1.5 fl oz | 123 | 0 | 0 | 0 | 0 | 0 | 0 | 0 |
| beer, ale | 12 fl oz | 147 | 1 | 13 | n/a | n/a | 0 | 0 | 34 |
| beer, amber | 12 fl oz | 169 | 2 | 14 | n/a | n/a | 0 | 0 | 44 |
| beer, amber bock | 12 fl oz | 166 | 1 | 15 | n/a | n/a | 0 | 0 | 9 |
| beer, black and tan | 12 fl oz | 174 | 2 | 18 | n/a | n/a | 0 | 0 | 9 |
| beer, dark | 12 fl oz | 150 | 1 | 13 | n/a | n/a | 0 | 0 | 34 |
| beer, dark, classic | 12 fl oz | 159 | 1 | 15 | n/a | n/a | 0 | 0 | 9 |
| beer, draft, genuine | 12 fl oz | 143 | 1 | 13 | n/a | n/a | 0 | 0 | 7 |
| beer, draft, genuine light | 12 fl oz | 110 | 1 | 7 | n/a | n/a | 0 | 0 | 6 |

## BEVERAGES (cont.)

| FOOD ITEM | SERVING SIZE | CALORIES | PRO (g) | CARB (g) | FIBER (g) | SUGAR (g) | FAT (g) | SAT FAT (g) | SOD (mg) |
|---|---|---|---|---|---|---|---|---|---|
| beer, draft, golden | 12 fl oz | 151 | 2 | 13 | n/a | n/a | 0 | 0 | 9 |
| beer, draft, golden light | 12 fl oz | 110 | 1 | 7 | n/a | n/a | 0 | 0 | 9 |
| beer, draft, hamms golden | 12 fl oz | 144 | 1 | 12 | n/a | n/a | 0 | 0 | 7 |
| beer, lager | 12 fl oz | 102 | 1 | 6 | 1 | 0 | 0 | 0 | 14 |
| beer, light | 12 fl oz | 110 | 1 | 7 | 0 | n/a | 0 | 0 | 11 |
| beer, maize | 12 fl oz | 176 | 3 | 19 | 1 | n/a | 1 | n/a | n/a |
| beer, nonalcoholic (near beer) | 12 fl oz | 32 | 1 | 5 | 0 | n/a | 0 | 0 | 18 |
| beer, nonalcoholic, O'Doul's | 12 fl oz | 70 | 1 | 15 | n/a | n/a | 0 | 0 | 9 |
| beer, pale ale | 12 fl oz | 179 | 2 | 17 | n/a | n/a | 0 | 0 | 9 |
| beer, porter | 12 fl oz | 190 | 3 | 20 | n | n/a | 0 | 0 | 9 |
| beer, private reserve | 12 fl oz | 128 | 1 | 9 | n/a | n/a | 0 | 0 | 35 |
| beer, black and tan | 12 fl oz | 174 | 2 | 18 | n/a | n/a | 0 | 0 | 9 |
| black Russian cocktail | 1.5 fl oz | 115 | 0 | 8 | 0 | 6 | 0 | 0 | 2 |
| Bloody Mary | 8 fl oz | 50 | 1 | 8 | 1 | 5 | 0 | 0 | 1211 |
| bourbon, 80 proof | 1.5 fl oz | 98 | 0 | 0 | 0 | 0 | 0 | 0 | 0 |
| bourbon, 86 proof | 1.5 fl oz | 104 | 0 | 0 | 0 | 0 | 0 | 0 | 0 |
| bourbon, 90 proof | 1.5 fl oz | 110 | 0 | 0 | 0 | 0 | 0 | 0 | 0 |
| bourbon, 94 proof | 1.5 fl oz | 115 | 0 | 0 | 0 | 0 | 0 | 0 | 0 |
| bourbon, 100 proof | 1.5 fl oz | 125 | 0 | 0 | 0 | 0 | 0 | 0 | 0 |
| brandy, 80 proof | 1.5 fl oz | 96 | 0 | 0 | 0 | 0 | 0 | 0 | 0 |
| brandy, 86 proof | 1.5 fl oz | 104 | 0 | 0 | 0 | 0 | 0 | 0 | 0 |
| brandy, 90 proof | 1.5 fl oz | 110 | 0 | 0 | 0 | 0 | 0 | 0 | 0 |
| brandy, 94 proof | 1.5 fl oz | 115 | 0 | 0 | 0 | 0 | 0 | 0 | 0 |
| brandy, 100 proof | 1.5 fl oz | 123 | 0 | 0 | 0 | 0 | 0 | 0 | 0 |
| coffee and cream liqueur | 1.5 fl oz | 153 | 1 | 10 | 0 | 9 | 7 | 5 | 43 |
| coffee liqueur, 53 proof | 1.5 fl oz | 175 | 0 | 24 | 0 | 24 | 0 | 0 | 4 |
| coffee liqueur, 63 proof | 1.5 fl oz | 161 | 0 | 17 | 0 | 17 | 0 | 0 | 4 |
| crème de menthe | 1.5 fl oz | 187 | 0 | 21 | 0 | 21 | 0 | 0 | 3 |
| daiquiri | 8 fl oz | 185 | 0 | 47 | 1 | 46 | 0 | 0 | 231 |
| Gibson cocktail | 1.5 fl oz | 95 | 0 | 0 | 0 | n/a | 0 | 0 | 1 |
| gin, 80 proof | 1.5 fl oz | 96 | 0 | 0 | 0 | 0 | 0 | 0 | 0 |

| FOOD ITEM | SERVING SIZE | CALORIES | PRO (g) | CARB (g) | FIBER (g) | SUGAR (g) | FAT (g) | SAT FAT (g) | SOD (mg) |
|---|---|---|---|---|---|---|---|---|---|
| **Alcohol (cont.)** | | | | | | | | | |
| gin, 86 proof | 1.5 fl oz | 104 | 0 | 0 | 0 | 0 | 0 | 0 | 0 |
| gin, 90 proof | 1.5 fl oz | 112 | 0 | 0 | 0 | 0 | 0 | 0 | 1 |
| gin, 94 proof | 1.5 fl oz | 115 | 0 | 0 | 0 | 0 | 0 | 0 | 0 |
| gin, 100 proof | 1.5 fl oz | 123 | 0 | 0 | 0 | 0 | 0 | 0 | 0 |
| gin and tonic cocktail | 6 fl oz | 117 | 0 | 6 | 0 | 6 | 0 | 0 | 5 |
| gin fizz cocktail | 6 fl oz | 105 | 0 | 4 | 0 | 4 | 0 | 0 | 29 |
| Harvey Wallbanger | 6 fl oz | 145 | 1 | 15 | 0 | 15 | 0 | 0 | 2 |
| highball cocktail | 6 fl oz | 111 | 0 | 0 | 0 | 0 | 0 | 0 | 27 |
| hot buttered rum cocktail | 6 fl oz | 214 | 0 | 3 | 0 | n/a | 8 | 5 | 5 |
| lager, honey beer | 12 fl oz | 172 | 2 | 17 | n/a | n/a | 0 | 0 | 9 |
| Long Island iced tea | 6 fl oz | 142 | 0 | 11 | 0 | n/a | 0 | 0 | 7 |
| mai tai | 1.5 fl oz | 103 | 0 | 10 | 0 | 9 | 0 | 0 | 4 |
| Manhattan cocktail | 6 fl oz | 213 | 0 | 6 | 0 | 6 | 0 | 0 | 5 |
| margarita | 1.5 fl oz | 94 | 0 | 6 | 0 | 6 | 0 | 0 | 2 |
| martini | 1.5 fl oz | 103 | 0 | 1 | 0 | 0 | 0 | 0 | 1 |
| mint julep cocktail | 1.5 fl oz | 102 | 0 | 3 | 0 | 3 | 0 | 0 | 0 |
| piña colada | 1.5 fl oz | 82 | 0 | 11 | 0 | n/a | 1 | 1 | 3 |
| rum, 80 proof | 1.5 fl oz | 96 | 0 | 0 | 0 | 0 | 0 | 0 | 0 |
| rum, 86 proof | 1.5 fl oz | 104 | 0 | 0 | 0 | 0 | 0 | 0 | 0 |
| rum, 90 proof | 1.5 fl oz | 110 | 0 | 0 | 0 | 0 | 0 | 0 | 0 |
| rum, 94 proof | 1.5 fl oz | 115 | 0 | 0 | 0 | 0 | 0 | 0 | 0 |
| rum, 100 proof | 1.5 fl oz | 123 | 0 | 0 | 0 | 0 | 0 | 0 | 0 |
| sangria | 5 fl oz | 98 | 0 | 13 | 0 | n/a | 0 | 0 | 10 |
| screwdriver | 6 fl oz | 145 | 1 | 15 | 0 | 15 | 0 | 0 | 2 |
| Singapore sling cocktail | 6 fl oz | 172 | 0 | 10 | 0 | 10 | 0 | 0 | 25 |
| sloe gin fizz | 6 fl oz | 93 | 0 | 2 | 0 | n/a | 0 | 0 | 29 |
| Stolichnaya Citrona malt beverage | 6 fl oz | 120 | 0 | 18 | n/a | n/a | 0 | 0 | 149 |
| tequila, 80 proof | 1.5 fl oz | 96 | 0 | 0 | 0 | 0 | 0 | 0 | 0 |
| tequila, 86 proof | 1.5 fl oz | 104 | 0 | 0 | 0 | 0 | 0 | 0 | 0 |

| FOOD ITEM | SERVING SIZE | CALORIES | PRO (g) | CARB (g) | FIBER (g) | SUGAR (g) | FAT (g) | SAT FAT (g) | SOD (mg) |
|---|---|---|---|---|---|---|---|---|---|
| tequila, 90 proof | 1.5 fl oz | 110 | 0 | 0 | 0 | 0 | 0 | 0 | 0 |
| tequila, 94 proof | 1.5 fl oz | 115 | 0 | 0 | 0 | 0 | 0 | 0 | 0 |
| tequila, 100 proof | 1.5 fl oz | 123 | 0 | 0 | 0 | 0 | 0 | 0 | 0 |
| tequila sunrise | 6 fl oz | 187 | 1 | 14 | 0 | 14 | 0 | 0 | 7 |
| Tom Collins cocktail | 6 fl oz | 69 | 0 | 5 | 0 | 4 | 0 | 0 | 27 |
| vodka, 80 proof | 1.5 fl oz | 96 | 0 | 0 | 0 | 0 | 0 | 0 | 0 |
| vodka, 86 proof | 1.5 fl oz | 104 | 0 | 0 | 0 | 0 | 0 | 0 | 0 |
| vodka, 90 proof | 1.5 fl oz | 110 | 0 | 0 | 0 | 0 | 0 | 0 | 0 |
| vodka, 94 proof | 1.5 fl oz | 115 | 0 | 0 | 0 | 0 | 0 | 0 | 0 |
| vodka, 100 proof | 1.5 fl oz | 123 | 0 | 0 | 0 | 0 | 0 | 0 | 0 |
| whiskey, 80 proof | 1.5 fl oz | 96 | 0 | 0 | 0 | 0 | 0 | 0 | 0 |
| whiskey, 86 proof | 1.5 fl oz | 104 | 0 | 0 | 0 | 0 | 0 | 0 | 0 |
| whiskey, 90 proof | 1.5 fl oz | 110 | 0 | 0 | 0 | 0 | 0 | 0 | 0 |
| whiskey, 94 proof | 1.5 fl oz | 115 | 0 | 0 | 0 | 0 | 0 | 0 | 0 |
| whiskey sour cocktail | 6 fl oz | 289 | 0 | 28 | 0 | 28 | 0 | 0 | 81 |
| white Russian | 1.5 fl oz | 109 | 0 | 7 | 0 | 6 | 1 | 0 | 3 |
| wine cooler | 5 fl oz | 71 | 0 | 8 | 0 | n/a | 0 | 0 | 12 |
| wine, dessert, dry | 5 fl oz | 224 | 0 | 17 | 0 | 2 | 0 | 0 | 13 |
| wine, dessert, sweet | 5 fl oz | 236 | 0 | 20 | 0 | 11 | 0 | 0 | 13 |
| wine, dessert, sweet Madeira | 5 fl oz | 236 | 0 | 20 | 0 | 11 | 0 | 0 | 13 |
| wine, dry, burgundy | 5 fl oz | 102 | 0 | 2 | n/a | n/a | 0 | 0 | 12 |
| wine, dry, claret | 5 fl oz | 102 | 0 | 2 | n/a | n/a | 0 | 0 | 12 |
| wine, dry, sherry | 5 fl oz | 102 | 0 | 2 | n/a | n/a | 0 | 0 | 12 |
| wine, Japanese rice | 5 fl oz | 195 | 1 | 7 | 0 | 0 | 0 | 0 | 3 |
| wine, light | 5 fl oz | 74 | 0 | 2 | 0 | 2 | 0 | 0 | 10 |
| wine, Marsala | 5 fl oz | 236 | 0 | 20 | 0 | 11 | 0 | 0 | 13 |
| wine, mirin | 5 fl oz | 336 | 1 | 47 | 0 | 47 | 0 | 0 | n/a |
| wine, nonalcoholic, light | 5 fl oz | 9 | 0 | 2 | 0 | 2 | 0 | 0 | 10 |
| wine, plum | 5 fl oz | 229 | 0 | 26 | 0 | 26 | 0 | n/a | n/a |
| wine, port | 5 fl oz | 236 | 0 | 20 | 0 | 11 | 0 | 0 | 13 |
| wine, red | 5 fl oz | 125 | 0 | 4 | 0 | 1 | 0 | 0 | 6 |

| FOOD ITEM | SERVING SIZE | CALORIES | PRO (g) | CARB (g) | FIBER (g) | SUGAR (g) | FAT (g) | SAT FAT (g) | SOD (mg) |
|---|---|---|---|---|---|---|---|---|---|
| **Alcohol (cont.)** | | | | | | | | | |
| wine, red, Barbera | 5 fl oz | 126 | 0 | 4 | n/a | n/a | 0 | 0 | n/a |
| wine, red, Carignane | 5 fl oz | 112 | 0 | 4 | n/a | n/a | 0 | 0 | n/a |
| wine, red, claret | 5 fl oz | 123 | 0 | 4 | n/a | n/a | 0 | 0 | n/a |
| wine, red, Gamay | 5 fl oz | 116 | 0 | 4 | n/a | n/a | 0 | 0 | n/a |
| wine, red, Merlot | 5 fl oz | 123 | 0 | 4 | 0 | 1 | 0 | 0 | 6 |
| wine, red, Pinot Noir | 5 fl oz | 83 | 0 | 2 | n | n/a | 0 | 0 | n/a |
| wine, red, Syrah | 5 fl oz | 123 | 0 | 4 | n/a | n/a | 0 | 0 | n/a |
| wine, red, Zinfandel | 5 fl oz | 131 | 0 | 4 | n/a | n/a | 0 | 0 | n/a |
| wine, rice (sake) | 5 fl oz | 195 | 1 | 7 | 0 | 0 | 0 | 0 | 3 |
| wine, white, Chenin Blanc | 5 fl oz | 120 | 0 | 5 | n/a | n/a | 0 | 0 | n/a |
| wine, white, Gewürztraminer | 5 fl oz | 121 | 0 | 4 | n/a | n/a | 0 | 0 | n/a |
| wine, white, late harvest | 5 fl oz | 174 | 0 | 21 | n/a | n/a | 0 | 0 | n/a |
| wine, white, medium | 5 fl oz | 122 | 0 | 4 | 0 | 1 | 0 | 0 | 7 |
| wine, white, Pinot Grigio | 5 fl oz | 123 | 0 | 3 | n/a | n/a | 0 | 0 | n/a |
| wine, white Sauvignon Blanc | 5 fl oz | 120 | 0 | 3 | n | n/a | 0 | 0 | n/a |
| wine, white, Sémillon | 5 fl oz | 122 | 0 | 5 | n | n/a | 0 | 0 | n/a |
| wine, white, vermouth | 5 fl oz | 230 | 0 | 18 | n/a | n/a | 0 | 0 | 14 |
| wine spritzer | 5 fl oz | 59 | 0 | 1 | 0 | n/a | 0 | 0 | 19 |
| **Coffee and Tea** | | | | | | | | | |
| cappuccino, instant, with sugar, dry | 1 tbsp | 86 | 1 | 18 | 0 | 15 | 1 | 1 | 38 |
| cappuccino, with fat-free milk | 8 fl oz | 53 | 5 | 7 | 0 | 7 | 0 | 0 | 73 |
| cappuccino, with low-fat milk | 8 fl oz | 73 | 5 | 7 | 0 | 7 | 2 | 2 | 73 |
| chai, Celestial Seasonings, original | 8 fl oz | 0 | 0 | 0 | 0 | 0 | 0 | 0 | 0 |
| chai, Celestial Seasonings, original, decaf | 8 fl oz | 0 | 0 | 0 | 0 | 0 | 0 | 0 | 0 |
| chai, Power Dream | 1 tbsp | 11 | 0 | 2 | 0 | 1 | 0 | 0 | 3 |
| chai, Silk Chai, with soy milk | 8 fl oz | 130 | 6 | 19 | 0 | 14 | 3.5 | 0.5 | 100 |
| coffee, brewed | 8 fl oz | 2 | 0 | 0 | 0 | 0 | 0 | 0 | 0 |
| coffee, decaf, brewed | 8 fl oz | 0 | 0 | 0 | 0 | 0 | 0 | 0 | 0 |

| FOOD ITEM | SERVING SIZE | CALORIES | PRO (g) | CARB (g) | FIBER (g) | SUGAR (g) | FAT (g) | SAT FAT (g) | SOD (mg) |
|---|---|---|---|---|---|---|---|---|---|
| coffee, iced latte, with fat-free milk | 8 fl oz | 47 | 5 | 7 | 0 | 6 | 0 | 0 | 67 |
| coffee, iced latte, with fat-free milk, double | 8 fl oz | 47 | 5 | 7 | 0 | 6 | 0 | 0 | 67 |
| coffee, iced latte, with low-fat milk | 8 fl oz | 60 | 5 | 7 | 0 | 6 | 2 | 1 | 67 |
| coffee, instant | 1 tbsp | 7 | 0 | 1 | 0 | 0 | 0 | 0 | 1 |
| coffee, instant, café Francais | 1 tbsp | 47 | 0 | 5 | 0 | 3 | 3 | 1 | 70 |
| coffee, instant, café Vienna | 1 tbsp | 53 | 1 | 9 | n/a | 7 | 2 | 0 | 83 |
| coffee, instant, café Vienna, sugar-free | 1 tbsp | 61 | 2 | 6 | n/a | 0 | 3 | 1 | 152 |
| coffee, instant, chai latte | 1 tbsp | 55 | 0 | 10 | n/a | 8 | 2 | 1 | 48 |
| coffee, instant, chai latte, sugar-free | 1 tbsp | 30 | 0 | 2 | 0 | 0 | 3 | 2 | 35 |
| coffee, instant, crème caramel | 1 tbsp | 66 | 0 | 11 | n/a | 9 | 2 | 0 | 52 |
| coffee, instant, decaf | 1 tbsp | 12 | 1 | 2 | 0 | 0 | 0 | 0 | 1 |
| coffee, instant, 50% less caffeine | 1 tbsp | 16 | 1 | 3 | 0 | 0 | 0 | 0 | 2 |
| coffee, instant, flavor coffee subs | 1 tbsp | 30 | 0 | 9 | n/a | n/a | 0 | 0 | 0 |
| coffee, instant, French vanilla, decaf | 1 tbsp | 45 | 1 | 8 | n/a | 5 | 2 | 0 | 41 |
| coffee, instant, hazelnut Belgian café | 1 tbsp | 53 | 1 | 9 | n/a | 7 | 2 | 0 | 45 |
| coffee, instant, mocha, fat-free, sugar-free | 1 tbsp | 19 | 0 | 4 | 0 | 0 | 0 | 0 | 26 |
| coffee, instant, mocha, no-fat and sugar, prepared | 1 tbsp | 50 | 0 | 10 | n/a | 0 | 0 | 0 | 71 |
| coffee, instant, substitute | 1 tbsp | 30 | 0 | 9 | n/a | n/a | 0 | 0 | 0 |
| coffee, instant, Swiss mocha, decaf, sugar-free, prepared | 1 tbsp | 30 | 0 | 2 | 0 | 0 | 2 | 2 | 30 |
| coffee, instant Swiss white chocolate | 1 tbsp | 53 | 0 | 9 | n/a | 7 | 2 | 0 | 23 |
| coffee, instant, Viennese chocolate café | 1 tbsp | 38 | 1 | 8 | n/a | 7 | 1 | 0 | 23 |
| coffee, instant, with chicory | 1 tbsp | 19 | 1 | 4 | 0 | n/a | 0 | 0 | 15 |
| coffee, latte, with fat-free milk | 8 fl oz | 47 | 5 | 7 | 0 | 6 | 0 | 0 | 67 |
| coffee, latte, with fat-free milk, decaf | 8 fl oz | 47 | 5 | 7 | 0 | 6 | 0 | 0 | 67 |
| coffee, latte, with low-fat milk | 8 fl oz | 60 | 5 | 7 | 0 | 6 | 2 | 1 | 67 |

| FOOD ITEM | SERVING SIZE | CALORIES | PRO (g) | CARB (g) | FIBER (g) | SUGAR (g) | FAT (g) | SAT FAT (g) | SOD (mg) |
|---|---|---|---|---|---|---|---|---|---|
| **Coffee and Tea (cont.)** | | | | | | | | | |
| coffee, latte, with low-fat milk, decaf | 8 fl oz | 60 | 5 | 7 | 0 | 6 | 2 | 1 | 67 |
| coffee, latte, with Silk soy milk | 8 fl oz | 170 | 5 | 29 | 0 | 23 | 4 | 0 | 50 |
| coffee, latte, with Silk soy milk, spicy | 8 fl oz | 145 | 6 | 20 | 0 | 18 | 4 | 0 | 145 |
| coffee, mocha, with fat-free milk | 8 fl oz | 120 | 8 | 22 | 1 | 19 | 1 | 0 | 100 |
| coffee, mocha, with fat-free milk, decaf | 8 fl oz | 120 | 8 | 22 | 1 | 19 | 1 | 0 | 100 |
| coffee, mocha, with low-fat milk | 8 fl oz | 200 | 8 | 22 | 1 | 19 | 10 | 6 | 107 |
| coffee, mocha, with low-fat milk, decaf | 8 fl oz | 200 | 8 | 22 | 1 | 19 | 10 | 6 | 107 |
| coffee, mocha, with soy milk | 8 fl oz | 140 | 6 | 20 | 1 | 15 | 4 | 0 | 50 |
| espresso | 4 fl oz | 11 | 0 | 2 | 0 | 2 | 0 | 0 | 17 |
| espresso, decaf | 4 fl oz | 11 | 0 | 2 | 0 | 2 | 0 | 0 | 17 |
| tea, black, decaf | 8 fl oz | 0 | 0 | 0 | 0 | 0 | 0 | 0 | 0 |
| tea, black, iced, unsweetened | 8 fl oz | 0 | 0 | 0 | 0 | 0 | 0 | 0 | 0 |
| tea, black, iced, unsweetened, decaf | 8 fl oz | 0 | 0 | 0 | 0 | 0 | 0 | 0 | 0 |
| tea, chamomile | 8 fl oz | 2 | 0 | 0 | 0 | 0 | 0 | 0 | 2 |
| tea, herbal | 8 fl oz | 2 | 0 | 0 | 0 | 0 | 0 | 0 | 2 |
| tea, mint | 8 fl oz | 0 | 0 | 0 | 0 | 0 | 0 | 0 | 0 |
| tea, mint, decaf | 8 fl oz | 0 | 0 | 0 | 0 | 0 | 0 | 0 | 0 |
| **Juice** | | | | | | | | | |
| aloe vera juice | 4 fl oz | 45 | 1 | 11 | 0 | 0 | 0 | 0 | 33 |
| apple cider | 4 fl oz | 60 | 0 | 15 | 0 | 13 | 0 | 0 | 13 |
| apple juice, unsweetened | 4 fl oz | 58 | 0 | 14 | 0 | 14 | 0 | 0 | 4 |
| apple juice, unsweetened, frozen | 4 fl oz | 56 | 0 | 14 | 0 | 13 | 0 | 0 | 8 |
| apple-cherry juice | 4 fl oz | 58 | 0 | 15 | 1 | n/a | 0 | 0 | 3 |
| apple-cherry juice, infants' | 4 fl oz | 60 | 0 | 14 | n/a | 13 | 0 | 0 | 5 |
| apple-cranberry juice | 4 fl oz | 70 | 0 | 17 | 0 | 16 | 0 | 0 | 16 |
| apple-grape juice | 4 fl oz | 64 | 0 | 16 | 0 | 16 | 0 | 0 | 4 |

| FOOD ITEM | SERVING SIZE | CALORIES | PRO (g) | CARB (g) | FIBER (g) | SUGAR (g) | FAT (g) | SAT FAT (g) | SOD (mg) |
|---|---|---|---|---|---|---|---|---|---|
| apple-raspberry-blackberry juice | 4 fl oz | 56 | 0 | 15 | 0 | 13 | 0 | 0 | 9 |
| beetroot juice | 4 fl oz | 41 | 1 | 10 | n/a | n/a | 0 | 0 | 236 |
| blackberry juice | 4 fl oz | 44 | 0 | 9 | 0 | 9 | 1 | 0 | 1 |
| blackberry-lime juice | 4 fl oz | 58 | 0 | 14 | 0 | 14 | 0 | 0 | 0 |
| carrot juice | 4 fl oz | 47 | 1 | 11 | 1 | 5 | 0 | 0 | 34 |
| carrot tropical juice drink | 4 fl oz | 55 | 0 | 14 | 0 | 14 | 0 | 0 | 25 |
| cherry juice | 4 fl oz | 70 | 0 | 17 | 0 | 16 | 0 | 0 | 8 |
| clam and tomato juice | 4 fl oz | 58 | 1 | 13 | 0 | 4 | 0 | 0 | 437 |
| cranberry juice, unsweetened | 4 fl oz | 58 | 0 | 15 | 0 | 15 | 0 | 0 | 3 |
| cranberry juice cocktail | 4 fl oz | 68 | 0 | 17 | 0 | 15 | 0 | 0 | 3 |
| cranberry juice cocktail, low-calorie | 4 fl oz | 23 | 0 | 6 | 0 | 5 | 0 | 0 | 4 |
| cranberry-apricot juice, low-calorie | 4 fl oz | 23 | 0 | 6 | 0 | 6 | 0 | 0 | 3 |
| grape juice, unsweetened | 4 fl oz | 77 | 1 | 19 | 0 | 19 | 0 | 0 | 4 |
| grape juice drink | 4 fl oz | 71 | 0 | 18 | 0 | 18 | 0 | 0 | 11 |
| grapefruit juice, unsweetened | 4 fl oz | 47 | 1 | 11 | 0 | 11 | 0 | 0 | 1 |
| grapefruit juice, unsweetened, frozen, from concentrate | 4 fl oz | 50 | 1 | 12 | 0 | 12 | 0 | 0 | 1 |
| grapefruit juice, white | 4 fl oz | 48 | 1 | 11 | 0 | 11 | 0 | 0 | 1 |
| guava juice drink | 4 fl oz | 66 | 0 | 17 | 1 | 16 | 0 | 0 | 4 |
| guava nectar | 4 fl oz | 74 | 0 | 19 | 1 | 18 | 0 | 0 | 3 |
| lemon juice | 4 fl oz | 30 | 0 | 10 | 0 | 3 | 0 | 0 | 1 |
| lime juice | 4 fl oz | 31 | 1 | 10 | 0 | 2 | 0 | 0 | 2 |
| mango nectar juice | 4 fl oz | 72 | 0 | 19 | 1 | 18 | 0 | 0 | 3 |
| orange juice | 4 fl oz | 56 | 1 | 13 | 0 | 10 | 0 | 0 | 1 |
| orange juice, frozen, from concentrate | 4 fl oz | 56 | 1 | 13 | 0 | 10 | 0 | 0 | 1 |
| orange juice, ruby red | 4 fl oz | 58 | 1 | 14 | 0 | 12 | 0 | 0 | 0 |
| orange juice, Tropicana | 4 fl oz | 51 | 1 | 12 | 0 | 10 | 0 | 0 | 0 |
| orange-pineapple juice | 4 fl oz | 55 | 1 | 14 | 0 | 12 | 0 | 0 | 8 |
| orange-strawberry-banana juice | 4 fl oz | 55 | 1 | 14 | 0 | 12 | 0 | 0 | 3 |

| FOOD ITEM | SERVING SIZE | CALORIES | PRO (g) | CARB (g) | FIBER (g) | SUGAR (g) | FAT (g) | SAT FAT (g) | SOD (mg) |
|---|---|---|---|---|---|---|---|---|---|
| **Juice (cont.)** | | | | | | | | | |
| passion fruit concentrate | 1 oz | 58 | 2 | 10 | n/a | 10 | 1 | 0 | 21 |
| passion fruit juice, purple | 4 fl oz | 63 | 0 | 17 | 0 | 17 | 0 | 0 | 7 |
| passion fruit juice, yellow | 4 fl oz | 60 | 1 | 14 | 0 | n/a | 0 | 0 | 6 |
| passion fruit-apple-carrot juice | 4 fl oz | 60 | 1 | 14 | n/a | n/a | 0 | 0 | 48 |
| pineapple juice, canned, unsweetened | 4 fl oz | 66 | 0 | 160 | 0 | 12 | 0 | 0 | 3 |
| pineapple juice, unsweetened, frozen, from concentrate | 4 fl oz | 65 | 1 | 16 | 0 | 16 | 0 | 0 | 1 |
| pink grapefruit juice | 4 fl oz | 48 | 1 | 11 | 0 | n/a | 0 | 0 | 1 |
| pink grapefruit juice, canned, unsweetened | 4 fl oz | 47 | 1 | 11 | 0 | 11 | 0 | 0 | 1 |
| pink grapefruit juice, light | 4 fl oz | 18 | 0 | 5 | 0 | 3 | 0 | 0 | 10 |
| pomegranate juice | 4 fl oz | 70 | 1 | 18 | 0 | 17 | 0 | 0 | 15 |
| pomegranate juice concentrate | 1 fl oz | 80 | 0 | 22 | 0 | 20 | 0 | 0 | 0 |
| pomegranate-blueberry juice | 4 fl oz | 70 | 1 | 17 | 0 | 12 | 0 | 0 | 23 |
| pomegranate-cherry juice | 4 fl oz | 70 | 1 | 17 | 0 | 14 | 0 | 0 | 18 |
| pomegranate-mango juice | 4 fl oz | 70 | 1 | 17 | 0 | 14 | 0 | 0 | 35 |
| pomegranate-tangerine juice | 4 fl oz | 75 | 1 | 19 | 0 | 16 | 0 | 0 | 38 |
| prune juice, canned | 4 fl oz | 90 | 1 | 22 | 1 | 21 | 0 | 0 | 5 |
| prune juice, with pulp | 4 fl oz | 85 | 1 | 21 | 2 | 8 | 0 | 0 | 18 |
| prune juice concentrate | 1 fl oz | 77 | 1 | 19 | 1 | n/a | 0 | 0 | 9 |
| raspberry juice | 4 fl oz | 36 | 0 | 9 | 0 | 9 | 0 | 0 | 4 |
| raspberry juice concentrate | 1 fl oz | 68 | 1 | 16 | 0 | 13 | 0 | 0 | 18 |
| spinach juice | 4 fl oz | 7 | 2 | 1 | n/a | n/a | 0 | 0 | 86 |
| strawberry juice | 4 fl oz | 34 | 1 | 8 | 0 | 8 | 0 | 0 | 1 |
| strawberry-orange juice | 4 fl oz | 69 | 1 | 16 | 0 | 14 | 0 | 0 | 13 |
| tangerine juice | 4 fl oz | 53 | 1 | 12 | 0 | 12 | 0 | 0 | 1 |
| tangerine juice, canned | 4 fl oz | 62 | 1 | 15 | 0 | 15 | 0 | 0 | 1 |
| tangerine-orange juice | 4 fl oz | 55 | 1 | 13 | 0 | 11 | 0 | 0 | 0 |
| tomato juice, canned | 4 fl oz | 21 | 1 | 5 | 0 | 4 | 0 | 0 | 327 |

| FOOD ITEM | SERVING SIZE | CALORIES | PRO (g) | CARB (g) | FIBER (g) | SUGAR (g) | FAT (g) | SAT FAT (g) | SOD (mg) |
|---|---|---|---|---|---|---|---|---|---|
| tomato juice, canned, unsalted | 4 fl oz | 21 | 1 | 5 | 0 | 4 | 0 | 0 | 12 |
| tomato-vegetable juice, low-sodium | 4 fl oz | 25 | 1 | 5 | 1 | 4 | 0 | 0 | 70 |
| vegetable juice, V8 | 4 fl oz | 25 | 1 | 5 | 1 | 4 | 0 | 0 | 310 |
| vegetable juice, V8, picante | 4 fl oz | 25 | 1 | 5 | 1 | 4 | 0 | 0 | 340 |
| vegetable juice, V8, spicy hot | 4 fl oz | 25 | 1 | 5 | 1 | 4 | 0 | 0 | 360 |
| wheatgrass juice | 4 fl oz | 19 | 4 | 4 | 0 | 4 | 0 | 0 | 0 |
| **Milk and Nondairy** | | | | | | | | | |
| acidophilus fat-free milk | 1 cup | 110 | 9 | 13 | 0 | 12 | 2.5 | 1.5 | 130 |
| acidophilus reduced-fat 2% milk | 1 cup | 100 | 10 | 14 | 0 | 14 | 0 | 0 | 140 |
| buttermilk, cultured, low-fat | 1 cup | 110 | 9 | 13 | 0 | 12 | 3 | 2 | 270 |
| buttermilk, dried | 1 fl oz | 110 | 10 | 14 | 0 | 14 | 2 | 1 | 147 |
| diet shake, Slim-Fast, chocolate | 11-fl oz can | 220 | 10 | 40 | 5 | 34 | 3 | 1 | 220 |
| diet shake, Slim-Fast, chocolate royale | 11-fl oz can | 220 | 10 | 40 | 5 | 35 | 3 | 1 | 220 |
| diet shake, Slim-Fast, French vanilla | 11-fl oz can | 220 | 10 | 40 | 5 | 35 | 2.5 | 0.5 | 230 |
| diet shake, Slim-Fast High Protein, creamy chocolate | 11-fl oz can | 190 | 15 | 24 | 5 | 13 | 5 | 2 | 220 |
| diet shake, Slim-Fast High Protein, creamy coffee | 11-fl oz can | 190 | 15 | 23 | 5 | 13 | 5 | 2 | 200 |
| diet shake, Slim-Fast High Protein, creamy strawberry | 11-fl oz can | 190 | 15 | 23 | 5 | 13 | 5 | 2 | 200 |
| diet shake, Slim-Fast High Protein, creamy vanilla | 11-fl oz can | 190 | 15 | 23 | 5 | 13 | 5 | 2 | 200 |
| diet shake, Slim-Fast Optima, cappuccino | 11-fl oz can | 180 | 10 | 25 | 5 | 18 | 6 | 0.5 | 200 |
| diet shake, Slim-Fast Optima, chocolate royale | 11-fl oz can | 190 | 10 | 24 | 5 | 18 | 6 | 2.5 | 200 |
| diet shake, Slim-Fast Optima, French vanilla | 11-fl oz can | 180 | 10 | 24 | 5 | 17 | 6 | 2.5 | 200 |
| diet shake, Slim-Fast Optima, milk chocolate | 11-fl oz can | 190 | 10 | 25 | 5 | 18 | 6 | 2.5 | 200 |
| diet shake, Slim-Fast Optima, strawberry and cream | 11-fl oz can | 180 | 10 | 23 | 5 | 17 | 5 | 2 | 200 |
| evaporated milk, fat-free | 4 fl oz | 88 | 7 | 14 | 0 | 14 | 0 | 0 | 142 |
| evaporated milk, fat-free, canned | 4 fl oz | 88 | 9 | 13 | 0 | 13 | 0 | 0 | 130 |

| FOOD ITEM | SERVING SIZE | CALORIES | PRO (g) | CARB (g) | FIBER (g) | SUGAR (g) | FAT (g) | SAT FAT (g) | SOD (mg) |
|---|---|---|---|---|---|---|---|---|---|
| **Milk and Nondairy (cont.)** | | | | | | | | | |
| evaporated milk, reduced-fat 2% | 4 fl oz | 104 | 9 | 13 | 0 | 13 | 2 | 1 | 128 |
| half-and-half, fat-free | 1 fl oz | 37 | 1 | 1 | 0 | 1 | 0 | 0 | 14 |
| hot cocoa, sugar-free, with water | 8 fl oz | 66 | 3 | 12 | 1 | 8 | 1 | 0 | 202 |
| hot cocoa, with fat-free milk | 8 fl oz | 138 | 8 | 27 | 1 | n/a | 1 | 1 | 146 |
| hot cocoa, with low-fat milk | 8 fl oz | 158 | 8 | 27 | 1 | n/a | 3 | 2 | 144 |
| hot cocoa, with water | 8 fl oz | 125 | 2 | 26 | 1 | 23 | 1 | 1 | 161 |
| hot cocoa, with whole milk | 8 fl oz | 193 | 7 | 27 | 1 | n/a | 8 | 5 | 141 |
| milk, fat-free | 1 cup | 90 | 9 | 13 | 0 | 12 | 0 | 0 | 130 |
| milk, lactose-reduced 1% | 1 cup | 103 | 8 | 12 | 0 | 12 | 3 | 2 | 124 |
| milk, lactose-reduced 1%, Lactaid | 1 cup | 103 | 8 | 12 | 0 | 12 | 3 | 2 | 125 |
| milk, low-fat 1% | 1 cup | 118 | 10 | 14 | 0 | 11 | 3 | 2 | 143 |
| milk, reduced-fat 2% | 1 cup | 122 | 8 | 11 | 0 | 11 | 5 | 3 | 100 |
| milk, whole | 1 cup | 146 | 8 | 11 | 0 | 11 | 8 | 5 | 98 |
| nondairy milk, Almond Breeze | 1 cup | 63 | 1 | 8 | 1 | 7 | 3 | 0 | 153 |
| nondairy milk, Almond Breeze, chocolate | 1 cup | 120 | 1 | 21 | 1 | 20 | 3 | 0 | 160 |
| nondairy milk, Almond Breeze, vanilla | 1 cup | 94 | 1 | 16 | 1 | 14 | 3 | 0 | 154 |
| protein drink, Myoplex Carb Sense, chocolate | 1 packet | 140 | 25 | 6 | 3 | 0 | 3.5 | 2.5 | 360 |
| protein drink, Myoplex Carb Sense, ready-to-drink, chocolate fudge | 1 drink | 150 | 25 | 5 | 2 | <1 | 3.5 | 0 | 350 |
| protein drink, Myoplex Carb Sense, ready-to-drink, strawberry cream | 1 drink | 150 | 25 | 5 | 2 | 1 | 3.5 | 1 | 340 |
| protein drink, Myoplex Carb Sense, ready to-drink, vanilla | 1 drink | 150 | 25 | 5 | 2 | 1 | 3.5 | 0 | 350 |
| protein drink, Myoplex Carb Sense, vanilla | 1 packet | 140 | 25 | 5 | 3 | 0 | 3.5 | 2.5 | 330 |
| rice milk | 1 cup | 144 | 3 | 28 | 2 | n/a | 2 | 0 | 86 |
| rice milk, Better Than Milk, vanilla, dry | 1 fl oz | 107 | 1 | 25 | 0 | 21 | 0 | 0 | 134 |
| rice milk, Imagine foods | 1 cup | 120 | 1 | 25 | n/a | 11 | 2 | 0 | 90 |

| FOOD ITEM | SERVING SIZE | CALORIES | PRO (g) | CARB (g) | FIBER (g) | SUGAR (g) | FAT (g) | SAT FAT (g) | SOD (mg) |
|---|---|---|---|---|---|---|---|---|---|
| rice milk, Rice Dream, carob | 1 cup | 150 | 1 | 32 | n/a | 24 | 2.5 | 0 | 100 |
| rice milk, Rice Dream, vanilla | 1 cup | 130 | 1 | 28 | n/a | 12 | 2 | 0 | 90 |
| rice milk, Rice Dream, enriched, chocolate | 1 cup | 170 | 1 | 36 | 0 | 25 | 3 | 0 | 115 |
| rice milk, Rice Dream, enriched, original | 1 cup | 120 | 1 | 25 | 0 | 11 | 2 | 0 | 90 |
| rice milk, Rice Dream, enriched, vanilla | 1 cup | 130 | 1 | 28 | 0 | 12 | 2 | 0 | 90 |
| rice milk, Rice Dream Heartwise, enriched, original | 1 cup | 130 | 1 | 27 | 3 | 9 | 2 | 0 | 80 |
| rice milk, WN, enriched, plain | 1 cup | 100 | 1 | 18 | 0 | 14 | 3 | 0 | 60 |
| rice milk, WN, enriched, vanilla | 1 cup | 120 | 1 | 22 | 0 | 17 | 3 | 0 | 65 |
| Silk Nog with soy milk, low-fat | 1 cup | 180 | 6 | 30 | n/a | 24 | 2 | n/a | 150 |
| soy and rice beverage, EdenBlend | 1 cup | 120 | 7 | 18 | 1 | 8 | 3 | 1 | 90 |
| soy drink, So Good Soy Drink | 1 cup | 158 | 8 | 13 | 2 | 5 | 8 | 1 | 92 |
| soy milk | 1 cup | 127 | 11 | 12 | 3 | 1 | 5 | 1 | 135 |
| soy milk, Better Than Milk, chocolate, dry | 1 fl oz | 116 | 1 | 22 | 0 | 14 | 2 | 0 | 204 |
| soy milk, Better Than Milk, original, dry | 1 fl oz | 107 | 1 | 25 | 0 | 20 | 0 | 0 | 134 |
| soy milk, Better Than Milk, vanilla, dry | 1 fl oz | 134 | 3 | 15 | 0 | 3 | 7 | 1 | 172 |
| soy milk, Silk, chocolate | 1 cup | 140 | 5 | 23 | 2 | 19 | 3.5 | 0.5 | 100 |
| soy milk, Silk, chocolate, light | 1 cup | 120 | 5 | 22 | 2 | 19 | 1.5 | 0 | 100 |
| soy milk, Silk, coffee latte | 11 fl oz | 200 | 7 | 34 | 1 | 29 | 4.5 | 1 | 140 |
| soy milk, Silk, enhanced | 1 cup | 110 | 7 | 8 | 1 | 6 | 5 | 0.5 | 120 |
| soy milk, Silk, original, light | 1 cup | 70 | 6 | 8 | 1 | 6 | 2 | 0 | 120 |
| soy milk, Silk, plain, organic | 1 cup | 100 | 7 | 8 | 0 | 4 | 4 | 0 | 75 |
| soy milk, Silk, spice latte | 11 fl oz | 190 | 8 | 27 | 1 | 23 | 5 | 1 | 160 |
| soy milk, Silk, unsweetened | 1 cup | 80 | 7 | 4 | 1 | 1 | 4 | 0.5 | 85 |
| soy milk, Silk, vanilla | 1 cup | 100 | 6 | 10 | 1 | 7 | 3.5 | 0.5 | 95 |
| soy milk, Silk, vanilla, light | 1 cup | 80 | 6 | 10 | 1 | 7 | 2 | 0 | 95 |

| FOOD ITEM | SERVING SIZE | CALORIES | PRO (g) | CARB (g) | FIBER (g) | SUGAR (g) | FAT (g) | SAT FAT (g) | SOD (mg) |
|---|---|---|---|---|---|---|---|---|---|
| **Milk and Nondairy (cont.)** | | | | | | | | | |
| soy milk, Silk, very vanilla | 1 cup | 130 | 6 | 19 | 1 | 16 | 4 | 0.5 | 140 |
| soy milk, Soy Dream, carob | 1 cup | 152 | 7 | 22 | n/a | 13 | 4 | 0.5 | 140 |
| soy milk, Soy Dream, original | 1 cup | 132 | 7 | 17 | n/a | 9 | 4 | 0.5 | 140 |
| soy milk, Soy Dream, vanilla | 1 cup | 204 | 7 | 36 | n/a | 22 | 3.5 | 0.5 | 160 |
| soy milk, Soy Dream, enriched, chocolate | 1 cup | 208 | 7 | 37 | 1 | 24 | 3.5 | 0.5 | 160 |
| soy milk, Soy Dream, enriched, original | 1 cup | 132 | 7 | 17 | 0 | 9 | 4 | 0.5 | 140 |
| soy milk, Soy Dream, enriched, vanilla | 1 cup | 152 | 7 | 22 | 0 | 22 | 4 | 0.5 | 140 |
| soy milk beverage, Vitasoy, carob | 1 cup | 210 | 8 | 32 | n/a | n/a | 6 | 1 | 160 |
| soy milk beverage, Vitasoy, original, light | 1 cup | 90 | 4 | 15 | n/a | n/a | 2 | 0 | 95 |
| soy milk beverage, Vitasoy, rich cocoa | 1 cup | 210 | 8 | 32 | n/a | n/a | 6 | 1 | 180 |
| soy milk beverage, Vitasoy, vanilla, light | 1 cup | 110 | 4 | 20 | n/a | n/a | 2 | 0 | 95 |
| soy milk beverage, Vitasoy, vanilla delight | 1 cup | 190 | 7 | 27 | n/a | n/a | 6 | 1 | 130 |
| soy milk creamer, Silk, French vanilla | 1 fl oz | 35 | 0 | 5 | 0 | 5 | 2 | 0 | 9 |
| soy milk creamer, Silk, hazelnut | 1 fl oz | 28 | 0 | 2 | 0 | 0 | 2 | 0 | 9 |
| soy milk creamer, Silk, plain | 1 fl oz | 28 | 0 | 2 | 0 | 0 | 2 | 0 | 9 |
| **Soda and Water** | | | | | | | | | |
| Aquafina water | 8 fl oz | 0 | 0 | 0 | 0 | 0 | 0 | 0 | 0 |
| Calistoga water | 8 fl oz | 0 | 0 | 0 | 0 | 0 | 0 | 0 | 0 |
| Coca-Cola Zero | 8 fl oz | 1 | n/a | 0 | n/a | n/a | n/a | n/a | 28 |
| Crystal Light, bottled, Lemon Tea | 8 fl oz | 5 | 0 | 0 | n/a | 0 | 0 | n/a | 15 |
| Crystal Light, bottled, Lemonade | 8 fl oz | 5 | 0 | 0 | n/a | 0 | 0 | n/a | 15 |
| Crystal Light, bottled, Pink Lemonade | 8 fl oz | 5 | 0 | 0 | n/a | 0 | 0 | n/a | 15 |
| Crystal Light, bottled, Raspberry Ice | 8 fl oz | 5 | 0 | 0 | n/a | 0 | 0 | n/a | 15 |
| Crystal Light, bottled, Strawberry Kiwi | 8 fl oz | 5 | 0 | 0 | n/a | 0 | 0 | n/a | 15 |
| Crystal Light, bottled, Sunrise Classic Orange | 8 fl oz | 5 | 0 | 0 | n/a | 0 | 0 | n/a | 15 |

| FOOD ITEM | SERVING SIZE | CALORIES | PRO (g) | CARB (g) | FIBER (g) | SUGAR (g) | FAT (g) | SAT FAT (g) | SOD (mg) |
|---|---|---|---|---|---|---|---|---|---|
| Crystal Light Decaffeinated Iced Tea | 1 g | 5 | 0 | 0 | n/a | 0 | 0 | n/a | 0 |
| Crystal Light Iced Tea | 1 g | 5 | 0 | 0 | n/a | 0 | 0 | n/a | 0 |
| Crystal Light Lemonade | 2 g | 5 | 0 | 0 | n/a | 0 | 0 | n/a | 35 |
| Crystal Light Peach Tea | 1 g | 5 | 0 | 0 | n/a | 0 | 0 | n/a | 0 |
| Crystal Light Pineapple Orange | 1 g | 5 | 0 | 0 | n/a | 0 | 0 | n/a | 0 |
| Crystal Light Pink Lemonade | 2 g | 5 | 0 | 0 | n/a | 0 | 0 | n/a | 0 |
| Crystal Light Raspberry Lemonade | 2 g | 5 | 0 | 0 | n/a | 0 | 0 | n/a | 0 |
| Crystal Light Raspberry Ice | 1 g | 5 | 0 | 0 | n/a | 0 | 0 | n/a | 0 |
| Crystal Light Raspberry Tea | 1 g | 5 | 0 | 0 | n/a | 0 | 0 | n/a | 0 |
| Crystal Light Strawberry Kiwi | 1 g | 5 | 0 | 0 | n/a | 0 | 0 | n/a | 0 |
| Crystal Light Strawberry Orange Banana | 1 g | 5 | 0 | 0 | n/a | 0 | 0 | n/a | 0 |
| Crystal Light Sunrise Classic Orange | 2 g | 5 | 0 | 0 | n/a | 0 | 0 | n/a | 0 |
| Crystal Light Sunrise Ruby Red Grapefruit | 2 g | 5 | 0 | 0 | n/a | 0 | 0 | n/a | 0 |
| Diet 7UP | 8 fl oz | 0 | 0 | 0 | 0 | 0 | 0 | 0 | 35 |
| Diet A&W Cream | 8 fl oz | 0 | 0 | 0 | 0 | 0 | 0 | 0 | 45 |
| Diet A&W Root Beer | 8 fl oz | 0 | 0 | 0 | 0 | 0 | 0 | 0 | 45 |
| Diet Barq's Red Crème Soda | 8 fl oz | 4 | 0 | 0 | 0 | 0 | 0 | 0 | 19 |
| Diet Barq's Root Beer | 8 fl oz | 1 | 0 | 0 | 0 | 0 | 0 | 0 | 24 |
| Diet Cherry 7Up | 8 fl oz | 0 | 0 | 0 | 0 | 0 | 0 | 0 | 35 |
| Diet Cherry Coke | 8 fl oz | 1 | 0 | 0 | 0 | 0 | 0 | 0 | 4 |
| Diet Coke | 8 fl oz | 1 | 0 | 0 | 0 | 0 | 0 | 0 | 4 |
| Diet Coke, Caffeine-free | 8 fl oz | 1 | 0 | 0 | 0 | 0 | 0 | 0 | 4 |
| Diet Coke, with Lime | 8 fl oz | 2 | n/a | 0 | n/a | n/a | n/a | n/a | 28 |
| Diet Coke, with Splenda | 8 fl oz | 1 | n/a | 0 | n/a | n/a | n/a | n/a | 28 |
| Diet Dr Pepper | 8 fl oz | 0 | 0 | 0 | 0 | 0 | 0 | 0 | 35 |
| Diet Dr Pepper, Caffeine-free | 8 fl oz | 0 | 0 | 0 | 0 | 0 | 0 | 0 | 35 |
| Diet Hires Root Beer | 8 fl oz | 0 | 0 | 0 | 0 | 0 | 0 | 0 | 70 |
| Diet IBC Root Beer | 8 fl oz | 0 | 0 | 0 | 0 | 0 | 0 | 0 | 75 |

| FOOD ITEM | SERVING SIZE | CALORIES | PRO (g) | CARB (g) | FIBER (g) | SUGAR (g) | FAT (g) | SAT FAT (g) | SOD (mg) |
|---|---|---|---|---|---|---|---|---|---|
| **Soda and Water (cont.)** | | | | | | | | | |
| Diet Mountain Dew | 8 fl oz | 0 | 0 | 0 | 0 | 0 | 0 | 0 | 23 |
| Diet Mr. Pibb | 8 fl oz | 1 | 0 | 0 | 0 | 0 | 0 | 0 | 2 |
| Diet Mug Root Beer | 8 fl oz | 0 | 0 | 0 | n/a | 0 | 0 | n/a | 25 |
| Diet Pepsi | 8 fl oz | 0 | 0 | 0 | 0 | 0 | 0 | 0 | 23 |
| Diet Pepsi Lime | 8 fl oz | 0 | 0 | 0 | n/a | 0 | 0 | n/a | 25 |
| Diet Pepsi Twist | 8 fl oz | 0 | 0 | 0 | n/a | 0 | 0 | n/a | 25 |
| Diet Rite Pure Zero Cola | 8 fl oz | 0 | 0 | 0 | n/a | n/a | 0 | n/a | 0 |
| Diet Rite Pure Zero Red Raspberry | 8 fl oz | 0 | 0 | 0 | n/a | n/a | 0 | n/a | 0 |
| Diet Rite Pure Zero Tangerine | 8 fl oz | 0 | 0 | 0 | n/a | n/a | 0 | n/a | 0 |
| Diet Rite Pure Zero White Grape | 8 fl oz | 0 | 0 | 0 | n/a | n/a | 0 | n/a | 0 |
| Diet Snapple Apple | 8 fl oz | 15 | 0 | 4 | n/a | 3 | 0 | n/a | 10 |
| Diet Snapple Cran Raspberry | 8 fl oz | 10 | 0 | 2 | n/a | 2 | 0 | n/a | 10 |
| Diet Snapple Lemon Tea | 8 fl oz | 10 | 0 | 1 | n/a | 0 | 0 | n/a | 10 |
| Diet Snapple Lemonade Iced Tea | 8 fl oz | 10 | 0 | 2 | n/a | 1 | 0 | n/a | 15 |
| Diet Snapple Lime Green Tea | 8 fl oz | 0 | 0 | 1 | n/a | 0 | 0 | n/a | 10 |
| Diet Snapple Orange Carrot | 8 fl oz | 10 | 0 | 3 | n/a | 1 | 0 | n/a | 10 |
| Diet Snapple Peach Tea | 8 fl oz | 0 | 0 | 1 | n/a | 0 | 0 | n/a | 10 |
| Diet Snapple Pink Lemonade | 8 fl oz | 10 | 0 | 2 | n/a | 2 | 0 | n/a | 10 |
| Diet Sprite | 8 fl oz | 3 | 0 | 0 | 0 | 0 | 0 | 0 | 0 |
| Diet Squirt | 8 fl oz | 0 | 0 | 0 | 0 | 0 | 0 | 0 | 15 |
| Diet Squirt Ruby Red | 8 fl oz | 5 | 0 | 1 | 0 | 1 | 0 | 0 | 20 |
| Diet Sunkist orange soda | 8 fl oz | 0 | 0 | 0 | 0 | 0 | 0 | 0 | 130 |
| Diet Vernors Ginger Ale | 8 fl oz | 0 | 0 | 0 | 0 | 0 | 0 | 0 | 15 |
| Distilled water | 8 fl oz | 0 | 0 | 0 | 0 | 0 | 0 | 0 | 0 |
| Evian water | 8 fl oz | 0 | 0 | 0 | 0 | 0 | 0 | 0 | 0 |
| Fresca Sparkling Black Cherry Citrus | 8 fl oz | 20 | 0 | 5 | n/a | 5 | 0 | n/a | 0 |
| Fresca Sparkling Citrus | 8 fl oz | 3 | 0 | 0 | 0 | 0 | 0 | 0 | 1 |

| FOOD ITEM | SERVING SIZE | CALORIES | PRO (g) | CARB (g) | FIBER (g) | SUGAR (g) | FAT (g) | SAT FAT (g) | SOD (mg) |
|---|---|---|---|---|---|---|---|---|---|
| Fresca Sparkling Peach Citrus | 8 fl oz | 20 | 0 | 5 | n/a | 5 | 0 | n/a | 0 |
| Glaceau Fruit Water, grape | 8 fl oz | 20 | 0 | 5 | n/a | 5 | 0 | n/a | 0 |
| Glaceau Fruit Water, lime | 8 fl oz | 20 | 0 | 5 | n/a | 5 | 0 | n/a | 0 |
| Glaceau Fruit Water, peach | 8 fl oz | 20 | 0 | 5 | n/a | 5 | 0 | n/a | 0 |
| Glaceau Fruit Water, raspberry | 8 fl oz | 20 | 0 | 5 | n/a | 5 | 0 | n/a | 0 |
| LaCroix Natural Spring Water | 8 fl oz | 0 | 0 | 0 | 0 | 0 | 0 | 0 | 5 |
| Le Nature's Ice Water, lemon-lime | 8 fl oz | 0 | 0 | 0 | n/a | 0 | 0 | n/a | 0 |
| Le Nature's Ice Water, squeeze of lemon | 8 fl oz | 0 | 0 | 1 | n/a | 1 | 0 | n/a | 0 |
| Le Nature's Ice Water, tropical mandarin mist | 8 fl oz | 0 | 0 | 1 | n/a | 1 | 0 | n/a | 0 |
| Mt. Shasta Spring Water | 8 fl oz | 0 | 0 | 0 | 0 | 0 | 0 | 0 | 5 |
| O Water, lemon lime | 8 fl oz | 0 | 0 | 0 | n/a | n/a | 0 | n/a | 0 |
| O Water, mandarin | 8 fl oz | 0 | 0 | 0 | n/a | n/a | 0 | n/a | 0 |
| O Water, mango orange | 8 fl oz | 0 | 0 | 0 | n/a | n/a | 0 | n/a | 0 |
| O Water, peach | 8 fl oz | 0 | 0 | 0 | n/a | n/a | 0 | n/a | 0 |
| O Water, plain | 8 fl oz | 0 | 0 | 0 | n/a | n/a | 0 | n/a | 0 |
| O Water, strawberry | 8 fl oz | 0 | 0 | 0 | n/a | n/a | 0 | n/a | 0 |
| O Water, wild berry | 8 fl oz | 0 | 0 | 0 | n/a | n/a | 0 | n/a | 0 |
| Pepsi One | 8 fl oz | 1 | 0 | 0 | n/a | 0 | 0 | n/a | 25 |
| Perrier | 8 fl oz | 0 | 0 | 0 | 0 | 0 | 0 | 0 | 2 |
| Poland Spring water | 8 fl oz | 0 | 0 | 0 | n/a | n/a | 0 | n/a | 2 |
| Sierra Mist Free | 8 fl oz | 0 | 0 | 0 | n/a | 0 | 0 | n/a | 25 |

## BREADS AND CRACKERS

| FOOD ITEM | SERVING SIZE | CALORIES | PRO (g) | CARB (g) | FIBER (g) | SUGAR (g) | FAT (g) | SAT FAT (g) | SOD (mg) |
|---|---|---|---|---|---|---|---|---|---|
| bagel, blueberry | 1 oz | 73 | 3 | 15 | 0 | 3 | 0 | 0 | 119 |
| bagel, cinnamon raisin | 1 oz | 77 | 3 | 16 | 1 | 2 | 0 | 0 | 91 |
| bagel, egg | 1 oz | 78 | 3 | 15 | 1 | n/a | 1 | 0 | 143 |
| bagel, onion | 1 oz | 78 | 3 | 15 | 1 | n/a | 0 | 0 | 151 |

| FOOD ITEM | SERVING SIZE | CALORIES | PRO (g) | CARB (g) | FIBER (g) | SUGAR (g) | FAT (g) | SAT FAT (g) | SOD (mg) |
|---|---|---|---|---|---|---|---|---|---|
| bagel, plain | 1 oz | 81 | 3 | 16 | 1 | 2 | 0 | 0 | 136 |
| bagel, poppy seed | 1 oz | 78 | 3 | 15 | 1 | n/a | 0 | 0 | 151 |
| bagel, whole grain | 1 oz | (75) | 3 | 16 | 3 | 1 | 0 | 0 | 153 |
| biscuit, buttermilk | ½ of 2.5" biscuit | 105 | 2 | 13 | 1 | 1 | 5 | 1 | 174 |
| biscuit, mixed grain | ½ of 2.5" biscuit | 58 | 1 | 10 | n/a | n/a | 1 | 0 | 147 |
| biscuit, plain | ½ of 2.5" biscuit | 64 | 1 | 9 | 9 | 1 | 3 | 0 | 184 |
| bread, banana | ½ slice (1 oz) | 98 | 1 | 16 | 0 | n/a | 3 | 1 | 91 |
| bread, Boston brown | 1 slice (1.6 oz) | 88 | 2 | 19 | 2 | 1 | 1 | 0 | 284 |
| bread, cracked wheat | 1 slice (1 oz) | 65 | 2 | 12 | 1 | n/a | 1 | 0 | 135 |
| bread, egg | 1 slice (1 oz) | 113 | 4 | 19 | 1 | 1 | 2 | 1 | 197 |
| bread, Ezekiel 4:9, Cinnamon Raisin Sprouted Grain | 1 slice (34 g) | 80 | 4 | 18 | 2 | n/a | 0 | 0 | 65 |
| bread, Ezekiel 4:9, Low-Sodium Sprouted Grain | 1 slice (34 g) | 80 | 4 | 15 | 3 | n/a | 1 | 0 | 0 |
| bread, Ezekiel 4:9, Sesame Sprouted Grain | 1 slice (34 g) | 80 | 4 | 14 | 3 | n/a | 1 | 0 | 80 |
| bread, Ezekiel 4:9, Sprouted Grain Bread | 1 slice (34 g) | 80 | 4 | 15 | 3 | n/a | 1 | 0 | 75 |
| bread, French | 1 slice (1 oz) | 86 | 3 | 16 | 1 | 0 | 1 | 0 | 192 |
| bread, Irish soda | 1 oz | 82 | 2 | 16 | 1 | n/a | 1 | 0 | 113 |
| bread, oat bran | 1 slice (1 oz) | 71 | 3 | 12 | 1 | 2 | 1 | 0 | 122 |
| bread, oat bran, reduced-calorie | 2 slices (2 oz) | 92 | 4 | 19 | 6 | 2 | 1 | 0 | 161 |
| bread, oatmeal | 1 slice (1 oz) | 73 | 2 | 13 | 1 | 2 | 1 | 0 | 162 |
| bread, oatmeal, reduced-calorie | 2 slices (2 oz) | 97 | 4 | 20 | n/a | n/a | 2 | 0 | 178 |
| bread, pita, white | ½ of 6.5" pita (1 oz) | 83 | 3 | 17 | 1 | 0 | 0 | 0 | 161 |
| bread, pita, whole wheat | ½ of 6.5" pita (1 oz) | 85 | 3 | 18 | 2 | 0 | 1 | 0 | 170 |
| bread, protein | 1 slice (1 oz) | 47 | 2 | 8 | 1 | 0 | 0 | 0 | 104 |

| FOOD ITEM | SERVING SIZE | CALORIES | PRO (g) | CARB (g) | FIBER (g) | SUGAR (g) | FAT (g) | SAT FAT (g) | SOD (mg) |
|---|---|---|---|---|---|---|---|---|---|
| bread, pumpernickel | 1 slice (1 oz) | 65 | 2 | 12 | 2 | 0 | 1 | 0 | 174 |
| bread, raisin | 1 slice (1 oz) | 71 | 2 | 14 | 1 | 1 | 1 | 0 | 101 |
| bread, rice bran | 1 slice (1 oz) | 66 | 2 | 12 | 1 | 1 | 1 | 0 | 119 |
| bread, rye | 1 slice (1 oz) | 82 | 3 | 15 | 2 | 1 | 1 | 0 | 211 |
| bread, 7 grain | 1 slice (1 oz) | 65 | 3 | 12 | 2 | 3 | 1 | 0 | 127 |
| bread, wheat, reduced-calorie | 2 slices (2 oz) | 80 | 4 | 18 | 7 | 3 | 1 | 0 | 240 |
| bread, wheat bran | 1 slice (1 oz) | 89 | 3 | 17 | 1 | 3 | 1 | 0 | 175 |
| bread, wheat germ | 1 slice (1 oz) | 73 | 3 | 14 | 1 | 1 | 1 | 0 | 155 |
| bread, wheatberry | 1 slice (1 oz) | 65 | 2 | 12 | 1 | 1 | 1 | 0 | 133 |
| bread, white | 1 slice (1 oz) | 67 | 2 | 13 | 1 | 1 | 1 | 0 | 170 |
| bread, white, reduced-calorie | 2 slices (2 oz) | 95 | 4 | 20 | 4 | 2 | 1 | 0 | 208 |
| bread, whole grain | 1 slice (1 oz) | 65 | 3 | 12 | 2 | 3 | 1 | 0 | 127 |
| bread, whole wheat | 1 slice (1 oz) | 69 | 3 | 13 | 2 | 2 | 1 | 0 | 148 |
| bread crumbs, dry | 1 oz | 112 | 4 | 20 | 1 | 2 | 2 | 0 | 208 |
| bread crumbs, fresh | 1 oz | 75 | 2 | 14 | 1 | 1 | 1 | 0 | 193 |
| bread crumbs, seasoned | 1 oz | 109 | 4 | 19 | 1 | 2 | 2 | 0 | 499 |
| bread stick | 1 oz | 82 | 2 | 14 | 1 | 0 | 2 | 0 | 131 |
| bread stuffing | 1 oz | 50 | 1 | 6 | 1 | 1 | 2 | 0 | 154 |
| corn bread | 1 oz | 89 | 2 | 14 | 1 | n/a | 3 | 1 | 221 |
| corn bread stuffing | 1 oz | 51 | 1 | 6 | 1 | 1 | 2 | 1 | 129 |
| cracker, cheese | 0.75 oz | 107 | 2 | 12 | 1 | 0 | 5 | 2 | 212 |
| cracker, cheese, low-sodium | 0.75 oz | 107 | 2 | 12 | 1 | 1 | 5 | 2 | 97 |
| cracker, crispbread, rye | 0.75 oz | 78 | 2 | 17 | 4 | 0 | 0 | 0 | 56 |
| cracker, crispbread, rye, low-sodium | 0.75 oz | 78 | 2 | 17 | 4 | 1 | 0 | 0 | 56 |
| cracker, graham | 0.75 oz | 89 | 1 | 16 | 1 | 7 | 2 | 0 | 127 |

| FOOD ITEM | SERVING SIZE | CALORIES | PRO (g) | CARB (g) | FIBER (g) | SUGAR (g) | FAT (g) | SAT FAT (g) | SOD (mg) |
|---|---|---|---|---|---|---|---|---|---|
| cracker, graham, low-fat | 0.75 oz | 82 | 1 | 17 | 1 | 5 | 1 | 0 | 130 |
| cracker, Health Valley, low-fat oat bran graham | 0.75 oz | 91 | 2 | 17 | 2 | 2 | 2 | 0 | 61 |
| cracker, Health Valley, low-fat whole wheat | 0.75 oz | 91 | 3 | 15 | 2 | 2 | 2 | 0 | 61 |
| cracker, Kashi TLC, Original 7 Grain | 0.75 oz | 92 | 2 | 16 | 1 | 2 | 2 | 0 | 113 |
| cracker, matzo, egg | 0.75 oz | 83 | 3 | 17 | 1 | n/a | 0 | 0 | 4 |
| cracker, matzo, egg, and onion | 0.75 oz | 83 | 2 | 16 | 1 | n/a | 1 | 0 | 61 |
| cracker, matzo, plain | 0.75 oz | 84 | 2 | 18 | 1 | 0 | 0 | 0 | 0 |
| cracker, matzo, whole wheat | 0.75 oz | 75 | 3 | 17 | 3 | n/a | 0 | 0 | 0 |
| cracker, melba toast, plain | 0.75 oz | 83 | 3 | 16 | 1 | 0 | 1 | 0 | 176 |
| cracker, melba toast, rye | 0.75 oz | 83 | 2 | 16 | 2 | n/a | 1 | 0 | 191 |
| cracker, melba toast, wheat | 0.75 oz | 80 | 3 | 16 | 2 | n/a | 0 | 0 | 178 |
| cracker, milk | 0.75 oz | 97 | 2 | 15 | 0 | 4 | 3 | 1 | 126 |
| cracker, rye wafer | 0.75 oz | 71 | 2 | 17 | 5 | 0 | 0 | 0 | 169 |
| cracker, saltine | 0.75 oz | 91 | 2 | 15 | 1 | 0 | 2 | 0 | 228 |
| cracker, saltine, fat-free | 0.75 oz | 85 | 1 | 17 | 0 | 0 | 0 | 0 | 241 |
| cracker, saltine, low-sodium | 0.75 oz | 92 | 2 | 15 | 1 | 0 | 3 | 1 | 135 |
| cracker, saltine, low-sodium, fat-free | 0.75 oz | 84 | 2 | 18 | 1 | 0 | 0 | 0 | 135 |
| cracker, stoned wheat, low-fat | 0.75 oz | 91 | 3 | 15 | 2 | 2 | 2 | 0 | 213 |
| cracker, Triscuit | 0.75 oz | 93 | 2 | 15 | 2 | 0 | 4 | 1 | 138 |
| cracker, Wasa, fiber rye crisp | 1 oz | 104 | 2 | 23 | 5 | 2 | 0 | 0 | 75 |
| cracker, wheat | 0.75 oz | 94 | 2 | 15 | 2 | 0 | 4 | 1 | 140 |
| cracker, wheat, low-salt | 0.75 oz | 94 | 2 | 15 | 2 | 0 | 4 | 1 | 53 |
| cracker, Wheat Thins | 0.75 oz | 92 | 2 | 15 | 2 | 0 | 4 | 1 | 128 |
| crispbread, Wasa, multi-grain | 1 slice (14 g) | 45 | 2 | 10 | 2 | 0 | 0 | 0 | 80 |
| crispbread, Wasa, oat | 1 slice (16 g) | 60 | 2 | 11 | 2 | 0 | 1 | 0 | 95 |
| crispbread, Wasa, rye, fiber | 1 slice (10 g) | 30 | 1 | 7 | 2 | 0 | 1 | 0 | 50 |

| FOOD ITEM | SERVING SIZE | CALORIES | PRO (g) | CARB (g) | FIBER (g) | SUGAR (g) | FAT (g) | SAT FAT (g) | SOD (mg) |
|---|---|---|---|---|---|---|---|---|---|
| crispbread, Wasa, rye, hearty | 1 slice (14 g) | 45 | 1 | 11 | 2 | 0 | 0 | 0 | 70 |
| crispbread, Wasa, rye, light | 2 slices (17 g) | 60 | 2 | 14 | 3 | 0 | 0 | 0 | 70 |
| crispbread, Wasa, sourdough rye | 1 slice (11 g) | 35 | 1 | 9 | 2 | 0 | 0 | 0 | 45 |
| crispbread, Wasa, sesame | 1 slice (14 g) | 60 | 2 | 9 | <1 | 0 | 2 | 0 | 70 |
| crispbread, Wasa, 7-grain light | 3 slices (16 g) | 60 | 2 | 13 | 1 | <1 | 0 | 0 | 35 |
| croissant | ½ medium | 116 | 2 | 13 | 1 | 3 | 6 | 3 | 212 |
| croissant, cheese | ½ medium | 118 | 3 | 13 | 1 | 3 | 6 | 3 | 158 |
| croissant, chocolate | ½ medium | 117 | 2 | 12 | 1 | n/a | 7 | 4 | 188 |
| English muffin | ½ (1 oz) | 65 | 3 | 13 | 1 | 1 | 0 | 0 | 121 |
| English muffin, cinnamon raisin | ½ (1 oz) | 68 | 2 | 14 | 1 | 4 | 1 | 0 | 95 |
| English muffin, granola | ½ (1 oz) | 78 | 3 | 15 | 1 | 0 | 0 | 0 | 137 |
| English muffin, whole wheat | ½ (1 oz) | 67 | 3 | 13 | 2 | 3 | 1 | 0 | 210 |
| French toast | ½ slice (1 oz) | 74 | 3 | 8 | 0 | n/a | 4 | 1 | 156 |
| hush puppy | 1 oz | 93 | 2 | 13 | 1 | n/a | 4 | 1 | 351 |
| muffin, blueberry | ½ (1 oz) | 79 | 2 | 14 | 1 | 6 | 2 | 0 | 127 |
| muffin, bran | ½ (1 oz) | 107 | 2 | 14 | 1 | 13 | 5 | 1 | 98 |
| muffin, corn | ½ (1 oz) | 87 | 2 | 15 | 1 | 2 | 2 | 0 | 148 |
| muffin, oat bran | ½ (1 oz) | 77 | 2 | 14 | 1 | 2 | 2 | 0 | 112 |
| muffin, plain, low-fat | ½ (1 oz) | 75 | 1 | 16 | 1 | 11 | 0 | 0 | 185 |
| muffin, wheat bran | ½ (1 oz) | 53 | 1 | 10 | 1 | 3 | 2 | 0 | 89 |
| pancake, blueberry | ½ of 6" pancake (1 oz) | 85 | 2 | 11 | 0 | n/a | 4 | 1 | 159 |
| pancake, buckwheat | ½ of 5" pancake (1 oz) | 57 | 2 | 11 | 1 | 1 | 1 | 0 | 168 |
| pancake, buttermilk | 1 4" pancake (1 oz) | 81 | 2 | 14 | 1 | 4 | 2 | 0 | 182 |
| pancake, cornmeal | 1 4" pancake (1 oz) | 43 | 1 | 7 | 0 | 1 | 1 | 0 | 52 |

| FOOD ITEM | SERVING SIZE | CALORIES | PRO (g) | CARB (g) | FIBER (g) | SUGAR (g) | FAT (g) | SAT FAT (g) | SOD (mg) |
|---|---|---|---|---|---|---|---|---|---|
| pancake, plain | 1 4" pancake (1 oz) | 74 | 2 | 14 | 0 | n/a | 1 | 0 | 239 |
| pancake, whole wheat | ½ of a 5" pancake (1 oz) | 50 | 2 | 10 | 1 | 1 | 0 | 0 | 107 |
| pappadam cracker (not fried) | 1 (10 g) | 37 | 3 | 6 | 2 | 0 | 0 | 0 | 175 |
| phyllo dough | 1 oz | 85 | 2 | 15 | 1 | 0 | 2 | 0 | 137 |
| popover | ½ (1 oz) | 94 | 3 | 9 | 0 | 1 | 5 | 2 | 75 |
| roll, cinnamon | ½ of a 2.75" roll (1 oz) | 112 | 2 | 15 | 1 | 10 | 5 | 1 | 115 |
| roll, dinner, bran | 1 (1 oz) | 76 | 3 | 14 | 1 | 1 | 2 | 0 | 136 |
| roll, dinner, plain | 1 (1 oz) | 84 | 2 | 14 | 1 | 1 | 2 | 0 | 146 |
| roll, dinner, rye | 1 (1 oz) | 81 | 3 | 15 | 1 | 0 | 1 | 0 | 253 |
| roll, dinner, wheat | 1 (1 oz) | 77 | 2 | 13 | 1 | 0 | 2 | 0 | 96 |
| roll, dinner, whole wheat | 1 (1 oz) | 75 | 2 | 14 | 2 | 2 | 1 | 0 | 136 |
| roll, French | 1 (1 oz) | 105 | 3 | 19 | 1 | 0 | 2 | 0 | 231 |
| roll, hamburger bun | ½ (1 oz) | 60 | 3 | 11 | 1 | 2 | 1 | 1 | 110 |
| roll, hard | ½ (1 oz) | 84 | 3 | 15 | 1 | 1 | 1 | 0 | 155 |
| roll, hotdog bun | ½ (1 oz) | 60 | 2 | 11 | 0 | 1 | 1 | 0 | 103 |
| roll, kaiser | ½ (1 oz) | 84 | 3 | 15 | 1 | 1 | 1 | 0 | 155 |
| roll, pumpernickel | 1 (1 oz) | 78 | 3 | 15 | 2 | 0 | 1 | 0 | 159 |
| roll, sweet | 1 (1 oz) | 110 | 3 | 16 | 0 | 5 | 4 | 1 | 140 |
| roll, whole-wheat bun | ½ (1 oz) | 57 | 2 | 11 | 2 | 2 | 1 | 0 | 102 |
| scone, Health Valley, blueberry, fat-free | 1 | 180 | 4 | 43 | 5 | 18 | 0 | 0 | 190 |
| scone, Health Valley, cinnamon-raisin, fat-free | 1 | 180 | 4 | 43 | 5 | 18 | 0 | 0 | 190 |
| scone, Health Valley, cranberry-orange, fat-free | 1 | 180 | 4 | 43 | 5 | 18 | 0 | 0 | 190 |
| scone, whole wheat | 1 | 357 | 9 | 48 | 1 | 5 | 15 | 5 | 406 |
| taco shell, baked | 1 5" shell (0.5 oz) | 62 | 1 | 8 | 1 | 0 | 3 | 0 | 49 |
| taco shell, fried | 1 5" shell (0.5 oz) | 50 | 1 | 7 | 0 | 0 | 2 | 1 | 45 |
| toaster pastry, apple | ½ (1 oz) | 102 | 1 | 18 | 1 | 6 | 3 | 0 | 109 |

| FOOD ITEM | SERVING SIZE | CALORIES | PRO (g) | CARB (g) | FIBER (g) | SUGAR (g) | FAT (g) | SAT FAT (g) | SOD (mg) |
|---|---|---|---|---|---|---|---|---|---|
| toaster pastry, blueberry | ½ (1 oz) | 102 | 1 | 18 | 1 | 6 | 3 | 0 | 109 |
| toaster pastry, brown sugar cinnamon | ½ (1 oz) | 103 | 1 | 17 | 0 | n/a | 4 | 1 | 106 |
| toaster pastry, cherry | ½ (1 oz) | 102 | 1 | 19 | 1 | 6 | 3 | 0 | 109 |
| toaster pops, Amy's Organics, apple | ½ | 75 | 2 | 13 | 0 | 4 | 2 | 0 | 55 |
| toaster pops, Amy's Organics, cheese | ½ | 75 | 3 | 12 | 0 | 1 | 3 | 1 | 110 |
| toaster pops, Amy's Organics, strawberry | ½ | 75 | 2 | 13 | 0 | 4 | 2 | 0 | 55 |
| tortilla, corn | 1 6" tortilla | 57 | 1 | 12 | 2 | 0 | 1 | 0 | 12 |
| tortilla, Ezekiel 4:9, Organic Sprouted Corn Tortilla | 2 | 120 | 2 | 25 | 4 | 0 | 1 | 0 | 0 |
| tortilla, Ezekiel 4:9, Sprouted Grain Tortillas | 1 | 150 | 6 | 24 | 5 | n/a | 3.5 | n/a | 140 |
| tortilla, flour | 1 6" tortilla | 100 | 3 | 16 | 1 | 1 | 2 | 1 | 204 |
| tortilla, flour | 1 10" tortilla | 225 | 6 | 37 | 2 | 1 | 6 | 1 | 458 |
| tortilla, Tortilla Factory, low-carb, low-fat | 1 large | 80 | 8 | 19 | 14 | 1 | 3 | 0 | 300 |
| tortilla, Tortilla Factory, low-carb, low-fat green onion | 1 small | 50 | 5 | 11 | 8 | 0 | 2 | 0 | 180 |
| tortilla, Tortilla Factory, low-carb, low-fat, wheat | 1 small | 60 | 7 | 8 | 6 | 0 | 3 | 0 | 150 |
| tortilla, wheat | 1 6" tortilla (1 oz) | 73 | 3 | 20 | 2 | n/a | 0 | 0 | 171 |
| tortilla, wheat | 1 11" tortilla (3.5 oz) | 175 | 8 | 33 | 2 | n/a | 3 | 1 | 84 |
| waffle, Eggo, blueberry, low-fat | 1 (1 oz) | 95 | 2 | 15 | 1 | 4 | 3 | 1 | 185 |
| waffle, Eggo, nutri-grain, low-fat | 1 (1 oz) | 90 | 3 | 14 | 2 | 2 | 3 | 1 | 210 |
| waffle, Eggo, oat | 1 (1 oz) | 69 | 2 | 13 | 1 | 1 | 1 | 0 | 135 |
| waffle, plain | 1 (1 oz) | 84 | 2 | 13 | 1 | 1 | 3 | 0 | 193 |
| waffle, Special K, low-carb | 1 (1 oz) | 95 | 8 | 8 | 4 | 1 | 6 | 1 | 175 |

# CEREALS

| FOOD ITEM | SERVING SIZE | CALORIES | PRO (g) | CARB (g) | FIBER (g) | SUGAR (g) | FAT (g) | SAT FAT (g) | SOD (mg) |
|---|---|---|---|---|---|---|---|---|---|
| All-Bran cereal | ⅓ cup | 51 | 3 | 15 | 6 | 3 | 1 | 0 | 48 |
| All-Bran Buds cereal | ¼ cup | 57 | 2 | 18 | 10 | 6 | 0 | 0 | 154 |
| All-Bran Extra Fiber cereal | ⅓ cup | 38 | 2 | 15 | 10 | 0 | 1 | 0 | 95 |
| Alpen cereal | ¼ cup | 100 | 3 | 21 | 3 | 6 | 1 | 0 | 60 |
| Alpen cereal, no sugar added | ¼ cup | 75 | 3 | 15 | 1 | 3 | 1 | 0 | 11 |
| Alti Plano Gold, quinoa instant hot cereal, chai almond | 1 packet | 210 | 5 | 33 | 5 | 14 | 7 | 0 | 200 |
| Alti Plano Gold, quinoa instant hot cereal, oaxacan chocolate | 1 packet | 170 | 6 | 30 | 5 | 9 | 3 | 0 | 120 |
| Alti Plano Gold, quinoa instant hot cereal, orange date | 1 packet | 180 | 4 | 36 | 6 | 20 | 3 | 0 | 200 |
| Alti Plano Gold, quinoa instant hot cereal, regular, organic | 1 packet | 190 | 6 | 32 | 7 | 1 | 3 | 0 | 5 |
| Alti Plano Gold, quinoa instant hot cereal, spiced apple raisin | 1 packet | 160 | 6 | 35 | 5 | 12 | 2 | 0 | 110 |
| Basic 4 cereal | ¼ cup | 50 | 1 | 11 | 1 | 3 | 1 | 0 | 79 |
| blue corn flakes cereal | ½ cup | 67 | 2 | 16 | 3 | 3 | 0 | 0 | 7 |
| Bob's Red Mill 5-Grain Rolled hot cereal, dry | ⅓ cup | 120 | 5 | 25 | 5 | 1 | 1 | 0 | 0 |
| Bob's Red Mill 8-Grain Wheatless Cereal, dry | ¼ cup | 110 | 4 | 20 | 3 | 0 | 2 | 1 | 5 |
| Bob's Red Mill 10-Grain hot cereal, dry | ¼ cup | 180 | 6 | 35 | 3 | 0 | 3 | 0 | 5 |
| Bob's Red Mill Creamy Buckwheat hot cereal, organic, dry | ¼ cup | 140 | 5 | 30 | 3 | 0 | 1 | 0 | 0 |
| Bob's Red Mill Organic High Fiber hot cereal, dry | ⅓ cup | 150 | 8 | 27 | 10 | 0 | 5 | 0 | 330 |
| Bob's Red Mill Right Stuff 6-Grain Hot Cereal with Flaxseed, dry | ¼ cup | 140 | 6 | 27 | 4 | 0 | 2 | 0 | 0 |
| bran flake cereal with raisins | ⅓ cup | 62 | 2 | 15 | 2 | 6 | 0 | 0 | 96 |
| brown rice, crispy | ½ cup | 62 | 1 | 14 | 1 | 1 | 1 | 0 | 2 |
| buckwheat hot cereal, dry | 2 tbsp | 110 | 3 | 21 | 3 | 0 | 0 | 0 | 0 |
| Cheerios | ½ cup | 55 | 2 | 11 | 2 | 1 | 1 | 0 | 107 |
| Cheerios, multigrain | ½ cup | 54 | 1 | 12 | 1 | 3 | 1 | 0 | 100 |
| Complete All-Bran Oat Bran Flakes cereal | ½ cup | 70 | 2 | 15 | 3 | 4 | 1 | 0 | 140 |

| FOOD ITEM | SERVING SIZE | CALORIES | PRO (g) | CARB (g) | FIBER (g) | SUGAR (g) | FAT (g) | SAT FAT (g) | SOD (mg) |
|---|---|---|---|---|---|---|---|---|---|
| Complete All-Bran Wheat Bran Flakes cereal | ½ cup | 61 | 2 | 15 | 3 | 3 | 0 | 0 | 138 |
| Corn Flakes cereal | ½ cup | 51 | 1 | 12 | 0 | 1 | 0 | 0 | 101 |
| corn grits, white | ½ cup | 71 | 2 | 16 | 0 | 0 | 0 | 0 | 2 |
| corn grits, white, quick, cooked | ½ cup | 71 | 2 | 16 | 0 | 0 | 0 | 0 | 2 |
| corn grits, white, quick, uncooked | 2 tbsp | 72 | 2 | 16 | 0 | 0 | 0 | 0 | 0 |
| corn grits, white, regular, uncooked | 2 tbsp | 72 | 2 | 16 | 0 | 0 | 0 | 0 | 0 |
| corn grits, yellow | ½ cup | 71 | 2 | 16 | 0 | 0 | 0 | 0 | 2 |
| corn grits, yellow, quick, cooked | ½ cup | 71 | 2 | 16 | 0 | 0 | 0 | 0 | 2 |
| corn grits, yellow, quick, uncooked | 2 tbsp | 72 | 2 | 16 | 0 | 0 | 0 | 0 | 0 |
| corn grits, yellow, regular, uncooked | 2 tbsp | 72 | 2 | 16 | 0 | 0 | 0 | 0 | 0 |
| Cracklin' Oat Bran cereal | ¼ cup | 74 | 1 | 13 | 2 | 6 | 3 | 1 | 57 |
| Cream of Rice, cooked | ½ cup | 63 | 1 | 14 | 0 | 0 | 0 | 0 | 1 |
| Cream of Rice, uncooked | 2 tbsp | 80 | 1 | 18 | 0 | 0 | 0 | 0 | 1 |
| Crispix cereal | ½ cup | 55 | 1 | 12 | 0 | 2 | 0 | 0 | 111 |
| Ezekial 4:9 Sprouted Grain Cereal, almond | ½ cup | 200 | 8 | 38 | 6 | < 1 | 3 | 0 | 190 |
| Ezekial 4:9 Sprouted Grain Cereal, cinnamon raisin | ½ cup | 190 | 7 | 41 | 5 | 8 | 1 | 0 | 160 |
| Ezekial 4:9 Sprouted Grain Cereal, golden flax | ½ cup | 180 | 8 | 37 | 6 | 0 | 2.5 | 0 | 190 |
| Ezekial 4:9 Sprouted Grain Cereal, original | ½ cup | 190 | 8 | 41 | 5 | 0 | 1 | 0 | 200 |
| familia, uncooked | 2 tbsp | 59 | 1 | 11 | 1 | 4 | 1 | 0 | 8 |
| Farina, apple cereal, uncooked | 1 packet | 132 | 2 | 29 | 1 | n/a | 0 | 0 | 241 |
| Farina, banana cereal, dry | 1 packet | 132 | 2 | 29 | 1 | n/a | 0 | 0 | 241 |
| Farina, banana cereal, with water | 1 packet | 132 | 2 | 29 | 0 | n/a | 0 | 0 | 242 |
| Farina, wheat cereal | ½ cup | 56 | 2 | 12 | 0 | 0 | 0 | 0 | 2 |
| Farina wheat cereal, uncooked | 2 tbsp | 65 | 2 | 14 | 1 | 0 | 0 | 0 | 1 |
| Fiber One | ½ cup | 59 | 2 | 24 | 14 | 0 | 1 | 0 | 129 |
| flax + 4-grain hot cereal, uncooked | ¼ cup | 70 | 3 | 14 | 5 | 0 | 1 | 0 | 0 |
| granola, homemade | ¼ cup | 149 | 5 | 16 | 3 | 7 | 1 | 0 | 7 |

| FOOD ITEM | SERVING SIZE | CALORIES | PRO (g) | CARB (g) | FIBER (g) | SUGAR (g) | FAT (g) | SAT FAT (g) | SOD (mg) |
|---|---|---|---|---|---|---|---|---|---|
| granola, with raisins, low-fat | ¼ cup | 79 | 2 | 16 | 1 | 7 | 1 | 0 | 77 |
| granola, with raisins and dates, Sun Country | ¼ cup | 68 | 2 | 11 | 1 | 3 | 2 | 0 | 4 |
| Grape-Nuts cereal | ¼ cup | 104 | 3 | 24 | 3 | 3 | 1 | 0 | 177 |
| Grape-Nuts flakes | ½ cup | 71 | 2 | 16 | 2 | 3 | 1 | 0 | 93 |
| Harmony cereal | 1 oz | 103 | 3 | 22 | 1 | 7 | 1 | 0 | 183 |
| hominy grits, dry | 2 tbsp | 70 | 2 | 16 | 1 | 0 | 0 | 0 | 0 |
| Honey Crunch N Oats cereal | ½ cup | 80 | 1 | 16 | 1 | 4 | 1 | 0 | 90 |
| honey crunch wheat germ | 2 tbsp | 63 | 4 | 10 | 2 | 4 | 1 | 0 | 2 |
| Honey Nut Cheerios | ½ cup | 56 | 1 | 12 | 1 | 5 | 1 | 0 | 135 |
| Irish oats, uncooked | 2 tbsp | 74 | 3 | 14 | 2 | 0 | 1 | 0 | 1 |
| Just Right Fruit & Nut cereal | ⅓ cup | 67 | 1 | 15 | 1 | 5 | 1 | 0 | 84 |
| Kashi 7-Whole Grain Nuggets | ½ cup | 210 | 7 | 47 | 7 | 3 | 2 | 0 | 260 |
| Kashi 7-Whole Grain Puffs | ½ cup | 70 | 2 | 15 | 1 | 0 | 0 | 0 | 0 |
| Kashi GoLean cereal | ½ cup | 70 | 7 | 15 | 5 | 3 | 1 | 0 | 85 |
| Kashi GoLean Crunch cereal | ½ cup | 95 | 5 | 18 | 4 | 6 | 2 | 0 | 48 |
| Kashi Good Friends cereal | ½ cup | 85 | 3 | 22 | 6 | 5 | 1 | 0 | 65 |
| Kashi Heart to Heart cereal | ¾ cup | 110 | 4 | 25 | 5 | 5 | 2 | 0 | 90 |
| Kashi Heart to Heart Oatmeal Raisin Spice | 1 packet | 150 | 3 | 33 | 4 | 16 | 2 | 0 | 100 |
| Kashi Organic Promise Autumn Wheat | ½ cup | 95 | 3 | 23 | 3 | 4 | 0 | 0 | 0 |
| Kashi Organic Promise Cinnamon Harvest | ½ cup | 95 | 2 | 22 | 3 | 4 | 1 | 0 | 0 |
| Kashi Organic Promise Strawberry Fields | ½ cup | 60 | 1 | 14 | 1 | 5 | 0 | 0 | 100 |
| Kix | ½ cup | 43 | 1 | 10 | 0 | 1 | 0 | 0 | 100 |
| Malt-O-Meal, chocolate | ½ cup | 61 | 2 | 13 | 0 | n/a | 0 | 0 | 1 |
| Malt-O-Meal, chocolate, cooked, with salt | ½ cup | 61 | 2 | 13 | 0 | n/a | 0 | 0 | 162 |
| Maltex hot cereal | ⅓ cup | 57 | 2 | 12 | 1 | 0 | 0 | 0 | 4 |
| Maltex hot cereal, cooked, with salt | ⅓ cup | 57 | 2 | 12 | 1 | 0 | 0 | 0 | 57 |
| Maltex hot cereal, dry | 2 tbsp | 66 | 2 | 15 | 1 | 0 | 0 | 0 | 3 |
| Maypo hot cereal | ½ cup | 85 | 3 | 16 | 3 | 7 | 1 | 0 | 5 |
| Maypo hot cereal, uncooked | 3 tbsp | 68 | 2 | 13 | 2 | 6 | 1 | 0 | 3 |

| FOOD ITEM | SERVING SIZE | CALORIES | PRO (g) | CARB (g) | FIBER (g) | SUGAR (g) | FAT (g) | SAT FAT (g) | SOD (mg) |
|---|---|---|---|---|---|---|---|---|---|
| muesli, dried fruit and nuts | ¼ cup | 72 | 2 | 17 | 2 | 7 | 1 | 0 | 49 |
| muesli, strawberry pecan | ¼ cup | 53 | 1 | 11 | 1 | 4 | 1 | 0 | 43 |
| Multi-Bran Chex | ⅓ cup | 55 | 1 | 14 | 2 | 4 | 0 | 0 | 107 |
| MultiGrain Cheerios | ½ cup | 54 | 1 | 12 | 1 | 3 | 1 | 0 | 100 |
| multi-grain hot cereal | ½ cup | 101 | 3 | 20 | 2 | 1 | 1 | 0 | 1 |
| multi-grain oatmeal | ½ cup | 71 | 2 | 16 | 3 | 0 | 1 | 0 | 4 |
| multi grain oatmeal, uncooked | ¼ cup | 67 | 2 | 15 | 2 | 0 | 1 | 0 | 1 |
| oat bran | ¼ cup | 58 | 4 | 16 | 4 | 0 | 2 | 0 | 1 |
| oat bran flakes | ⅓ cup | 55 | 2 | 12 | 2 | 3 | 0 | 0 | 6 |
| oatmeal, old-fashioned, dry | ¼ cup | 74 | 3 | 14 | 2 | 0 | 2 | 0 | 1 |
| Oatmeal Raisin Crisp | ⅓ cup | 68 | 2 | 15 | 1 | 6 | 1 | 0 | 0 |
| 100% Bran Cereal | ¼ cup | 63 | 3 | 17 | 6 | 5 | 0 | 0 | 92 |
| Product 19 | ½ cup | 50 | 1 | 12 | 0 | 2 | 0 | 0 | 104 |
| Puffed Millet | ½ cup | 1 | 8 | 0 | 0 | 0 | 0 | 1 | 0 |
| Puffed Rice | ½ cup | 30 | 1 | 7 | 0 | 0 | 0 | 0 | 0 |
| Puffed Wheat | ½ cup | 25 | 1 | 6 | 1 | 0 | 0 | 0 | 0 |
| Raisin Bran | ⅓ cup | 65 | 2 | 16 | 2 | 7 | 1 | 0 | 120 |
| Raisin Bran Crunch | ⅓ cup | 62 | 1 | 15 | 1 | 7 | 0 | 0 | 70 |
| Raisin Nut Bran | ⅓ cup | 70 | 2 | 14 | 2 | 5 | 1 | 0 | 83 |
| Rice Chex | ½ cup | 47 | 1 | 11 | 0 | 1 | 0 | 0 | 117 |
| Rice Krispies | ½ cup | 51 | 1 | 11 | 0 | 1 | 0 | 0 | 125 |
| roman meal plain, dry | 3 tbsp | 56 | 3 | 13 | 3 | n/a | 0 | 0 | 1 |
| roman meal, with oats, cooked, with water, with salt | ½ cup | 85 | 4 | 17 | 4 | n/a | 1 | 0 | 270 |
| roman meal, with oats, uncooked | 3 tbsp | 64 | 3 | 13 | 3 | 0 | 1 | 0 | 4 |
| shredded wheat cereal | 1 single serve box | 85 | 3 | 21 | 3 | 0 | 0 | 0 | 2 |
| Shredded Wheat 'N Bran | ½ cup | 79 | 3 | 19 | 3 | 0 | 0 | 0 | 1 |
| Shredded Wheat Spoon Size | ⅓ cup | 55 | 2 | 14 | 2 | 0 | 0 | 0 | 1 |
| Smart Start Antioxidants | ⅓ cup | 63 | 1 | 14 | 1 | 9 | 0 | 0 | 93 |
| Smart Start Healthy Heart | ⅓ cup | 61 | 2 | 13 | 1 | 5 | 1 | 0 | 37 |
| Special K | ½ cup | 59 | 3 | 11 | 0 | 2 | 0 | 0 | 112 |

| FOOD ITEM | SERVING SIZE | CALORIES | PRO (g) | CARB (g) | FIBER (g) | SUGAR (g) | FAT (g) | SAT FAT (g) | SOD (mg) |
|---|---|---|---|---|---|---|---|---|---|
| Special K Low Carb Lifestyle Protein Plus | ½ cup | 67 | 7 | 9 | 3 | 1 | 2 | 0 | 73 |
| steel cut oats, organic, uncooked | 2 tbsp | 70 | 3 | 14 | 2 | 0 | 1 | 0 | 0 |
| Sunrise | 0.5 oz | 54 | 1 | 12 | 1 | 5 | 0 | 0 | 86 |
| Total cereal | ½ cup | 65 | 2 | 15 | 2 | 3 | 0 | 0 | 128 |
| Total Raisin Bran | ⅓ cup | 57 | 1 | 14 | 2 | 7 | 0 | 0 | 80 |
| Uncle Sam cereal | ⅓ cup | 79 | 3 | 12 | 4 | 0 | 2 | 0 | 38 |
| Uncle Sam cereal with Mixed Berries | ¼ cup | 55 | 2 | 10 | 3 | 0 | 1 | 0 | 25 |
| wheat and malt barley flake cereal | ½ cup | 71 | 2 | 16 | 2 | 3 | 1 | 0 | 93 |
| wheat bran | ¼ cup | 31 | 2 | 9 | 6 | 0 | 1 | 0 | 0 |
| Wheat Chex | ½ cup | 52 | 2 | 12 | 2 | 2 | 0 | 0 | 134 |
| wheat germ | 2 tbsp | 4 | 6 | 2 | n/a | 1 | 0 | 1 | n/a |
| Wheat N Raisins cereal | ¼ cup | 46 | 1 | 11 | 1 | 5 | 0 | 0 | 1 |
| Wheatena, cooked without salt | ½ cup | 68 | 2 | 14 | 3 | 0 | 1 | 0 | 2 |
| Wheatena, cooked with salt | ½ cup | 72 | 2 | 14 | 2 | 0 | 1 | 0 | 289 |
| Wheatena, uncooked | 2 tbsp | 62 | 2 | 13 | 2 | 0 | 1 | 0 | 2 |
| Wheaties | ½ cup | 53 | 2 | 12 | 2 | 2 | 0 | 0 | 109 |

## CHEESE

| FOOD ITEM | SERVING SIZE | CALORIES | PRO (g) | CARB (g) | FIBER (g) | SUGAR (g) | FAT (g) | SAT FAT (g) | SOD (mg) |
|---|---|---|---|---|---|---|---|---|---|
| American, pasteurized process, fat-free | 1" cube | 24 | 4 | 2 | 0 | 2 | 0 | 0 | 244 |
| American, pasteurized process, low-fat | 1" cube | 32 | 4 | 1 | 0 | 0 | 1 | 1 | 257 |
| American, pasteurized process, low-sodium | 1" cube | 68 | 4 | 0 | 0 | 0 | 6 | 4 | 1 |
| American, soy, substitute | 1 piece (0.7 oz) | 35 | 4 | 0 | 0 | 0 | 2 | 0 | 290 |
| American cheese food | 1 oz | 94 | 6 | 2 | 0 | n/a | 7 | 4 | 274 |
| American cheese food, low-fat | 1" cube | 32 | 4 | 1 | 0 | 0 | 1 | 1 | 257 |
| blue, crumbled | 1 tbsp | 30 | 2 | 0 | 0 | 0 | 2 | 2 | 118 |
| Brie | 1" cube | 57 | 4 | 0 | 0 | 0 | 5 | 3 | 107 |
| Camembert | 1" cube | 51 | 3 | 0 | 0 | 0 | 4 | 3 | 143 |

| FOOD ITEM | SERVING SIZE | CALORIES | PRO (g) | CARB (g) | FIBER (g) | SUGAR (g) | FAT (g) | SAT FAT (g) | SOD (mg) |
|---|---|---|---|---|---|---|---|---|---|
| Cheddar | 1" cube | 69 | 4 | 0 | 0 | 0 | 6 | 4 | 106 |
| Cheddar, fat-free | 1" cube | 40 | 8 | 1 | 0 | 1 | 0 | 0 | 220 |
| Cheddar, fat-free, natural, shredded | 2 tbsp | 23 | 5 | 1 | 0 | 0 | 0 | 0 | 110 |
| Cheddar, low-fat | 1" cube | 30 | 4 | 0 | 0 | 0 | 1 | 1 | 106 |
| Cheddar, low-sodium | 1 oz | 113 | 7 | 1 | 0 | 0 | 9 | 6 | 6 |
| Cheddar, low-sodium, shredded | 1 tbsp | 28 | 2 | 0 | 0 | 0 | 2 | 1 | 1 |
| Cheddar, soy substitute | 1 piece (0.7 oz) | 35 | 4 | 1 | 1 | 0 | 2 | 0 | 280 |
| Cheddar, soy substitute, shreds, Melissa's | 1 oz | 63 | 7 | 2 | 1 | 0 | 0 | 0 | 190 |
| Cheddar, string | 1 (1 oz) | 50 | 8 | 1 | 0 | 0 | 2 | 1 | 220 |
| Cheddar, string, fat-free | 1 (1 oz) | 40 | 8 | 1 | 0 | 1 | 0 | 0 | 220 |
| Cheddar, string, low-fat | 1 (1 oz) | 106 | 6 | 0 | 0 | 0 | 9 | 6 | 220 |
| cheese topping, vegetarian, soy substitute | 1 tbsp | 22.5 | 3 | 1 | n/a | n/a | 1 | 0 | 120 |
| Colby | 1" cube | 68 | 4 | 0 | 0 | 0 | 6 | 3 | 104 |
| cottage cheese, fat-free | 4 oz | 80 | 11 | 7 | 0 | 4 | 0 | 0 | 380 |
| cottage cheese, fat-free, large curd, dry | ½ cup | 96 | 20 | 2 | 0 | 2 | 0 | 0 | 15 |
| cottage cheese, fat-free, small curd, dry | ½ cup | 96 | 20 | 2 | 0 | 2 | 0 | 0 | 15 |
| cottage cheese, large or small curd | ¼ cup | 58 | 7 | 2 | 0 | 0 | 3 | 2 | 228 |
| cottage cheese, low-fat 1%, lactose-reduced | ¼ cup | 41 | 7 | 2 | 0 | 2 | 1 | 0 | 229 |
| cottage cheese, low-fat 1%, no sodium added | ¼ cup | 38 | 6 | 2 | 0 | 2 | 1 | 0 | 7 |
| cottage cheese, low-fat 1%, with vegetables | ¼ cup | 38 | 6 | 2 | 0 | 2 | 1 | 0 | 228 |
| cottage cheese, low-fat 2% | ¼ cup | 50 | 7 | 3 | 0 | 3 | 1 | 1 | 235 |
| cottage cheese, soy substitute | ¼ cup | 85 | 7 | 4 | 0 | 1 | 5 | 1 | 11 |
| cottage cheese, with fruit | ¼ cup | 55 | 6 | 3 | 0 | 1 | 2 | 1 | 194 |
| cream cheese | 2 tbsp | 101 | 2 | 1 | 0 | 0 | 10 | 6 | 86 |
| cream cheese, Better Than Plain Cream Cheese Substitute | 1 oz | 80 | 1 | 1 | 0 | 0 | 8 | 2 | 135 |
| cream cheese, fat-free | 2 tbsp | 28 | 4 | 2 | 0 | 0 | 0 | 0 | 158 |
| cream cheese, fat-free, brick | 1 oz | 30 | 4 | 2 | 0 | 1 | 0 | 0 | 140 |

| FOOD ITEM | SERVING SIZE | CALORIES | PRO (g) | CARB (g) | FIBER (g) | SUGAR (g) | FAT (g) | SAT FAT (g) | SOD (mg) |
|---|---|---|---|---|---|---|---|---|---|
| cream cheese, fat-free, garden vegetable | 2 tbsp | 30 | 5 | 2 | 0 | 1 | 0 | 0 | 220 |
| cream cheese, fat-free, garlic and herb | 2 tbsp | 25 | 4 | 2 | 1 | 0 | 0 | 0 | 200 |
| cream cheese, fat-free, plain | 2 tbsp | 25 | 4 | 2 | 1 | 0 | 0 | 0 | 200 |
| cream cheese, fat-free, soft | 2 tbsp | 30 | 5 | 2 | 0 | 1 | 0 | 0 | 200 |
| cream cheese, fat-free, soft, strawberry | 2 tbsp | 45 | 4 | 6 | 0 | 5 | 0 | 0 | 190 |
| cream cheese, fat-free, strawberry | 2 tbsp | 35 | 4 | 5 | 1 | 0 | 0 | 0 | 200 |
| cream cheese, low-fat | 2 tbsp | 69 | 3 | 2 | 0 | 0 | 5 | 3 | 89 |
| cream cheese, whipped | 2 tbsp | 70 | 2 | 1 | 0 | 0 | 7 | 4 | 59 |
| cream cheese, whipped, low-fat | 2 tbsp | 46 | 2 | 1 | 0 | 0 | 4 | 2 | 59 |
| cream cheese, whipped, with smoked salmon | 2 tbsp | 70 | 2 | 1 | 0 | 1 | 6 | 4 | 140 |
| Edam | 0.5 oz | 51 | 4 | 0 | 0 | 0 | 4 | 2 | 137 |
| feta | 1" cube | 45 | 2 | 1 | 0 | 1 | 4 | 3 | 190 |
| feta, low-fat | 1.25" cube | 50 | 6 | 1 | 0 | 0 | 3 | 2 | 370 |
| fontina | 1" cube | 58 | 4 | 0 | 0 | 0 | 5 | 3 | 120 |
| goat, hard | 1 oz | 128 | 9 | 1 | 0 | 1 | 10 | 7 | 98 |
| goat, semi soft | 1 oz | 103 | 6 | 10 | 0 | 1 | 8 | 6 | 146 |
| goat, soft | 1 oz | 76 | 5 | 0 | 0 | 0 | 6 | 4 | 104 |
| Gouda | 1 oz | 101 | 7 | 1 | 0 | 1 | 8 | 5 | 232 |
| Gruyère | 1" cube | 62 | 4 | 0 | 0 | 0 | 5 | 3 | 50 |
| Jalapeño Jack, soy substitute | 1 piece (0.7 oz) | 35 | 4 | 0 | 0 | 0 | 2 | 0 | 250 |
| Laughing Cow, light, garlic and herb | 1 piece | 35 | 2.5 | 1 | 0 | 1 | 2 | 1 | 260 |
| Laughing Cow, light, Swiss original | 1 piece | 35 | 2.5 | 1 | 0 | 1 | 2 | 1 | 260 |
| Laughing Cow, light, toasted onion | 1 piece | 35 | 2.5 | 1 | 0 | 1 | 2 | 1 | 260 |
| Mexican queso anejo | 2 tbsp | 62 | 4 | 1 | 0 | n/a | 5 | 3 | 187 |
| Mexican queso asadero | 1" cube | 64 | 4 | 1 | 0 | 1 | 5 | 3 | 118 |
| Mexican queso chihuahua | 1" cube | 64 | 4 | 1 | 0 | 1 | 5 | 3 | 105 |
| mild Mexican cheese, fat-free | 1" cube | 40 | 8 | 1 | 0 | 1 | 0 | 0 | 220 |
| Monterey Jack, fat-free | 1" cube | 40 | 8 | 1 | 0 | 1 | 0 | 0 | 220 |

## CHEESE (cont.)

| FOOD ITEM | SERVING SIZE | CALORIES | PRO (g) | CARB (g) | FIBER (g) | SUGAR (g) | FAT (g) | SAT FAT (g) | SOD (mg) |
|---|---|---|---|---|---|---|---|---|---|
| Monterey Jack, low-fat | 1" cube | 53 | 5 | 0 | 0 | 0 | 4 | 2 | 96 |
| mozzarella, fat-free, shredded | 1 oz | 42 | 9 | 1 | 1 | 0 | 0 | 0 | 211 |
| mozzarella, low-sodium | 1" cube | 50 | 5 | 1 | 0 | 0 | 3 | 2 | 3 |
| mozzarella, part-skim | 1" cube | 53 | 5 | 1 | 0 | 0 | 4 | 2 | 93 |
| mozzarella, part-skim, low moisture | 1 oz | 86 | 7 | 1 | 0 | 0 | 6 | 4 | 150 |
| mozzarella, soy cheese substitute | 1 piece (0.7 oz) | 30 | 4 | 0 | 0 | 0 | 2 | 0 | 270 |
| mozzarella, soy cheese substitute, shreds, Melissa's | 1 oz | 63 | 7 | 2 | 1 | 0 | 3 | 0 | 190 |
| mozzarella, string | 1 | 50 | 8 | 1 | 0 | 0 | 2 | 1 | 220 |
| mozzarella, string, reduced-fat | 1 | 50 | 6 | 1 | 0 | 0 | 3 | 2 | 180 |
| mozzarella cheese substitute | 1" cube | 44 | 2 | 4 | 0 | 4 | 2 | 1 | 121 |
| Muenster | 1" cube | 64 | 4 | 0 | 0 | 0 | 5 | 3 | 110 |
| Muenster, low-fat | 1" cube | 49 | 4 | 1 | 0 | 1 | 3 | 2 | 108 |
| Neufchâtel | 1 oz | 74 | 3 | 1 | 0 | 0 | 7 | 4 | 113 |
| Parmesan, grated | 2 tbsp | 40 | 4 | 0 | 0 | 0 | 3 | 2 | 120 |
| Parmesan, hard | 1" cube | 40 | 4 | 0 | 0 | 0 | 3 | 2 | 165 |
| Parmesan, low-sodium | 2 tbsp | 57 | 5 | 0 | 0 | 0 | 4 | 2 | 8 |
| Parmesan, shredded | 2 tbsp | 42 | 4 | 0 | 0 | n/a | 3 | 2 | 170 |
| Parmesan-style grated topping, reduced-fat, Kraft | 5 g | 20 | 1 | 2 | 0 | 0 | 1 | 0 | 75 |
| pepper Jack, fat-free | 1" cube | 40 | 8 | 1 | 0 | 1 | 0 | 0 | 220 |
| provolone | 1" cube | 60 | 4 | 0 | 0 | 0 | 5 | 3 | 149 |
| ricotta | ¼ cup | 108 | 7 | 2 | 0 | 0 | 8 | 5 | 52 |
| ricotta, fat-free | ¼ cup | 50 | 5 | 5 | 0 | 2 | 0 | 0 | 65 |
| ricotta, low-fat | ¼ cup | 86 | 7 | 3 | 0 | 0 | 5 | 3 | 78 |
| Romano | 2 tbsp | 70 | 6 | 0 | 0 | 0 | 5 | 3 | 260 |
| Roquefort | 1 oz | 105 | 6 | 1 | 0 | n/a | 9 | 5 | 513 |
| SmartBeat Fat-Free Cheese Substitute | 1 slice | 25 | 4 | 3 | 0 | 2 | 0 | 0 | 180 |
| soy cheese, chunk, Melissa's | 1 oz | 63 | 7 | 2 | 1 | 0 | 3 | 0 | 190 |
| soy cheese, slices, Melissa's | 1 slice (⅔ oz) | 45 | 3 | 3 | 0 | 0 | 2 | 0 | 180 |

## CHEESE (cont.)

| FOOD ITEM | SERVING SIZE | CALORIES | PRO (g) | CARB (g) | FIBER (g) | SUGAR (g) | FAT (g) | SAT FAT (g) | SOD (mg) |
|---|---|---|---|---|---|---|---|---|---|
| Swiss | 1" cube | 57 | 4 | 1 | 0 | 0 | 4 | 3 | 29 |
| Swiss, fat-free | 1" cube | 40 | 8 | 1 | 0 | 1 | 0 | 0 | 220 |
| Swiss, low-fat | 1" cube | 27 | 4 | 1 | 0 | 0 | 1 | 1 | 39 |
| Swiss, low-fat, singles | 1 | 40 | 5 | 2 | 0 | 1 | 1 | 1 | 200 |
| Swiss, pasteurized process | 1" cube | 60 | 4 | 0 | 0 | 0 | 4 | 3 | 245 |
| Swiss, pasteurized process, low-fat | 1" cube | 31 | 5 | 1 | 0 | 0 | 1 | 1 | 257 |
| Swiss, soy substitute | 1 piece (0.7 oz) | 35 | 4 | 1 | 0 | 0 | 2 | 0 | n/a |
| Swiss cheese food | 1 oz | 92 | 6 | 1 | 0 | n/a | 7 | 4 | 440 |

## CONDIMENTS, DRESSINGS, MARINADES, AND SPREADS

| FOOD ITEM | SERVING SIZE | CALORIES | PRO (g) | CARB (g) | FIBER (g) | SUGAR (g) | FAT (g) | SAT FAT (g) | SOD (mg) |
|---|---|---|---|---|---|---|---|---|---|
| barbecue sauce | 1 tbsp | 12 | 0 | 2 | 0 | 1 | 0 | 0 | 127 |
| barbecue sauce, Carb Control, low sugar | 1 tbsp | 5 | 0 | 2 | 0 | 0 | 0 | 0 | 170 |
| barbecue sauce, Steel's Gourmet, sugar-free | 2 tbsp | 15 | 0 | 2 | 0 | 0 | 0 | 0 | 200 |
| barbecue sauce, Steel's Gourmet, sugar-free, chipotle | 2 tbsp | 15 | 0 | 2 | 0 | 0 | 0 | 0 | 200 |
| basil pesto, Melissa's | 1 tbsp | 85 | 3 | 1 | 0 | 0 | 8 | 1 | 58 |
| capers, drained | 1 tbsp | 2 | 0 | 0 | 0 | 0 | 0 | 0 | 255 |
| cocktail sauce, Steel's Gourmet, no sugar added | 4 tbsp | 30 | 2 | 5 | 0 | 3 | 0 | 0 | 220 |
| dijon horseradish | 1 tbsp | 60 | 0 | 1 | 0 | 0 | 7 | 1 | 107 |
| dressing, bacon and tomato | 1 tbsp | 49 | 0 | 0 | 0 | 0 | 5 | 1 | 163 |
| dressing, bacon and tomato, low-calorie | 1 tbsp | 32 | 0 | 0 | 0 | 0 | 3 | 1 | 176 |
| dressing, balsamic vinaigrette | 1 tbsp | 45 | 0 | 2 | 0 | 2 | 4 | 1 | 150 |
| dressing, balsamic vinaigrette, Newman's Own, Lighten Up Balsamic Vinaigrette | 1 tbsp | 21 | 0 | 1 | 0 | 1 | 2 | 0 | 228 |
| dressing, balsamic vinegar | 1 tbsp | 18 | 0 | 4 | 0 | 4 | 0 | 0 | 230 |
| dressing, blue cheese | 1 tbsp | 77 | 1 | 1 | 0 | 1 | 8 | 2 | 167 |
| dressing, blue cheese, fat-free | 1 tbsp | 20 | 0 | 4 | 1 | 2 | 0 | 0 | 136 |

| FOOD ITEM | SERVING SIZE | CALORIES | PRO (g) | CARB (g) | FIBER (g) | SUGAR (g) | FAT (g) | SAT FAT (g) | SOD (mg) |
|---|---|---|---|---|---|---|---|---|---|
| dressing, blue cheese, low-calorie | 1 tbsp | 15 | 1 | 0 | 0 | 0 | 1 | 0 | 180 |
| dressing, blue cheese, reduced-calorie | 1 tbsp | 14 | 0 | 2 | 0 | 1 | 0 | 0 | 258 |
| dressing, buttermilk, light | 1 tbsp | 32 | 0 | 2 | 0 | 0 | 2 | 0 | 132 |
| dressing, Caesar | 1 tbsp | 78 | 0 | 0 | 0 | 0 | 8 | 1 | 158 |
| dressing, Caesar, fat-free | 1 tbsp | 23 | 1 | 6 | 1 | 1 | 0 | 0 | 180 |
| dressing, Caesar, Galeos | 1 tbsp | 14 | 1 | 1 | 1 | 0 | 1 | 0 | 56 |
| dressing, Caesar, Good Life Foods Classic Caesar | 1 tbsp | 45 | 0 | 0 | 0 | 0 | 4 | 1 | 110 |
| dressing, Caesar, low-calorie | 1 tbsp | 17 | 0 | 3 | 0 | 2 | 1 | 0 | 162 |
| dressing, Caesar, low-fat | 1 tbsp | 17 | 0 | 3 | 0 | 2 | 1 | 0 | 162 |
| dressing, Catalina, fat-free | 1 tbsp | 18 | 0 | 4 | 1 | 4 | 0 | 0 | 160 |
| dressing, coleslaw | 1 tbsp | 62 | 0 | 4 | 0 | 3 | 5 | 1 | 114 |
| dressing, coleslaw, reduced-fat | 1 tbsp | 56 | 0 | 7 | 0 | 7 | 3 | 1 | 272 |
| dressing, creamy dill, fat-free, organic | 1 tbsp | 13 | 1 | 2 | 0 | 1 | 0 | 0 | 95 |
| dressing, creamy French, light | 1 tbsp | 45 | 1 | 4 | 0 | 3 | 3 | 0 | 140 |
| dressing, creamy garlic, fat-free, organic | 1 tbsp | 10 | 0 | 2 | 0 | 2 | 0 | 0 | 90 |
| dressing, creamy Italian, fat-free | 1 tbsp | 25 | 0 | 6 | 1 | 2 | 0 | 0 | 165 |
| dressing, creamy Parmesan, low-fat | 1 tbsp | 23 | 0 | 4 | 0 | 2 | 1 | 0 | 135 |
| dressing, creamy sour cream buttermilk, low-calorie | 1 tbsp | 18 | 0 | 3 | 0 | 1 | 0 | 0 | 170 |
| dressing, cucumber ranch | 1 tbsp | 70 | 0 | 1 | 0 | 1 | 8 | 1 | 110 |
| dressing, cucumber ranch, one-third less fat | 1 tbsp | 30 | 0 | 1 | 0 | 1 | 3 | 1 | 240 |
| dressing, dijon vinaigrette, Good Life Foods | 1 tbsp | 50 | 0 | 0 | 0 | 0 | 4 | 1 | 90 |
| dressing, dijonnaise, Galeos | 1 tbsp | 19 | 1 | 1 | 1 | 1 | 2 | 0 | 35 |
| dressing, French | 1 tbsp | 79 | 0 | 2 | 0 | 2 | 7 | 1 | 130 |
| dressing, French, fat-free | 1 tbsp | 21 | 0 | 5 | 0 | 3 | 0 | 0 | 128 |
| dressing, French, low-calorie | 1 tbsp | 38 | 0 | 5 | 0 | 3 | 2 | 0 | 131 |
| dressing, French, low-calorie, low-sodium | 1 tbsp | 18 | 0 | 2 | n/a | n/a | 1 | 0 | |

| FOOD ITEM | SERVING SIZE | CALORIES | PRO (g) | CARB (g) | FIBER (g) | SUGAR (g) | FAT (g) | SAT FAT (g) | SOD (mg) |
|---|---|---|---|---|---|---|---|---|---|
| dressing, French, reduced-calorie | 1 tbsp | 32 | 0 | 4 | 0 | 4 | 2 | 0 | 160 |
| dressing, garlic ranch | 1 tbsp | 90 | 0 | 1 | 0 | 1 | 10 | 2 | 135 |
| dressing, garlic ranch fat-free | 1 tbsp | 23 | 0 | 6 | 1 | 1 | 0 | 0 | 160 |
| dressing, ginger lime, Steel's Gourmet Sweet Ginger Lime Sugar-Free | 1 tbsp | 68 | 0 | 1 | 1 | 0 | 7 | 0 | 0 |
| dressing, ginger soy, Good Life Foods | 1 tbsp | 30 | 0 | 0 | 0 | 0 | 3 | 0 | 145 |
| dressing, ginger wasabi, Galeos | 1 tbsp | 14 | 1 | 1 | 1 | 0 | 1 | 0 | 42 |
| dressing, Greek vinaigrette | 1 tbsp | 55 | 0 | 13 | 0 | 1 | 6 | 1 | 160 |
| dressing, green goddess | 1 tbsp | 64 | 0 | 1 | 0 | 1 | 7 | 1 | 130 |
| dressing, honey dijon, fat-free | 1 tbsp | 25 | 1 | 5 | 1 | 2 | 0 | 0 | 170 |
| dressing, honey dijon, low-fat | 1 tbsp | 18 | 0 | 2 | 0 | 2 | 1 | 0 | 100 |
| dressing, honey mustard | 1 tbsp | 51 | 0 | 7 | 0 | 7 | 3 | 0 | 37 |
| dressing, honey mustard, fat-free | 1 tbsp | 10 | 0 | 3 | 0 | 2 | 0 | 0 | 140 |
| dressing, honey mustard, Steel's Gourmet, Honey Mustard Sugar-Free | 1 tbsp | 90 | 0 | 0 | 0 | 0 | 7 | 1 | 125 |
| dressing, Italian, diet, low-sodium | 1 tbsp | 12 | 0 | 1 | n/a | n/a | 1 | n/a | 18 |
| dressing, Italian, fat-free | 1 tbsp | 7 | 0 | 1 | 0 | 1 | 0 | 0 | 158 |
| dressing, Italian, Light Done Right | 1 tbsp | 26 | 0 | 1 | 1 | 2 | 0 | 0 | 114 |
| dressing, Italian, olive oil, reduced-fat | 1 tbsp | 23 | 0 | 1 | 0 | 1 | 2 | 0 | 230 |
| dressing, Italian, pesto | 1 tbsp | 35 | 1 | 3 | 0 | 1 | 3 | 0 | 135 |
| dressing, Italian, reduced-calorie | 1 tbsp | 28 | 0 | 1 | 0 | 0 | 3 | 0 | 199 |
| dressing, mayonnaise, fat-free | 1 tbsp | 13 | 0 | 2 | 0 | 2 | 0 | 0 | 126 |
| dressing, Miracle Whip, fat-free | 1 tbsp | 13 | 0 | 2 | 0 | 2 | 0 | 0 | 126 |
| dressing, oil-free, low-calorie | 1 tbsp | 4 | 0 | 1 | 0 | 1 | 0 | 0 | 256 |
| dressing, oil and vinegar, Good Life Foods | 1 tbsp | 50 | 0 | 0 | 0 | 0 | 5 | 1 | 125 |
| dressing, onion garlic, fat-free, organic | 1 tbsp | 8 | 0 | 2 | 0 | 1 | 0 | 0 | 95 |
| dressing, peanut | 1 tbsp | 53 | 1 | 3 | 0 | 3 | 4 | 4 | 1 |

| FOOD ITEM | SERVING SIZE | CALORIES | PRO (g) | CARB (g) | FIBER (g) | SUGAR (g) | FAT (g) | SAT FAT (g) | SOD (mg) |
|---|---|---|---|---|---|---|---|---|---|
| dressing, peppercorn | 1 tbsp | 76 | 0 | 0 | 0 | 0 | 8 | 1 | 143 |
| dressing, peppercorn ranch, low-fat | 1 tbsp | 25 | 1 | 2 | 0 | 2 | 2 | 1 | 110 |
| dressing, poppy seed | 1 tbsp | 65 | 0 | 4 | 0 | 4 | 5 | 5 | 1 |
| dressing, porcini mushroom vinaigrette, organic | 1 tbsp | 35 | 1 | 1 | 0 | 1 | 3 | 1 | 120 |
| dressing, ranch | 1 tbsp | 69 | 0 | 1 | 0 | 0 | 7 | 1 | 116 |
| dressing, ranch, Bernstein's Light Fantastic Parmesan Garlic Ranch | 1 tbsp | 25 | 0 | 3 | 0 | 1 | 1 | 0 | 165 |
| dressing, ranch, fat-free | 1 tbsp | 17 | 0 | 4 | 0 | 1 | 0 | 0 | 107 |
| dressing, ranch, Good Life Foods Buttermilk Ranch | 1 tbsp | 50 | 0 | 0 | 0 | 0 | 5 | 1 | 140 |
| dressing, ranch, light | 1 tbsp | 40 | 0 | 2 | 0 | 1 | 4 | 0 | 150 |
| dressing, ranch, Light Done Right | 1 tbsp | 38 | 0 | 2 | 0 | 1 | 3 | 0 | 151 |
| dressing, ranch, low-fat | 1 tbsp | 23 | 0 | 4 | 0 | 2 | 1 | 0 | 165 |
| dressing, ranch, one-third less fat | 1 tbsp | 50 | 0 | 3 | 0 | 1 | 5 | 1 | 160 |
| dressing, ranch, reduced-fat | 1 tbsp | 31 | 0 | 2 | 0 | 0 | 2 | 0 | 132 |
| dressing, red wine vinaigrette, fat-free | 1 tbsp | 8 | 0 | 2 | 0 | 2 | 0 | 0 | 200 |
| dressing, Roka blue cheese, light | 1 tbsp | 35 | 1 | 2 | 0 | 1 | 3 | 1 | 145 |
| dressing, Roquefort, fat-free | 1 tbsp | 20 | 0 | 4 | 1 | 2 | 0 | 0 | 136 |
| dressing, Roquefort, reduced-calorie | 1 tbsp | 14 | 0 | 2 | 0 | 1 | 0 | 0 | 258 |
| dressing, roasted red pepper | 1 tbsp | 18 | 0 | 2 | 0 | 2 | 1 | 0 | 170 |
| dressing, Russian, low-calorie | 1 tbsp | 23 | 0 | 5 | 0 | 4 | 1 | 0 | 141 |
| dressing, sesame seed | 1 tbsp | 68 | 0 | 1 | 0 | 1 | 7 | 1 | 153 |
| dressing, sesame seed, Galeos | 1 tbsp | 22 | 1 | 1 | 1 | 1 | 2 | 0 | 35 |
| dressing, shiitake sesame, Good Life Foods | 1 tbsp | 55 | 0 | 0 | 0 | 0 | 6 | 1 | 150 |
| dressing, sun-dried tomato | 1 tbsp | 30 | 0 | 2 | 0 | 2 | 0 | 3 | 0 |
| dressing, tahini sesame | 1 tbsp | 55 | 2 | 4 | 1 | 1 | 4 | 1 | 55 |
| dressing, Thousand Island | 1 tbsp | 58 | 0 | 2 | 0 | 2 | 5 | 1 | 135 |
| dressing, Thousand Island, fat-free | 1 tbsp | 21 | 0 | 5 | 1 | 3 | 0 | 0 | 117 |

| FOOD ITEM | SERVING SIZE | CALORIES | PRO (g) | CARB (g) | FIBER (g) | SUGAR (g) | FAT (g) | SAT FAT (g) | SOD (mg) |
|---|---|---|---|---|---|---|---|---|---|
| dressing, Thousand Island, low-calorie | 1 tbsp | 31 | 0 | 3 | 0 | 3 | 2 | 0 | 127 |
| dressing, Thousand Island, low-sodium | 1 tbsp | 18 | 0 | 2 | n/a | n/a | 1 | n/a | 18 |
| dressing, toasted sesame, fat-free, organic | 1 tbsp | 8 | 0 | 2 | 0 | 1 | 0 | 0 | 110 |
| dressing, yogurt | 1 tbsp | 11 | 0 | 1 | 0 | 1 | 1 | 0 | 6 |
| dressing, zesty Italian, fat-free | 1 tbsp | 18 | 0 | 4 | 0 | 2 | 0 | 0 | 140 |
| dressing, zesty Italian, low-fat | 1 tbsp | 15 | 0 | 1 | 0 | 0 | 1 | 0 | 110 |
| dressing, zesty raspberry vinaigrette, fat-free | 1 tbsp | 18 | 0 | 4 | 0 | 3 | 0 | 0 | 18 |
| dressing mix, Caesar, dry | 1 packet | 120 | 0 | 16 | 0 | 0 | 0 | 0 | 2400 |
| dressing mix, cheese garlic, dry | 1 packet | 40 | 0 | 8 | 0 | 0 | 0 | 0 | 2640 |
| dressing mix, garlic herb, dry | 1 packet | 40 | 0 | 8 | 0 | 8 | 0 | 0 | 2720 |
| dressing mix, honey mustard, dry | 1 packet | 140 | 0 | 35 | 0 | 28 | 0 | 0 | 1960 |
| dressing mix, Italian, dry | 1 packet | 80 | 0 | 24 | n/a | 16 | 0 | 0 | 2320 |
| dressing mix, Italian, fat-free, dry | 1 packet | 80 | 0 | 24 | n/a | 16 | 0 | 0 | 2320 |
| dressing mix, Italian, low-calorie, dry | 1 packet | 40 | 0 | 8 | 0 | 8 | 0 | 0 | 2240 |
| dressing mix, Italian, mild, dry | 1 packet | 80 | 0 | 16 | 0 | 16 | 0 | 0 | 2960 |
| dressing mix, Mexican spice, dry | 1 packet | 80 | 0 | 16 | 0 | 8 | 0 | 0 | 2480 |
| dressing mix, Oriental sesame, dry | 1 packet | 120 | 0 | 24 | n/a | 16 | 0 | 0 | 2880 |
| dressing mix, Parmesan Italian, dry | 1 packet | 80 | 0 | 16 | n/a | 8 | 0 | 0 | 2640 |
| dressing mix, pasta salad vinaigrette, dry | 1 packet | 94 | 0 | 13 | n/a | n/a | 0 | 0 | 3717 |
| dressing mix, ranch, dry | 1 packet | 89 | 0 | 18 | n/a | n/a | 0 | 0 | 1772 |
| dressing mix, roasted garlic, dry | 1 packet | 80 | 0 | 16 | n/a | 8 | 0 | 0 | 2720 |
| dressing mix, zesty herb, dry | 1 packet | 95 | 0 | 9 | n/a | n/a | 0 | 0 | 3024 |
| dressing mix, zesty Italian, dry | 1 packet | 40 | 0 | 8 | 0 | 8 | 0 | 0 | 1760 |
| fruit butter, apple | 1 tbsp | 31 | 0 | 8 | 0 | 6 | 0 | 0 | 3 |
| fruit butter, peach | 1 tbsp | 45 | 0 | 11 | 0 | 10 | 0 | 0 | 10 |
| fruit spread, apricot | 1 tbsp | 40 | 0 | 10 | n/a | 10 | 0 | 0 | 0 |

## CONDIMENTS, DRESSINGS, MARINADES, AND SPREADS (cont.)

| FOOD ITEM | SERVING SIZE | CALORIES | PRO (g) | CARB (g) | FIBER (g) | SUGAR (g) | FAT (g) | SAT FAT (g) | SOD (mg) |
|---|---|---|---|---|---|---|---|---|---|
| fruit spread, blackberry | 1 tbsp | 40 | 0 | 10 | n/a | 10 | 0 | 0 | 0 |
| fruit spread, blackberry, seedless | 1 tbsp | 40 | 0 | 10 | 0 | 8 | 0 | 0 | 0 |
| fruit spread, black cherry | 1 tbsp | 40 | 0 | 10 | 0 | 8 | 0 | 0 | 0 |
| fruit spread, blueberry | 1 tbsp | 40 | 0 | 10 | 0 | 10 | 0 | 0 | 0 |
| fruit spread, boysenberry | 1 tbsp | 40 | 0 | 10 | 0 | 8 | 0 | 0 | 0 |
| fruit spread, concord grape | 1 tbsp | 40 | 0 | 10 | 0 | 10 | 0 | 0 | 0 |
| fruit spread, harvest berry | 1 tbsp | 40 | 0 | 10 | 0 | 10 | 0 | 0 | 0 |
| fruit spread, orange marmalade | 1 tbsp | 40 | 0 | 10 | 0 | 8 | 0 | 0 | 0 |
| fruit spread, peach | 1 tbsp | 40 | 0 | 10 | 0 | 8 | 0 | 0 | 0 |
| fruit spread, plum marmalade (sapotes) | 1 oz | 38 | 1 | 10 | 1 | n/a | 0 | 0 | 3 |
| fruit spread, raspberry | 1 tbsp | 40 | 0 | 10 | 0 | 10 | 0 | 0 | 0 |
| fruit spread, raspberry, black, seedless | 1 tbsp | 40 | 0 | 10 | 0 | 8 | 0 | 0 | 0 |
| fruit spread, raspberry, red, seedless | 1 tbsp | 40 | 0 | 10 | 0 | 8 | 0 | 0 | 0 |
| fruit spread, strawberry, all-fruit | 1 tbsp | 40 | 0 | 10 | 0 | 8 | 0 | 0 | 0 |
| fruit spread, strawberry, seedless | 1 tbsp | 40 | 0 | 10 | 0 | 8 | 0 | 0 | 0 |
| garlic sauce, Melissa's Fire Roasted Garlic Sauce | 3 g | 5 | 0 | 1 | 0 | | 0 | 0 | 0 |
| guacamole salsa, AvoClassic | 2 tbsp | 30 | 0 | 2 | 1 | 0 | 2.5 | 0 | 75 |
| hoisin sauce, Steel's Gourmet, No Sugar Added | 2 tbsp | 15 | 1 | 2 | 1 | 1 | 0 | 0 | 310 |
| horseradish | 1 tbsp | 7 | 0 | 2 | 0 | 1 | 0 | 0 | 47 |
| horseradish, fresh | 1 tbsp | 9 | 0 | 2 | 0 | 0 | 0 | 0 | 1 |
| horseradish cream | 1 tbsp | 29 | 0 | 2 | 1 | 1 | 2 | 0 | 66 |
| horseradish mustard | 1 tbsp | 29 | 1 | 2 | 1 | 1 | 3 | 0 | 162 |
| horseradish sauce | 1 tbsp | 30 | 0 | 1 | 0 | n/a | 3 | 2 | 10 |
| jam | 1 tbsp | 56 | 0 | 14 | 0 | 10 | 0 | 0 | 6 |
| jam, apricot | 1 tbsp | 48 | 0 | 13 | 0 | 7 | 0 | 0 | 8 |
| jam, apricot, low-sugar | 1 tbsp | 25 | 0 | 6 | 0 | 5 | 0 | 0 | 0 |
| jam, apricot sugar-free | 1 tbsp | 10 | 0 | 5 | 0 | 0 | 0 | 0 | 0 |
| jam, artificial sweetened | 1 tbsp | 18 | 0 | 8 | 0 | 5 | 0 | 0 | 0 |
| jam, blackberry | 1 tbsp | 50 | 0 | 13 | 0 | 12 | 0 | 0 | 0 |

| FOOD ITEM | SERVING SIZE | CALORIES | PRO (g) | CARB (g) | FIBER (g) | SUGAR (g) | FAT (g) | SAT FAT (g) | SOD (mg) |
|---|---|---|---|---|---|---|---|---|---|
| jam, blueberry | 1 tbsp | 50 | 0 | 13 | 0 | 12 | 0 | 0 | 0 |
| jam, boysenberry, low-sugar | 1 tbsp | 25 | 0 | 6 | 0 | 5 | 0 | 0 | 0 |
| jam, boysenberry, sugar-free | 1 tbsp | 10 | 0 | 5 | 0 | 0 | 0 | 0 | 0 |
| jam, cherry | 1 tbsp | 50 | 0 | 13 | 0 | 12 | 0 | 0 | 0 |
| jam, concord grape | 1 tbsp | 50 | 0 | 13 | n/a | 0 | 0 | 0 | 0 |
| jam, concord grape, low-sugar | 1 tbsp | 25 | 0 | 6 | 0 | 5 | 0 | 0 | 0 |
| jam, concord grape, sugar-free | 1 tbsp | 10 | 0 | 5 | 0 | 0 | 0 | 0 | 0 |
| jam, grape | 1 packet | 30 | 0 | 7 | 0 | 6 | 0 | 0 | 0 |
| jam, kiwifruit | 1 tbsp | 35 | 0 | 9 | 1 | n/a | 0 | 0 | 0 |
| jam, marionberry, fruit sweetened | 1 tbsp | 25 | 0 | 7 | 1 | 6 | 0 | 0 | 3 |
| jam, orange, sugar-free | 1 tbsp | 10 | 0 | 5 | 0 | 0 | 0 | 0 | 0 |
| jam, orange marmalade, low-sugar | 1 tbsp | 25 | 0 | 6 | 0 | 5 | 0 | 0 | 0 |
| jam, peach | 1 tbsp | 50 | 0 | 13 | 0 | 12 | 0 | 0 | 0 |
| jam, pineapple | 1 tbsp | 50 | 0 | 13 | 0 | 12 | 0 | 0 | 0 |
| jam, plum | 1 tbsp | 50 | 0 | 13 | 0 | 12 | 0 | 0 | 0 |
| jam, raspberry | 1 tbsp | 50 | 0 | 13 | 0 | 12 | 0 | 0 | 0 |
| jam, raspberry, fruit sweetened | 1 tbsp | 25 | 0 | 7 | 1 | 6 | 0 | 0 | 3 |
| jam, red raspberry, low-sugar | 1 tbsp | 25 | 0 | 6 | 0 | 5 | 0 | 0 | 0 |
| jam, red raspberry, sugar-free | 1 tbsp | 10 | 0 | 5 | 0 | 0 | 0 | 0 | 0 |
| jam, reduced-sugar | 1 tbsp | 36 | 0 | 9 | 1 | 7 | 0 | 0 | 5 |
| jam, strawberry | 1 packet | 30 | 0 | 7 | 0 | 0 | 0 | 0 | 0 |
| jam, strawberry, fruit sweetened | 1 tbsp | 25 | 0 | 7 | 1 | 6 | 0 | 0 | 3 |
| jelly | 1 packet | 38 | 0 | 10 | 0 | 7 | 0 | 0 | 4 |
| jelly | 1 tbsp | 51 | 0 | 13 | 0 | 10 | 0 | 0 | 6 |
| jelly, apple | 1 tbsp | 50 | 0 | 13 | 0 | 12 | 0 | 0 | 0 |
| jelly, apple, reduced-calorie | 1 tbsp | 5 | 0 | 2 | 0 | 1 | 0 | 0 | 0 |
| jelly, blackberry | 1 tbsp | 50 | 0 | 13 | 0 | 12 | 0 | 0 | 0 |
| jelly, black raspberry | 1 tbsp | 50 | 0 | 13 | 0 | 12 | 0 | 0 | 0 |
| jelly, cherry | 1 tbsp | 50 | 0 | 13 | 0 | 12 | 0 | 0 | 0 |

| FOOD ITEM | SERVING SIZE | CALORIES | PRO (g) | CARB (g) | FIBER (g) | SUGAR (g) | FAT (g) | SAT FAT (g) | SOD (mg) |
|---|---|---|---|---|---|---|---|---|---|
| jelly, cinnamon apple | 1 tbsp | 50 | 0 | 13 | 0 | 12 | 0 | 0 | 0 |
| jelly, currant | 1 tbsp | 50 | 0 | 13 | 0 | 12 | 0 | 0 | 0 |
| jelly, dietetic | 1 tbsp | 6 | 0 | 11 | 0 | 0 | 0 | 0 | 0 |
| jelly, elderberry | 1 tbsp | 50 | 0 | 13 | 0 | 12 | 0 | 0 | 0 |
| jelly, fruit, reduced-calorie | 1 tbsp | 5 | 0 | 13 | 0 | 12 | 0 | 0 | 0 |
| jelly, grape | 1 packet | 40 | 0 | 10 | 0 | 6 | 0 | 0 | 5 |
| jelly, grape, reduced-calorie | 1 tbsp | 5 | 0 | 2 | 0 | 1 | 0 | 0 | 0 |
| jelly, guava | 1 tbsp | 50 | 0 | 13 | 0 | 12 | 0 | 0 | 0 |
| jelly, mint | 1 tbsp | 50 | 0 | 13 | 0 | 12 | 0 | 0 | 0 |
| jelly, mint apple | 1 tbsp | 50 | 0 | 13 | 0 | 12 | 0 | 0 | 0 |
| jelly, mixed fruit | 1 tbsp | 50 | 0 | 13 | 0 | 12 | 0 | 0 | 0 |
| jelly, quince | 1 tbsp | 50 | 0 | 13 | 0 | 12 | 0 | 0 | 0 |
| jelly, reduced-sugar | 1 tbsp | 34 | 0 | 9 | 0 | 9 | 0 | 0 | 0 |
| jelly, strawberry | 1 tbsp | 50 | 0 | 13 | 0 | 12 | 0 | 0 | 0 |
| ketchup | 1 packet | 6 | 0 | 2 | 0 | 1 | 0 | 0 | 67 |
| ketchup | 1 tbsp | 15 | 0 | 4 | 0 | 3 | 0 | 0 | 167 |
| ketchup, fruit-sweetened, unsalted | 1 tbsp | 10 | 0 | 3 | 0 | 2 | 0 | 0 | 5 |
| ketchup, low-sodium | 1 tbsp | 16 | 0 | 4 | 0 | 3 | 0 | 0 | 3 |
| ketchup, organic | 1 tbsp | 15 | 0 | 3 | 0 | 3 | 0 | 0 | 190 |
| ketchup, reduced-calorie | 1 tbsp | 5 | 0 | 1 | 0 | 0 | 0 | 0 | 0 |
| ketchup, Steel's Gourmet, Sugar-Free | 1 tbsp | 10 | 0 | 0 | 0 | 0 | 0 | 0 | 40 |
| ketchup, unsweetened | 1 tbsp | 5 | 0 | 1 | 0 | 0 | 0 | 0 | 60 |
| mango sauce, Steel's Gourmet Mango Curry Sauce Sugar-Free | 1 tbsp | 13 | 2 | 3 | 0 | 0 | 0 | 0 | 0 |
| mango sauce, Steel's Gourmet Mango Ginger Chutney No Sugar Added | 5 tbsp | 25 | 0 | 6 | 1 | 5 | 0 | 0 | 10 |
| marinade, Cajun | 1 tbsp | 60 | 0 | 2 | n/a | n/a | 5 | n/a | 230 |
| marinade, chicken | 1 tbsp | 20 | 0 | 4 | n/a | n/a | 0 | 0 | 116 |
| marinade, dijon | 1 tbsp | 45 | 0 | 1 | 0 | 1 | 5 | 1 | n/a |
| marinade, dijon mustard, Melissa's Good Life Foods | 1 tbsp | 45 | 0 | 1 | 0 | 0 | 5 | 1 | 140 |
| marinade, fajita | 1 tbsp | 23 | 0 | 3 | n/a | n/a | 0 | 0 | 435 |

| FOOD ITEM | SERVING SIZE | CALORIES | PRO (g) | CARB (g) | FIBER (g) | SUGAR (g) | FAT (g) | SAT FAT (g) | SOD (mg) |
|---|---|---|---|---|---|---|---|---|---|
| marinade, garlic | 1 tbsp | 25 | 1 | 5 | 0 | 3 | 0 | 0 | 730 |
| marinade, ginger teriyaki | 1 tbsp | 60 | 0 | 5 | n/a | n/a | 3 | n/a | 560 |
| marinade, herb garlic, Melissa's Good Life Foods | 1 tbsp | 50 | 0 | 1 | 0 | 0 | 5 | 1 | 110 |
| marinade, honey mustard | 1 tbsp | 25 | 0 | 4 | n/a | n/a | 0 | 0 | 60 |
| marinade, honey soy | 1 tbsp | 30 | 0 | 7 | n/a | n/a | 0 | 0 | 390 |
| marinade, hot wings, Melissa's Good Life Foods | 1 tbsp | 30 | 0 | 1 | 0 | 1 | 3 | 0 | 125 |
| marinade, Korean | 1 tbsp | 5 | 0 | 1 | 0 | n/a | 0 | 0 | 41 |
| marinade, lemon herb | 1 tbsp | 30 | 0 | 6 | n/a | n/a | 0 | 0 | 900 |
| marinade, lime cilantro, Melissa's Good Life Foods | 1 tbsp | 35 | 0 | 1 | 0 | 0 | 4 | 1 | 200 |
| marinade, mesquite | 1 tbsp | 10 | 0 | 1 | n/a | n/a | 1 | n/a | 250 |
| marinade, olive oil and vinegar, Melissa's Good Life Foods | 1 tbsp | 40 | 0 | 1 | 0 | 0 | 4 | 1 | 45 |
| marinade, roasted garlic | 1 tbsp | 15 | 0 | 3 | n/a | n/a | 0 | 0 | 130 |
| marinade, smoky chipotle, Melissa's Good Life Foods | 1 tbsp | 30 | 0 | 1 | 0 | 0 | 3 | 0 | 150 |
| marinade, Southwest | 1 tbsp | 23 | 0 | 3 | n/a | n/a | 0 | 0 | 66 |
| marinade, spicy Cajun | 1 tbsp | 5 | 0 | 1 | n/a | n/a | 0 | 0 | 230 |
| marinade, spicy Caribbean | 1 tbsp | 30 | 0 | 3 | n/a | n/a | 0 | 0 | 162 |
| marinade, steak | 1 tbsp | 20 | 0 | 4 | 0 | 0 | 0 | 0 | 184 |
| marinade, teriyaki, light | 1 tbsp | 25 | 1 | 5 | 0 | 3 | 0 | 0 | 220 |
| marinade, teriyaki, Melissa's Good Life Foods | 1 tbsp | 30 | 0 | 1 | 0 | 0 | 3 | 0 | 320 |
| marinade, Thai peanut, Melissa's Good Life Foods | 1 tbsp | 25 | 0 | 1 | 0 | 0 | 2 | 0 | 150 |
| marinade, white wine dijon | 1 tbsp | 10 | 0 | 1 | n/a | n/a | 0 | 0 | 125 |
| mayonnaise | 1 packet | 90 | 0 | 0 | 0 | 0 | 10 | 2 | 65 |
| mayonnaise, canola | 1 tbsp | 100 | 0 | 0 | 0 | 0 | 11 | 1 | 100 |
| mayonnaise, egg-free | 1 tbsp | 68 | 0 | 2 | 0 | 1 | 7 | 1 | 50 |
| mayonnaise, fat-free | 1 tbsp | 13 | 0 | 2 | 0 | 2 | 0 | 0 | 126 |
| mayonnaise, hot and spicy | 1 tbsp | 100 | 0 | 0 | 0 | 0 | 11 | 2 | 85 |
| mayonnaise, imitation with soybeans | 1 tbsp | 35 | 0 | 2 | 0 | 1 | 3 | 0 | 75 |
| mayonnaise, light | 1 tbsp | 46 | 0 | 1 | 0 | 1 | 5 | 1 | 95 |
| mayonnaise, light garlic | 1 tbsp | 50 | 0 | 1 | 0 | 0 | 5 | 1 | 120 |

| FOOD ITEM | SERVING SIZE | CALORIES | PRO (g) | CARB (g) | FIBER (g) | SUGAR (g) | FAT (g) | SAT FAT (g) | SOD (mg) |
|---|---|---|---|---|---|---|---|---|---|
| mayonnaise, light herb | 1 tbsp | 50 | 0 | 1 | 0 | 0 | 5 | 1 | 120 |
| mayonnaise, low-calorie, low-sodium | 1 tbsp | 32 | 0 | 2 | 0 | 1 | 3 | 0 | 15 |
| mayonnaise, no cholesterol | 1 tbsp | 103 | 0 | 0 | 0 | 0 | 12 | 2 | 73 |
| mayonnaise, omega-3 | 1 tbsp | 100 | 0 | 0 | 0 | 0 | 11 | 2 | 90 |
| mayonnaise, roasted garlic | 1 tbsp | 100 | 0 | 0 | 0 | 0 | 11 | 2 | 30 |
| mayonnaise, safflower | 1 tbsp | 105 | 0 | 0 | 0 | 0 | 12 | 2 | 73 |
| mayonnaise, soybean | 1 tbsp | 100 | 0 | 0 | 0 | 0 | 11 | 2 | 65 |
| mayonnaise, tofu | 1 tbsp | 48 | 1 | 1 | 0 | 0 | 5 | 0 | 116 |
| mayonnaise, unsalted | 1 tbsp | 99 | 0 | 0 | 0 | n/a | 11 | 2 | 4 |
| mayonnaise, wasabi | 1 tbsp | 100 | 0 | 0 | 0 | 0 | 11 | 2 | 65 |
| mustard | 1 tbsp | 10 | 1 | 1 | 0 | 0 | 0 | 0 | 168 |
| mustard, Asian | 1 tbsp | 15 | 0 | 0 | 0 | 0 | 0 | 0 | 330 |
| mustard, cranberry | 1 tbsp | 29 | 0 | 6 | 1 | 5 | 1 | 0 | 80 |
| mustard, creamy dill | 1 tbsp | 32 | 0 | 2 | 1 | 1 | 3 | 0 | 164 |
| mustard, deli | 1 tbsp | 12 | 0 | 0 | 0 | 0 | 0 | 0 | 195 |
| mustard, dijon coarse grain | 1 tbsp | 20 | 1 | 1 | 1 | 0 | 1 | 0 | 323 |
| mustard, dijonnaise | 1 tbsp | 15 | 0 | 3 | 0 | 0 | 0 | 0 | 210 |
| mustard, honey | 1 tbsp | 21 | 1 | 4 | 1 | 3 | 0 | 0 | 99 |
| mustard, Parisian Poupon | 1 tbsp | 10 | 0 | 2 | 0 | 0 | 1 | 0 | 152 |
| mustard, yellow | 1 tbsp | 10 | 1 | 1 | 0 | 0 | 0 | 0 | 168 |
| olives, black | 5 small | 18 | 0 | 1 | 1 | 0 | 2 | 0 | 140 |
| olives, black | 5 large | 25 | 0 | 1 | 1 | 0 | 2 | 0 | 192 |
| olives, black | 5 jumbo | 34 | 0 | 2 | 1 | 0 | 3 | 0 | 373 |
| olives, black | 5 super colossal | 62 | 1 | 4 | 2 | 0 | 5 | 1 | 682 |
| olives, black, nicoise, pitted | 5 | 53 | 0 | 2 | 0 | 0 | 5 | 1 | 306 |
| olives, black, sliced | 1 tbsp | 10 | 0 | 1 | 0 | 0 | 1 | 0 | 73 |
| olives, green, pickled | 5 | 41 | 0 | 1 | 1 | 0 | 4 | 1 | 441 |
| olives, green, queen | 5 | 50 | 0 | 3 | 0 | 0 | 5 | 0 | 550 |
| olives, green, stuffed manzanilla | 5 | 42 | 0 | 2 | 0 | 0 | 3 | 0 | 400 |
| olives, green, stuffed queen | 5 | 38 | 0 | 3 | 0 | 0 | 4 | 0 | 625 |
| pepperoncini, Greek | 1 oz | 8 | 0 | 1 | 0 | 0 | 0 | 0 | 369 |

| FOOD ITEM | SERVING SIZE | CALORIES | PRO (g) | CARB (g) | FIBER (g) | SUGAR (g) | FAT (g) | SAT FAT (g) | SOD (mg) |
|---|---|---|---|---|---|---|---|---|---|
| pepperoncini, Italian | 1 oz | 6 | 0 | 1 | 0 | 0 | 0 | 0 | 598 |
| pickle, bread butter | ¼ cup | 34 | 0 | 8 | 1 | 4 | 0 | 0 | 286 |
| pickle, dill | 1 small | 7 | 0 | 2 | 0 | 1 | 0 | 0 | 474 |
| pickle, dill | 1 medium | 12 | 0 | 3 | 1 | 2 | 0 | 0 | 833 |
| pickle, dill | 1 large | 24 | 1 | 6 | 2 | 4 | 0 | 0 | 1731 |
| pickle, dill, low-sodium | 1 medium | 12 | 0 | 3 | 1 | 1 | 0 | 0 | 12 |
| pickle, dill, slices | 3 | 7 | 0 | 2 | 0 | 1 | 0 | 0 | 497 |
| pickle, dill, slices, low-sodium | 10 | 11 | 0 | 2 | 1 | 1 | 0 | 0 | 11 |
| pickle, dill, spears | 3 | 16 | 1 | 4 | 1 | 3 | 0 | 0 | 1154 |
| pickle, garlic, whole | 1 | 10 | 0 | 2 | 0 | 0 | 0 | 0 | 540 |
| pickle, Japanese Tsukemono | ¼ cup | 7 | 0 | 1 | 1 | n/a | 0 | 0 | 180 |
| pickle, kosher dill | 1 medium | 20 | 0 | 3 | n/a | n/a | 0 | 0 | 660 |
| pickle, kosher dill, halves | 3 | 30 | 0 | 6 | n/a | n/a | 0 | 0 | 1980 |
| pickle, kosher dill, halves, low-sodium | 3 | 20 | 0 | 4 | 0 | 0 | 0 | 0 | 540 |
| pickle, kosher dill, slices | 3 | 8 | 0 | 2 | 0 | 0 | 0 | 0 | 630 |
| pickle, kosher dill, spears | 3 | 15 | 0 | 3 | 0 | 3 | 0 | 0 | 638 |
| pickle, sour | 3 small | 12 | 0 | 3 | 1 | 1 | 0 | 0 | 1341 |
| pickle, sour | 1 medium | 7 | 0 | 1 | 1 | 1 | 0 | 0 | 785 |
| pickle, sour | 1 large | 15 | 0 | 3 | 2 | 1 | 0 | 0 | 1631 |
| pickle, sour, slices | 10 | 8 | 0 | 2 | 1 | 1 | 0 | 0 | 846 |
| pickle, sour, spears | 3 | 10 | 0 | 2 | 1 | 1 | 0 | 0 | 1087 |
| pickle, sweet | 3 small | 53 | 0 | 14 | 1 | 7 | 0 | 0 | 423 |
| pickle, sweet | 1 medium | 29 | 0 | 8 | 0 | 4 | 0 | 0 | 235 |
| pickle, sweet | 1 large | 41 | 0 | 11 | 0 | 5 | 0 | 0 | 329 |
| pickle, sweet, low-sodium | 3 small | 55 | 0 | 15 | 1 | 7 | 0 | 0 | 8 |
| pickle, sweet, low-sodium | 1 medium | 43 | 0 | 12 | 0 | 5 | 0 | 0 | 6 |
| pickle, sweet, low-sodium | 1 large | 43 | 0 | 12 | 0 | 5 | 0 | 0 | 6 |
| pickle, sweet, slices | 5 | 41 | 0 | 11 | 0 | 5 | 0 | 0 | 329 |
| pickle, sweet, slices, low-sodium | 5 | 37 | 0 | 10 | 0 | 4 | 0 | 0 | 5 |
| pickle, zesty dill, whole | 1 | 12 | 0 | 2 | 0 | 2 | 0 | 0 | 649 |
| pickle relish, chow chow | 1 tbsp | 16 | 0 | 4 | n/a | n/a | 0 | n/a | 75 |

| FOOD ITEM | SERVING SIZE | CALORIES | PRO (g) | CARB (g) | FIBER (g) | SUGAR (g) | FAT (g) | SAT FAT (g) | SOD (mg) |
|---|---|---|---|---|---|---|---|---|---|
| pickle relish, hamburger | 1 tbsp | 19 | 0 | 5 | 0 | 5 | 0 | 0 | 164 |
| pickle relish, hot dog | 1 tbsp | 14 | 0 | 4 | 0 | 3 | 0 | 0 | 164 |
| pickle relish, sweet | 1 packet | 13 | 0 | 4 | 0 | 2 | 0 | 0 | 81 |
| pickled apple | 1 | 25 | 0 | 6 | 0 | n/a | 0 | 0 | 0 |
| pickled cauliflower flowerets | 3 | 35 | 1 | 8 | 2 | 6 | 0 | 0 | 15 |
| pickled chile pepper | 3 | 24 | 0 | 6 | 1 | 4 | 0 | 0 | 1 |
| pickled egg | 1 | 135 | 7 | 3 | 1 | 3 | 5 | 2 | 130 |
| pickled green tomato | ¼ cup | 13 | 0 | 3 | 0 | 2 | 0 | 0 | 44 |
| pickled jalapeño | 1 | 3 | 0 | 1 | 0 | 0 | 0 | 0 | 190 |
| pickled Japanese cabbage | ¼ cup | 11 | 1 | 2 | 1 | 0 | 0 | 0 | 104 |
| pickled mushroom cap | 3 | 4 | 0 | 1 | 0 | 0 | 0 | 0 | 1 |
| pickled okra | 3 | 10 | 1 | 2 | 1 | n/a | 0 | 0 | 2 |
| pickled radish | ¼ cup | 11 | 0 | 2 | 1 | 1 | 0 | 0 | 296 |
| pickled red cabbage | ¼ cup | 55 | 0 | 14 | 0 | 14 | 0 | 0 | 7 |
| pickled seaweed | ¼ cup | 57 | 0 | 15 | 0 | 0 | 0 | 0 | 55 |
| pickled string bean | ¼ cup | 10 | 1 | 2 | 1 | 1 | 0 | 0 | 2 |
| pickled sushi ginger | 1 tbsp | 20 | 0 | 4 | 0 | 2 | 0 | 0 | 100 |
| pickled turnip slice | 3 | 9 | 0 | 2 | 0 | 2 | 0 | 0 | 9 |
| pickled zucchini squash | ¼ cup | 15 | 0 | 4 | 1 | 3 | 0 | 0 | 1 |
| salsa | 1 tbsp | 4 | 0 | 1 | 0 | 1 | 0 | 0 | 97 |
| salsa, Amy's Organic Black Bean & Corn Salsa | 2 tbsp | 15 | 1 | 3 | 0 | 1 | 0 | 0 | 170 |
| salsa, Amy's Organic Fire Roasted Vegetable Salsa | 2 tbsp | 10 | 0 | 3 | 0 | 1 | 0 | 0 | 200 |
| salsa, Amy's Organic Medium Salsa | 2 tbsp | 10 | 0 | 2 | 0 | 1 | 0 | 0 | 190 |
| salsa, Amy's Organic Mild Salsa | 2 tbsp | 10 | 0 | 2 | 0 | 1 | 0 | 0 | 190 |
| salsa, Amy's Organic Spicy Chipotle Salsa | 2 tbsp | 10 | 0 | 2 | 0 | 1 | 0 | 0 | 160 |
| salsa, picante | 1 tbsp | 3 | 0 | 1 | n/a | n/a | 0 | 0 | 124 |
| salsa, red jalapeño | 1 tbsp | 5 | 0 | 1 | 0 | 0 | 0 | 0 | 109 |
| salsa, suprema | 1 tbsp | 4 | 0 | 1 | 0 | 0 | 0 | n/a | 83 |
| salsa, thick and chunky | 1 tbsp | 5 | 0 | 2 | 0 | 1 | 0 | 0 | 115 |
| soy sauce | 1 tbsp | 11 | 2 | 1 | 0 | 0 | 0 | 0 | 1005 |

| FOOD ITEM | SERVING SIZE | CALORIES | PRO (g) | CARB (g) | FIBER (g) | SUGAR (g) | FAT (g) | SAT FAT (g) | SOD (mg) |
|---|---|---|---|---|---|---|---|---|---|
| soy sauce, low-sodium | 1 tbsp | 9 | 1 | 1 | 0 | 0 | 0 | 0 | 533 |
| steak sauce | 1 tbsp | 5 | 0 | 1 | 0 | 0 | 0 | 0 | 200 |
| stir fry sauce, Melissa's | 1 tbsp | 25 | 0 | 6 | 0 | | 0 | 0 | 720 |
| stir fry sauce, Melissa's Good Life Foods Soy Ginger | 1 tbsp | 5 | 0 | 1 | 0 | 0 | 0 | 0 | 270 |
| stir fry sauce, Melissa's Good Life Foods Teriyaki | 1 tbsp | 20 | 0 | 1 | 0 | 0 | 2 | 0 | 290 |
| Tabasco sauce | 1 tbsp | 2 | 0 | 0 | 0 | n/a | 0 | 0 | 89 |
| tahini | 1 tbsp | 89 | 3 | 3 | 1 | n/a | 8 | 1 | 5 |
| tartar sauce | 1 tbsp | 70 | 0 | 1 | 0 | 0 | 8 | 1 | 76 |
| tartar sauce, low-calorie | 1 tbsp | 31 | 0 | 2 | 0 | 0 | 3 | 0 | 82 |
| tofu sauce, Melissa's Good Life Foods Ginger Teriyaki | 1 tbsp | 5 | 0 | 1 | 0 | 0 | 0 | 0 | 360 |
| tofu sauce, Melissa's Good Life Foods Madras Curry | 1 tbsp | 35 | 0 | 1 | 0 | 0 | 4 | 0 | 105 |
| tofu sauce, Melissa's Good Life Foods Smoky Chipotle | 1 tbsp | 5 | 0 | 1 | 0 | 0 | 0 | 0 | 200 |
| tofu sauce, Melissa's Good Life Foods Thai Peanut | 1 tbsp | 20 | 0 | 1 | 0 | 0 | 2 | 0 | 220 |
| vinaigrette, balsamic | 1 tbsp | 45 | 0 | 2 | 0 | 2 | 4 | 1 | 150 |
| vinaigrette, barbecue | 1 tbsp | 35 | 0 | 2 | 0 | 0 | 3 | 0 | 165 |
| vinaigrette, basil | 1 tbsp | 85 | 0 | 2 | 0 | 2 | 9 | 1 | 65 |
| vinaigrette, Greek | 1 tbsp | 55 | 0 | 13 | 0 | 1 | 6 | 1 | 160 |
| vinaigrette, herb | 1 tbsp | 70 | 0 | 1 | 0 | 0 | 8 | 1 | 125 |
| vinaigrette, herb, fat-free | 1 tbsp | 8 | 0 | 2 | 0 | 1 | 0 | 0 | 59 |
| vinaigrette, Italian | 1 tbsp | 25 | 0 | 2 | 0 | 1 | 2 | 0 | 210 |
| vinaigrette, red wine | 1 tbsp | 45 | 0 | 1 | 0 | 12 | 5 | 1 | 240 |
| vinaigrette, red wine, fat-free | 1 tbsp | 8 | 0 | 2 | 0 | 2 | 0 | 0 | 200 |
| vinaigrette, red wine, herb | 1 tbsp | 20 | 0 | 4 | 0 | 4 | 0 | 0 | 220 |
| vinegar, apple cider | 1 tbsp | 1 | 0 | 0 | 0 | 0 | 0 | 0 | 3 |
| vinegar, balsamic | 1 tbsp | 10 | 0 | 2 | n/a | 2 | 0 | 0 | 5 |
| vinegar, brown rice | 1 tbsp | 10 | 0 | 0 | 0 | 0 | 0 | 0 | 0 |
| vinegar, champagne | 1 tbsp | 5 | 0 | 2 | 0 | 0 | 0 | 0 | 1 |
| vinegar, cider | 1 tbsp | 3 | 0 | 0 | 0 | 0 | 0 | 0 | 1 |
| vinegar, distilled | 1 tbsp | 3 | 0 | 0 | 0 | 0 | 0 | 0 | 0 |
| vinegar, garlic wine | 1 tbsp | 0 | 0 | 0 | 0 | 0 | 0 | 0 | 0 |

| FOOD ITEM | SERVING SIZE | CALORIES | PRO (g) | CARB (g) | FIBER (g) | SUGAR (g) | FAT (g) | SAT FAT (g) | SOD (mg) |
|---|---|---|---|---|---|---|---|---|---|
| vinegar, golden balsamic | 1 tbsp | 6 | 0 | 2 | 0 | 0 | 0 | 0 | 5 |
| vinegar, Italian herb | 1 tbsp | 0 | 0 | 0 | 0 | 0 | 0 | 0 | 0 |
| vinegar, malt | 1 tbsp | 0 | 0 | 0 | 0 | 0 | 0 | 0 | 0 |
| vinegar, red wine organic | 1 tbsp | 0 | 0 | 1 | 0 | 0 | 0 | 0 | 5 |
| vinegar, rice | 1 tbsp | 0 | 0 | 0 | 0 | 0 | 0 | 0 | 1 |
| vinegar, rice seasoned | 1 tbsp | 12 | 0 | 3 | 0 | 3 | 0 | 0 | 297 |
| vinegar, tarragon | 1 tbsp | 0 | 0 | 0 | 0 | 0 | 0 | 0 | 0 |
| vinegar, tarragon malt | 1 tbsp | 3 | 0 | 1 | 0 | 0 | 0 | 0 | 1 |
| vinegar, white distilled | 1 tbsp | 0 | 0 | 0 | 0 | 0 | 0 | 0 | 0 |
| vinegar, white wine | 1 tbsp | 5 | 0 | 2 | 0 | 0 | 0 | 0 | 0 |
| wasabi | 1 tbsp | 2 | 0 | 0 | 0 | 0 | 0 | 0 | 0 |
| worcestershire sauce | 1 tbsp | 11 | 0 | 3 | 0 | 2 | 0 | 0 | 167 |
| worcestershire sauce, low-sodium | 1 tbsp | 5 | 0 | 1 | 0 | 1 | 0 | 0 | 20 |
| wrap dressing, Melissa's Good Life Foods Chipotle | 2 tbsp | 130 | 0 | 0 | 0 | 0 | 14 | 2 | 190 |
| wrap dressing, Melissa's Good Life Foods Ranch | 2 tbsp | 130 | 0 | 1 | 0 | 0 | 14 | 2 | 340 |
| wrap dressing, Melissa's Good Life Foods Sesame | 2 tbsp | 110 | 0 | 1 | 0 | 0 | 12 | 2 | 280 |

## DAIRY PRODUCTS

| FOOD ITEM | SERVING SIZE | CALORIES | PRO (g) | CARB (g) | FIBER (g) | SUGAR (g) | FAT (g) | SAT FAT (g) | SOD (mg) |
|---|---|---|---|---|---|---|---|---|---|
| cream, heavy | 1 tbsp | 51 | 0 | 0 | 0 | 0 | 6 | 3 | 6 |
| cream, heavy, whipped | 1 tbsp | 26 | 0 | 0 | 0 | 0 | 3 | 2 | 3 |
| cream, light | 1 tbsp | 29 | 0 | 1 | 0 | 0 | 3 | 2 | 6 |
| cream, sour | 1 tbsp | 31 | 0 | 1 | 0 | 0 | 3 | 2 | 8 |
| cream, sour, fat-free | 1 tbsp | 10 | 0 | 2 | 0 | 0 | 0 | 0 | 20 |
| cream, sour, imitation | 1 tbsp | 30 | 0 | 1 | 0 | 1 | 3 | 3 | 15 |
| cream, sour, light | 1 tbsp | 19 | 1 | 1 | 0 | 0 | 2 | 1 | 10 |
| cream, sour, reduced-fat | 1 tbsp | 26 | 1 | 1 | 0 | 0 | 2 | 1 | 10 |
| cream substitute, liquid | 1 tbsp | 20 | 0 | 2 | 0 | 2 | 1 | 0 | 11 |
| cream substitute, powdered | 1 tbsp | 32 | 0 | 3 | 0 | 3 | 2 | 2 | 11 |
| half-and-half | 1 tbsp | 20 | 0 | 1 | 0 | 0 | 2 | 1 | 6 |

| FOOD ITEM | SERVING SIZE | CALORIES | PRO (g) | CARB (g) | FIBER (g) | SUGAR (g) | FAT (g) | SAT FAT (g) | SOD (mg) |
|---|---|---|---|---|---|---|---|---|---|
| half-and-half, fat-free | 1 tbsp | 9 | 0 | 1 | 0 | 1 | 0 | 0 | 22 |
| kefir | 1 cup | 145 | 7 | 11 | 0 | 11 | 8 | n/a | 104 |
| topping, Cool Whip, extra creamy | 2 tbsp | 25 | 0 | 2 | n/a | 2 | 2 | 2 | 5 |
| topping, Cool Whip, fat-free | 2 tbsp | 15 | 0 | 3 | n/a | 1 | 0 | 0 | 5 |
| topping, Cool Whip, light | 2 tbsp | 20 | 0 | 3 | n/a | 1 | 1 | 1 | 0 |
| topping, Cool Whip, nondairy | 2 tbsp | 25 | 0 | 2 | n/a | 1 | 2 | 2 | 0 |
| topping, DairyWhip Whipped Cream, light | 2 tbsp | 10 | 0 | 1 | 0 | 1 | 1 | 1 | 0 |
| topping, dessert, pressurized | 2 tbsp | 23 | 0 | 1 | 0 | 1 | 2 | 2 | 5 |
| topping, dessert mix, prepared with ½ cup milk | 2 tbsp | 19 | 0 | 2 | 0 | 2 | 1 | 1 | 7 |
| topping, Reddi-Wip, fat-free | ½ oz | 21 | 0 | 4 | 0 | 2 | 1 | 0 | 10 |
| topping, whipped, dietetic | 2 tbsp | 10 | 0 | 1 | 0 | 1 | 1 | 0 | 11 |
| topping, whipped, fat-free | 2 tbsp | 15 | 0 | 2 | 0 | 2 | 0 | 0 | 5 |
| topping, whipped, Kraft | 2 tbsp | 20 | 0 | 1 | 0 | 1 | 2 | 1 | 0 |
| topping, whipped, low-fat | 2 tbsp | 21 | 0 | 2 | 0 | 2 | 1 | 1 | 7 |
| yogurt, apple, organic | 4 oz | 90 | 2 | 16 | 2 | 9 | 2 | n/a | 65 |
| yogurt, apricot-mango, low-fat | 4 oz | 120 | 5 | 22 | 0 | 20 | 1 | 1 | 64 |
| yogurt, banana, low-fat | 4 oz | 120 | 5 | 21 | 0 | 18 | 2 | 2 | 60 |
| yogurt, banana crème, low-fat | 4 oz | 113 | 3 | 22 | 0 | 18 | 1 | 1 | 53 |
| yogurt, berry-banana, low-fat | 4 oz | 113 | 3 | 22 | 0 | 18 | 1 | 1 | 53 |
| yogurt, black cherry, low-fat | 4 oz | 120 | 5 | 23 | 0 | 21 | 1 | 1 | 65 |
| yogurt, blueberry–French vanilla, low-fat | 4 oz | 120 | 5 | 24 | 0 | 21 | 1 | 0 | 70 |
| yogurt, blueberry mist, low-fat | 4 oz | 141 | 5 | 25 | 0 | 21 | 3 | 2 | 75 |
| yogurt, cherry cheesecake, low-fat | 4 oz | 120 | 5 | 23 | 0 | 21 | 1 | 0 | 77 |
| yogurt, cherry chiffon, low-fat | 4 oz | 140 | 5 | 25 | 0 | 21 | 3 | 2 | 25 |
| yogurt, chocolate, fat-free | 4 oz | 127 | 4 | 27 | 1 | 17 | 0 | 0 | 153 |
| yogurt, chocolate, low-fat | 4 oz | 110 | 4 | 21 | 0 | 17 | 1 | 1 | 52 |
| yogurt, coconut cream pie, low-fat | 4 oz | 127 | 3 | 23 | 0 | 18 | 2 | 1 | 57 |
| yogurt, coffee, fat-free | 4 oz | 103 | 6 | 20 | 0 | 20 | 0 | 0 | 78 |

| FOOD ITEM | SERVING SIZE | CALORIES | PRO (g) | CARB (g) | FIBER (g) | SUGAR (g) | FAT (g) | SAT FAT (g) | SOD (mg) |
|---|---|---|---|---|---|---|---|---|---|
| yogurt, creamy strawberry, fat-free | 4 oz | 62 | 4 | 11 | 0 | 9 | 0 | 0 | 51 |
| yogurt, fruit, fat-free | 4 oz | 107 | 5 | 22 | 0 | 22 | 0 | 0 | 66 |
| yogurt, fruit, fat-free, with low-calorie sweetener | 4 oz | 57 | 5 | 9 | 1 | 9 | 0 | 0 | 66 |
| yogurt, fruit and nuts, low-fat | 4 oz | 134 | 5 | 22 | 0 | 21 | 3 | 1 | 64 |
| yogurt, key lime pie, fat-free | 4 oz | 67 | 5 | 12 | 0 | 10 | 0 | 0 | 73 |
| yogurt, lemon, fat-free | 4 oz | 103 | 6 | 20 | 0 | 20 | 0 | 0 | 78 |
| yogurt, lemon, low-fat | 4 oz | 96 | 6 | 16 | 0 | 16 | 1 | 1 | 75 |
| yogurt, lemon chiffon, fat-free | 4 oz | 67 | 5 | 12 | 0 | 10 | 0 | 0 | 87 |
| yogurt, mandarin orange, fat-free | 4 oz | 60 | 4 | 10 | 0 | 7 | 0 | 0 | 65 |
| yogurt, mandarin orange, low-fat | 4 oz | 113 | 3 | 22 | 0 | 18 | 1 | 1 | 53 |
| yogurt, maple, low-fat | 4 oz | 96 | 6 | 16 | 0 | 16 | 1 | 1 | 75 |
| yogurt, marionberry, fat-free | 4 oz | 67 | 5 | 12 | 0 | 11 | 0 | 0 | 73 |
| yogurt, mixed berry, low-fat | 4 oz | 113 | 3 | 22 | 0 | 18 | 1 | 1 | 53 |
| yogurt, orange crème, low-fat | 4 oz | 127 | 5 | 21 | 0 | 19 | 2 | 1 | 67 |
| yogurt, peach cobbler, low-fat | 4 oz | 113 | 3 | 22 | 0 | 18 | 1 | 1 | 53 |
| yogurt, peaches and cream, fat-free | 4 oz | 67 | 5 | 12 | 0 | 11 | 0 | 0 | 73 |
| yogurt, piña colada, low-fat | 4 oz | 113 | 3 | 22 | 0 | 19 | 1 | 1 | 63 |
| yogurt, pineapple, low-fat | 4 oz | 113 | 3 | 22 | 0 | 18 | 1 | 1 | 53 |
| yogurt, plain | 4 oz | 69 | 4 | 5 | 0 | 5 | 4 | 2 | 52 |
| yogurt, plain, fat-free | 4 oz | 50 | 5 | 9 | 0 | 6 | 0 | 0 | 67 |
| yogurt, plain, high protein | 4 oz | 71 | 6 | 8 | 0 | 8 | 2 | 1 | 79 |
| yogurt, plain, low-fat | 4 oz | 80 | 7 | 10 | 0 | 9 | 1 | 1 | 95 |
| yogurt, raspberry, fat-free | 4 oz | 67 | 5 | 12 | 0 | 10 | 0 | 0 | 83 |
| yogurt, raspberry, low-fat | 4 oz | 120 | 5 | 22 | 0 | 19 | 1 | 1 | 85 |
| yogurt, raspberry cheesecake, low-fat | 4 oz | 125 | 5 | 21 | 0 | 19 | 2 | 1 | 67 |
| yogurt, strawberry, fat-free | 4 oz | 67 | 5 | 12 | 0 | 10 | 0 | 0 | 73 |
| yogurt, strawberry-banana, low-fat | 4 oz | 118 | 4 | 23 | 0 | 20 | 1 | 0 | 55 |
| yogurt, strawberry-banana split, low-fat | 4 oz | 120 | 4 | 24 | 0 | 19 | 1 | 1 | 50 |

| FOOD ITEM | SERVING SIZE | CALORIES | PRO (g) | CARB (g) | FIBER (g) | SUGAR (g) | FAT (g) | SAT FAT (g) | SOD (mg) |
|---|---|---|---|---|---|---|---|---|---|
| yogurt, strawberry cheesecake, low-fat | 4 oz | 120 | 3 | 24 | 0 | 19 | 1 | 1 | 50 |
| yogurt, strawberry-kiwi, low-fat | 4 oz | 120 | 5 | 22 | 0 | 20 | 1 | 1 | 75 |
| yogurt, triple cherry, low-fat | 4 oz | 120 | 4 | 23 | 0 | 19 | 2 | 1 | 55 |
| yogurt, vanilla, fat-free | 4 oz | 103 | 6 | 20 | 0 | 20 | 0 | 0 | 78 |
| yogurt, vanilla, fat-free with low-calorie sweetener | 4 oz | 49 | 4 | 9 | 0 | 9 | 0 | 0 | 67 |
| yogurt, vanilla, low-fat | 4 oz | 96 | 6 | 16 | 0 | 16 | 1 | 1 | 75 |
| yogurt, vanilla classic, low-fat | 4 oz | 90 | 4 | 16 | 0 | 13 | 1 | 1 | 60 |
| yogurt, very berry—watermelon, low-fat | 4 oz | 120 | 4 | 23 | 0 | 19 | 2 | 1 | 55 |
| yogurt, watermelon burst, low-fat | 4 oz | 120 | 4 | 23 | 0 | 19 | 2 | 1 | 55 |
| yogurt cheese | 1 oz | 22 | 2 | 3 | 0 | n/a | 0 | 0 | 22 |
| yogurt dressing | 2 tbsp | 23 | 1 | 2 | 0 | 2 | 1 | 1 | 12 |
| yogurt drink, cherry, low-fat | 4 oz | 102 | 5 | 18 | 0 | 17 | 2 | 1 | 62 |
| yogurt drink, raspberry, low-fat | 4 oz | 102 | 5 | 18 | 0 | 17 | 2 | 1 | 62 |
| yogurt drink, strawberry, low-fat | 4 oz | 102 | 5 | 18 | 0 | 17 | 2 | 1 | 62 |
| yogurt drink, tropical punch, low-fat | 4 oz | 102 | 5 | 18 | 0 | 17 | 2 | 1 | 62 |

## DESSERTS AND SWEET TREATS

| FOOD ITEM | SERVING SIZE | CALORIES | PRO (g) | CARB (g) | FIBER (g) | SUGAR (g) | FAT (g) | SAT FAT (g) | SOD (mg) |
|---|---|---|---|---|---|---|---|---|---|
| brownie | 2" square | 112 | 1 | 12 | 1 | n/a | 7 | 2 | 82 |
| brownie, fat-free | 2" square | 100 | 2 | 21 | 1 | 14 | 0 | 0 | 90 |
| brownie, low-fat | 2 oz | 107 | 5 | 19 | 1 | 16 | 1 | 1 | 75 |
| brownie, with nuts | 2 oz | 248 | 1 | 32 | 1 | 31 | 14 | 4 | 30 |
| cake, angel food | 1 slice | 120 | 3 | 27 | 0 | 20 | 0 | 0 | 200 |
| cake, apple | 1 piece | 313 | 3 | 52 | 2 | 36 | 12 | 2 | 141 |
| cake, carrot, with cream cheese frosting | 1 slice | 300 | 3 | 35 | 1 | 25 | 16 | 4 | 380 |
| cake, chocolate, with chocolate frosting | 1 slice | 300 | 3 | 47 | 1 | 37 | 11 | 3 | 290 |
| cake, chocolate, without frosting | 1 slice | 197 | 5 | 36 | 1 | 27 | 4 | 1 | 42 |

| FOOD ITEM | SERVING SIZE | CALORIES | PRO (g) | CARB (g) | FIBER (g) | SUGAR (g) | FAT (g) | SAT FAT (g) | SOD (mg) |
|---|---|---|---|---|---|---|---|---|---|
| cake, coffeecake | 1 oz | 124 | 1 | 22 | 1 | 12 | 3 | 1 | 169 |
| cake, German chocolate | 1 slice | 280 | 3 | 35 | 0 | 24 | 15 | 5 | 300 |
| cake, gingerbread | 8" square | 263 | 3 | 36 | 1 | n/a | 12 | 3 | 242 |
| cake, marble, with chocolate icing | 1 piece | 377 | 4 | 61 | 1 | 45 | 14 | 6 | 300 |
| cake, pineapple upside-down | 8" square | 367 | 4 | 58 | 1 | n/a | 14 | 3 | 367 |
| cake, pound, fat-free | 1 oz | 80 | 2 | 17 | 0 | 10 | 0 | 0 | 97 |
| cake, pound, made with butter | 1 piece | 290 | 5 | 39 | 1 | 21 | 13 | 7 | 280 |
| cake, shortcake | 2 oz | 200 | 2 | 34 | 2 | 34 | 6 | 4 | 110 |
| cake, snack, crème-filled chocolate | 1 | 188 | 2 | 30 | 0 | 17 | 7 | 1 | 213 |
| cake, snack, sponge with crème filling | 1 | 155 | 1 | 27 | 0 | 17 | 5 | 1 | 155 |
| cake, sponge | 1 slice | 187 | 5 | 36 | 0 | n/a | 3 | 1 | 144 |
| cake, white, with chocolate frosting | 1 slice | 428 | 2 | 75 | 1 | 67 | 14 | 7 | 356 |
| cake, white, without frosting | 1 piece | 264 | 4 | 42 | 1 | 26 | 9 | 2 | 242 |
| cake, yellow, with frosting | 1 piece | 245 | 4 | 36 | 0 | n/a | 10 | 3 | 233 |
| cake, yellow, without frosting | 1 piece | 320 | 3 | 41 | 1 | 29 | 17 | 7 | 260 |
| candy, 3 Musketeers | 1 fun size | 69 | 1 | 13 | 0 | 11 | 2 | 1 | 32 |
| candy, 5th Avenue | 1 fun size | 82 | 1 | 11 | 1 | 8 | 4 | 1 | 38 |
| candy, Almond Joy | 1 fun size | 95 | 1 | 12 | 1 | 10 | 5 | 3 | 218 |
| candy, Almond Roca | 1 piece | 48 | 1 | 7 | 0 | 7 | 2 | 1 | 20 |
| candy, Baby Ruth | 1 fun size | 65 | 1 | 9 | 0 | 7 | 4 | 2 | 30 |
| candy, Bit o Honey | 1 | 113 | 1 | 23 | 0 | 13 | 2 | 1 | 85 |
| candy, bittersweet chocolate bar | 1 fun size | 153 | 2 | 16 | 3 | 10 | 10 | 5 | 0 |
| candy, Butterfinger | 1 fun size | 100 | 1 | 15 | 0 | 11 | 4 | 2 | 45 |
| candy, butterscotch | 1 piece | 23 | 0 | 5 | 0 | 5 | 0 | 0 | 23 |
| candy, caramel chocolate with nuts | 0.5 oz | 66 | 1 | 8 | 1 | 6 | 3 | 1 | 3 |
| candy, caramel vanilla | 1 | 39 | 0 | 8 | 0 | 7 | 1 | 0 | 25 |
| candy, Caramello | 1.6 oz | 210 | 3 | 29 | 1 | 26 | 10 | 6 | 55 |
| candy, carob | 1 oz | 153 | 2 | 16 | 1 | 15 | 9 | 8 | 30 |
| candy, chocolate, sugar-free | 1 piece | 44 | 1 | 3 | 1 | n/a | 3 | 2 | 9 |

| FOOD ITEM | SERVING SIZE | CALORIES | PRO (g) | CARB (g) | FIBER (g) | SUGAR (g) | FAT (g) | SAT FAT (g) | SOD (mg) |
|---|---|---|---|---|---|---|---|---|---|
| candy, chocolate bar with almonds | 1 fun size | 60 | 1 | 5 | 0 | 4 | 4 | 2 | 5 |
| candy, chocolate-covered almond | 1 | 18 | 0 | 2 | 0 | 1 | 1 | 1 | 4 |
| candy, chocolate-covered coffee bean | 1 | 8 | 0 | 1 | 0 | 1 | 0 | 0 | 0 |
| candy, chocolate-covered peanut | 1 | 21 | 1 | 2 | 0 | 2 | 1 | 1 | 2 |
| candy chocolate-covered raisin | 1 | 5 | 0 | 1 | 0 | 1 | 0 | 0 | 1 |
| candy, fondant | 1 piece | 60 | 0 | 15 | 0 | 14 | 0 | 0 | 3 |
| candy, fudge | 1 piece | 70 | 0 | 13 | 0 | 13 | 2 | 1 | 8 |
| candy, fudge, with nuts | 1 piece | 88 | 1 | 13 | 0 | 12 | 4 | 1 | 8 |
| candy, Goobers | 1 oz | 145 | 4 | 14 | 2 | n/a | 10 | 3 | 12 |
| candy, gum drops | ¼ cup | 180 | 0 | 45 | 0 | 37 | 0 | 0 | 20 |
| candy, hard, sugar-free | 1 piece | 11 | 0 | 3 | 0 | 0 | 0 | 0 | 0 |
| candy, Heath bite | 1 piece | 14 | 0 | 2 | 0 | 2 | 1 | 0 | 6 |
| candy, Hershey's Kisses, dark chocolate | 1 piece | 26 | 0 | 3 | 0 | 2 | 1 | 1 | 0 |
| candy, Kit Kat bites | 1 | 13 | 0 | 2 | 0 | 1 | 1 | 0 | 2 |
| candy, licorice, black vine | 1 | 35 | 0 | 8 | 0 | 4 | 0 | 0 | 15 |
| candy, licorice, red vine | 1 | 35 | 0 | 9 | 0 | 5 | 0 | 0 | 5 |
| candy, M&M's Peanut | 1 fun size | 108 | 2 | 13 | 1 | 11 | 6 | 2 | 10 |
| candy, M&M's Plain | 1 fun size | 98 | 1 | 14 | 1 | 13 | 4 | 3 | 12 |
| candy, milk chocolate bar | 1 mini bar (0.25 oz) | 37 | 1 | 4 | 0 | 4 | 2 | 1 | 6 |
| candy, milk chocolate candy kiss with caramel | 1 | 23 | 0 | 3 | 0 | 3 | 1 | 1 | 8 |
| candy, Milky Way Midnight | 1 fun size | 81 | 1 | 13 | 0 | 11 | 3 | 2 | 41 |
| candy, Mounds bar | 1 fun size | 96 | 1 | 12 | 1 | 9 | 5 | 4 | 29 |
| candy, Nestle Crunch | 1 fun size | 50 | 1 | 6 | 0 | 6 | 3 | 2 | 15 |
| candy, Oh Henry! | 1 oz | 131 | 2 | 19 | 1 | 14 | 7 | 2 | 65 |
| candy, Peppermint Pattie | 1 fun size | 10 | 0 | 2 | 0 | 2 | 0 | 0 | 1 |
| candy, Reese's Peanut Butter Cups | 1 fun size | 36 | 1 | 4 | 0 | 3 | 2 | 1 | 22 |
| candy, Rolo | 1 piece | 14 | 0 | 2 | 0 | 2 | 1 | 0 | 6 |
| candy, Skittles | 1 oz | 115 | 0 | 26 | 0 | 22 | 1 | 0 | 5 |

| FOOD ITEM | SERVING SIZE | CALORIES | PRO (g) | CARB (g) | FIBER (g) | SUGAR (g) | FAT (g) | SAT FAT (g) | SOD (mg) |
|---|---|---|---|---|---|---|---|---|---|
| candy, Snickers | 1 fun size | 70 | 1 | 10 | 0 | 7 | 3 | 1 | 34 |
| candy, Starburst | 1 oz | 112 | 0 | 24 | 0 | 19 | 2 | 0 | 16 |
| candy, Tootsie Pop | 1 | 60 | 0 | 15 | 0 | 10 | 0 | 0 | 0 |
| candy, Twix | 1 oz | 156 | 2 | 16 | 1 | 15 | 9 | 1 | 75 |
| cheesecake | 1 piece | 309 | 8 | 30 | 0 | 21 | 18 | 9 | 227 |
| cheesecake, fat-free | 1 piece | 140 | 7 | 28 | 1 | 18 | 0 | 0 | 20 |
| chewing gumball | 1 oz | 120 | 0 | 34 | 0 | 24 | 0 | 0 | 0 |
| chocolate chips, milk chocolate | 1 tbsp | 56 | 1 | 6 | 0 | 5 | 3 | 1 | 8 |
| chocolate chips, semisweet | 1 tbsp | 50 | 0 | 7 | 1 | 6 | 3 | 2 | 1 |
| churro | 1 (45 g) | 170 | 2 | 22 | 0 | 9 | 8 | 2 | 140 |
| cookie, animal cracker | 1 | 8 | 0 | 1 | 0 | 0 | 0 | 0 | 10 |
| cookie, biscotti, chocolate-covered, sugar-free | 1 | 40 | 1 | 6 | 0 | 0 | 2 | 1 | 3 |
| cookie, butter | 0.5 oz | 75 | 1 | 10 | 0 | n/a | 4 | 1 | 68 |
| cookie, chocolate | 2.5 oz | 210 | 2 | 30 | 1 | 20 | 10 | 4 | 170 |
| cookie, chocolate chip | 0.5 oz | 78 | 1 | 9 | 0 | n/a | 5 | 2 | 55 |
| cookie, chocolate chip, sugar-free | 0.5 oz | 62 | 1 | 9 | 0 | 0 | 4 | 1 | 58 |
| cookie, chocolate sandwich, reduced-fat | 1 | 43 | 0 | 8 | 0 | 4 | 1 | 0 | 37 |
| cookie, chocolate sandwich, with cream filling | 1 | 47 | 1 | 7 | 0 | 4 | 2 | 0 | 49 |
| cookie, chocolate wafer | 1 | 28 | 0 | 5 | 0 | 2 | 1 | 0 | 46 |
| cookie, coconut macaroon | 1 | 97 | 1 | 17 | 0 | 17 | 3 | 3 | 59 |
| cookie, devil's food | 1 | 72 | 1 | 15 | n/a | n/a | 1 | 1 | 40 |
| cookie, devil's food, SnackWells Devil's Food Fat Free | 1 | 49 | 1 | 12 | 0 | 7 | 0 | 0 | 28 |
| cookie, fig bar | 1 | 56 | 1 | 11 | 1 | 7 | 1 | 0 | 56 |
| cookie, fig bar, whole grain | 1 | 60 | 1 | 13 | 1 | 8 | 0 | 0 | 25 |
| cookie, fortune | 1 | 30 | 0 | 7 | 0 | 4 | 0 | 0 | 22 |
| cookie, fudge and caramel | 1 small | 80 | 1 | 10 | 0 | 7 | 4 | 3 | 15 |
| cookie, gingersnap | 1 | 29 | 0 | 5 | 0 | 1 | 1 | 0 | 46 |
| cookie, graham cracker | 1 square | 30 | 0 | 5 | 0 | 2 | 1 | 0 | 42 |

| FOOD ITEM | SERVING SIZE | CALORIES | PRO (g) | CARB (g) | FIBER (g) | SUGAR (g) | FAT (g) | SAT FAT (g) | SOD (mg) |
|---|---|---|---|---|---|---|---|---|---|
| cookie, hermit | 1 | 95 | 1 | 17 | 1 | 8 | 3 | 1 | 147 |
| cookie, lemon sandwich | 1 | 156 | 1 | 8 | 1 | 3 | 2 | 0 | 27 |
| cookie, marshmallow pie dipped in chocolate | 1 | 164 | 2 | 26 | 1 | 17 | 7 | 2 | 66 |
| cookie, molasses | 1 | 65 | 1 | 11 | 0 | 3 | 2 | 0 | 69 |
| cookie, oatmeal | 1 | 106 | 2 | 17 | 1 | 8 | 4 | 1 | 87 |
| cookie, oatmeal, sugar-free | 1 | 50 | 1 | 7 | 1 | 0 | 2 | 1 | 53 |
| cookie, oatmeal raisin | 1 | 107 | 1 | 17 | 1 | 9 | 4 | 1 | 98 |
| cookie, peanut butter | 1 | 95 | 2 | 12 | 0 | n/a | 5 | 1 | 104 |
| cookie, peanut butter sandwich | 1 | 67 | 1 | 9 | 0 | 5 | 3 | 1 | 52 |
| cookie, raisin, soft | 1 (0.5 oz) | 60 | 1 | 10 | 0 | 7 | 2 | 1 | 51 |
| cookie, shortbread, reduced-fat | 1 (0.5 oz) | 80 | 1 | 11 | 0 | 4 | 4 | 1 | 65 |
| cookie, sugar | 1 | 98 | 1 | 17 | 0 | 8 | 3 | 1 | 162 |
| cookie, sugar, fat-free | 1 | 71 | 1 | 17 | 0 | 8 | 0 | 0 | 80 |
| cookie, sugar wafer | 1 | 34 | 0 | 4 | 0 | 3 | 2 | 0 | 7 |
| cookie, vanilla wafer | 1 | 18 | 0 | 3 | n/a | 1 | 1 | 0 | 15 |
| cream puff, chocolate with custard filling | 1 (3") | 293 | 7 | 27 | 1 | 7 | 18 | 5 | 377 |
| custard, made with 2% milk | ½ cup | 148 | 5 | 23 | 0 | n/a | 4 | 2 | 118 |
| custard, made with whole milk | ½ cup | 161 | 5 | 23 | 0 | n/a | 5 | 3 | 117 |
| doughnut, cake, chocolate | 1 | 204 | 2 | 21 | 1 | 10 | 13 | 3 | 184 |
| doughnut, cake, plain | 1 | 180 | 3 | 19 | 1 | 7 | 11 | 2 | 210 |
| doughnut, cake, sugared | 1 | 310 | 4 | 28 | 1 | 10 | 20 | 4 | 380 |
| doughnut, hole, cake, plain | 1 | 50 | 1 | 5 | 0 | 2 | 3 | 1 | 73 |
| doughnut, hole, raised, glazed | 1 | 53 | 1 | 9 | 0 | 5 | 2 | 0 | 43 |
| doughnut, raised, glazed | 1 | 160 | 3 | 23 | 1 | 5 | 7 | 2 | 200 |
| doughnut, raised, with cream filling | 1 | 320 | 4 | 39 | 1 | 19 | 16 | 4 | 250 |
| éclair, with custard and chocolate | 1 | 204 | 5 | 19 | 0 | 5 | 12 | 3 | 263 |
| flan | ½ cup | 137 | 4 | 25 | 0 | n/a | 2 | 1 | 150 |
| frozen yogurt, chocolate | ½ cup | 110 | 3 | 19 | 1 | 18 | 3 | 2 | 55 |
| frozen yogurt, chocolate, fat-free | ½ cup | 104 | 5 | 21 | 2 | 16 | 0 | 0 | 61 |

| FOOD ITEM | SERVING SIZE | CALORIES | PRO (g) | CARB (g) | FIBER (g) | SUGAR (g) | FAT (g) | SAT FAT (g) | SOD (mg) |
|---|---|---|---|---|---|---|---|---|---|
| frozen yogurt, coffee | ½ cup | 140 | 5 | 20 | 0 | 18 | 4 | 3 | 75 |
| frozen yogurt, dulce de leche, low-fat | ½ cup | 190 | 6 | 35 | 0 | 25 | 3 | 2 | 75 |
| frozen yogurt, strawberry, fat-free | ½ cup | 140 | 5 | 31 | 0 | 20 | 0 | 0 | 40 |
| frozen yogurt, strawberry-banana, low-fat | ½ cup | 160 | 3 | 30 | 1 | 27 | 2 | 1 | 25 |
| frozen yogurt, vanilla | ½ cup | 140 | 3 | 21 | 0 | 16 | 5 | 3 | 45 |
| frozen yogurt, vanilla, fat-free | ½ cup | 95 | 5 | 19 | 0 | 19 | 0 | 0 | 64 |
| frozen yogurt, vanilla, low-fat | ½ cup | 160 | 7 | 33 | 0 | 19 | 0 | 0 | 51 |
| frozen yogurt, vanilla and fruit, fat-free | ½ cup | 97 | 5 | 19 | 0 | 19 | 0 | 0 | 65 |
| gum, chewing, regular | 1 stick | 10 | 0 | 3 | 0 | 0 | 0 | 0 | 0 |
| ice cream, butter pecan | ½ cup | 170 | 3 | 14 | 0 | 13 | 12 | 5 | 110 |
| ice cream, chocolate | ½ cup | 188 | 3 | 15 | 1 | 13 | 13 | 8 | 42 |
| ice cream, chocolate, 98% fat-free | ½ cup | 92 | 3 | 21 | 4 | 14 | 1 | 1 | 51 |
| ice cream, chocolate, low-fat | ½ cup | 120 | 3 | 21 | 2 | 18 | 2 | 1 | 45 |
| ice cream, chocolate, sugar-free | ½ cup | 149 | 3 | 25 | 1 | 5 | 6 | 4 | 74 |
| ice cream, strawberry | ½ cup | 250 | 4 | 23 | 1 | 21 | 16 | 10 | 80 |
| ice cream, vanilla | ½ cup | 133 | 2 | 16 | 0 | 14 | 7 | 4 | 53 |
| ice cream, vanilla, fat-free | ½ cup | 135 | 4 | 29 | 1 | 6 | 0 | 0 | 95 |
| ice cream, vanilla, low-fat | ½ cup | 110 | 3 | 19 | 1 | 18 | 2 | 1 | 45 |
| ice cream, vanilla, sugar-free | ½ cup | 99 | 3 | 15 | 0 | 4 | 4 | 3 | 46 |
| ice cream cone, sugar cone | ½ cup | 40 | 1 | 8 | 0 | 3 | 0 | 0 | 32 |
| ice cream cone, wafer type | ½ cup | 17 | 0 | 3 | 0 | 0 | 0 | 0 | 6 |
| ice cream novelty, Creamsicle, cherry, sugar-free | 2 pops | 40 | 1 | 10 | 6 | 0 | 2 | 1.5 | 5 |
| ice cream novelty, Creamsicle, mixed berry, sugar-free | 2 pops | 40 | 1 | 10 | 6 | 0 | 2 | 1.5 | 5 |
| ice cream novelty, Creamsicle, orange, sugar-free | 2 pops | 40 | 1 | 10 | 6 | 0 | 2 | 1.5 | 5 |
| ice cream novelty, Dreamsicle | 1 | 91 | 2 | 18 | n/a | n/a | 2 | 1 | 43 |
| ice cream novelty, Drumstick | 1 | 159 | 3 | 18 | n/a | n/a | 9 | 4 | 44 |
| ice cream novelty, Fudgsicle, fat-free | 1 | 70 | 3 | 14 | 1 | 10 | 0 | 0 | 50 |

| FOOD ITEM | SERVING SIZE | CALORIES | PRO (g) | CARB (g) | FIBER (g) | SUGAR (g) | FAT (g) | SAT FAT (g) | SOD (mg) |
|---|---|---|---|---|---|---|---|---|---|
| ice cream novelty, Fudgsicle, sugar-free | 2 pops | 70 | 4 | 16 | 4 | 0 | 2 | 1 | 60 |
| ice cream novelty, Popsicle, Caribbean fruit punch, sugar-free | 1 | 15 | 0 | 4 | 0 | 0 | 0 | 0 | 0 |
| ice cream novelty, Popsicle, cherry, sugar-free | 1 | 15 | 0 | 4 | 0 | 0 | 0 | 0 | 0 |
| ice cream novelty, Popsicle, diet A&W Root Beer, sugar-free | 1 | 15 | 0 | 4 | 0 | 0 | 0 | 0 | 0 |
| ice cream novelty, Popsicle, diet Dr. Pepper, sugar-free | 1 | 15 | 0 | 3 | 0 | 0 | 0 | 0 | 0 |
| ice cream novelty, Popsicle, diet Orange Crush, sugar-free | 1 | 15 | 0 | 3 | 0 | 0 | 0 | 0 | 0 |
| ice cream novelty, Popsicle, grape, sugar-free | 1 | 15 | 0 | 4 | 0 | 0 | 0 | 0 | 0 |
| ice cream novelty, Popsicle, orange, sugar-free | 1 | 15 | 0 | 4 | 0 | 0 | 0 | 0 | 0 |
| ice cream novelty, Popsicle, Tropical Orange, sugar-free | 1 | 15 | 0 | 4 | 0 | 0 | 0 | 0 | 0 |
| ice cream novelty, Skinny Cow, fudge bar, fat-free | 1 | 100 | 4 | 21 | 0 | 18 | 0 | 0 | 60 |
| ice cream sandwich | 1 | 144 | 3 | 22 | 1 | 15 | 6 | 3 | 36 |
| ice cream sandwich, 98% fat-free | 1 | 135 | 4 | 28 | 3 | 14 | 2 | 0 | 22 |
| ice cream sandwich, low-fat | 1 | 130 | 3 | 27 | 1 | 14 | 1 | 1 | 150 |
| ice cream sandwich, Skinny Cow, mint, sugar-free | 1 | 140 | 4 | 30 | 5 | 5 | 2 | 1 | 120 |
| ice cream sandwich, Skinny Cow, vanilla, sugar-free | 1 | 140 | 4 | 30 | 5 | 4 | 2 | 1 | 115 |
| marshmallows | 1 | 23 | 0 | 6 | 0 | 4 | 0 | 0 | 6 |
| marshmallows, miniature | 10 | 22 | 0 | 6 | 0 | 4 | 0 | 0 | 6 |
| pastry, Danish, cheese | 1 | 266 | 6 | 26 | 1 | 5 | 16 | 5 | 320 |
| pastry, Danish, cinnamon | 1 | 279 | 5 | 30 | 1 | 17 | 16 | 4 | 236 |
| pastry, Danish, fruit | 1 | 335 | 5 | 45 | n/a | n/a | 16 | 3 | 333 |
| pastry, Danish, nut raisin | 1 | 280 | 5 | 30 | 1 | 17 | 16 | 4 | 236 |
| pie, apple | 1 piece | 277 | 2 | 40 | 2 | 18 | 13 | 4 | 311 |
| pie, banana cream | 1 piece | 387 | 6 | 47 | 1 | 23 | 20 | 5 | 346 |
| pie, blueberry | 1 piece | 271 | 2 | 41 | 1 | 15 | 12 | 2 | 380 |
| pie, Boston cream | 1 piece | 260 | 3 | 42 | 1 | 18 | 9 | 3 | 120 |

| FOOD ITEM | SERVING SIZE | CALORIES | PRO (g) | CARB (g) | FIBER (g) | SUGAR (g) | FAT (g) | SAT FAT (g) | SOD (mg) |
|---|---|---|---|---|---|---|---|---|---|
| pie, cherry | 1 piece | 304 | 2 | 47 | 1 | 17 | 13 | 3 | 288 |
| pie, cherry, fried | 1 piece | 404 | 4 | 55 | 3 | n/a | 21 | 3 | 479 |
| pie, chocolate crème | 1 piece | 280 | 4 | 36 | 1 | 21 | 14 | 4 | 300 |
| pie, coconut cream | 1 piece | 259 | 3 | 27 | 0 | n/a | 17 | 8 | 309 |
| pie, egg custard | 1 piece | 221 | 6 | 22 | 2 | 12 | 12 | 2 | 252 |
| pie, lemon | 1 piece | 189 | 4 | 34 | 0 | 31 | 5 | 2 | 74 |
| pie, lemon meringue | 1 piece | 303 | 2 | 53 | 1 | 37 | 10 | 2 | 165 |
| pie, mince | 1 piece | 477 | 4 | 79 | 4 | 47 | 18 | 4 | 419 |
| pie, mud | 1 piece | 244 | 3 | 37 | 2 | 28 | 10 | 7 | 113 |
| pie, peach | 1 piece | 261 | 2 | 38 | 1 | 18 | 12 | 2 | 316 |
| pie, pecan | 1 piece | 503 | 6 | 64 | n/a | n/a | 27 | 5 | 320 |
| pie, pumpkin | 1 piece | 316 | 7 | 41 | 4 | n/a | 14 | 5 | 349 |
| pie, sour cream–apple | 1 piece | 339 | 3 | 50 | 3 | n/a | 15 | 5 | 17 |
| pie, sweet potato | 1 piece | 295 | 6 | 36 | 2 | n/a | 14 | 3 | 54 |
| pie, vanilla cream | 1 piece | 350 | 6 | 41 | 1 | 21 | 18 | 5 | 328 |
| sherbet, lemon | ½ cup | 90 | 0 | 22 | 0 | 22 | 0 | 0 | 0 |
| sherbet, lime | ½ cup | 127 | 0 | 32 | 0 | 32 | 0 | 0 | 22 |
| sherbet, orange | ½ cup | 107 | 1 | 23 | 2 | 18 | 1 | 1 | 34 |
| sorbet, berry, Ben & Jerry's, Berried Treasure | ½ cup | 110 | 0 | 29 | 1 | 24 | 0 | 0 | 5 |
| sorbet, strawberry-kiwi, Ben & Jerry's, Strawberry Kiwi Swirl | ½ cup | 110 | 0 | 28 | 1 | 24 | 0 | 0 | 10 |
| sorbet, tropical fruit, Ben & Jerry's, Jamaican Me Crazy | ½ cup | 130 | 0 | 33 | 4 | 28 | 0 | 0 | 10 |
| syrup, butterscotch | 1 tbsp | 52 | 0 | 14 | 0 | n/a | 0 | 0 | 72 |
| syrup, caramel | 1 tbsp | 52 | 0 | 14 | 0 | n/a | 0 | 0 | 72 |
| syrup, chocolate | 1 tbsp | 50 | 1 | 12 | n/a | 10 | 0 | 0 | 13 |
| syrup, fudge | 1 tbsp | 67 | 1 | 12 | 1 | 6 | 2 | 1 | 66 |
| topping, marshmallow | 1 tbsp | 60 | 0 | 15 | 0 | 14 | 0 | 0 | 0 |
| topping, pineapple | 1 tbsp | 54 | 0 | 14 | 0 | 4 | 0 | 0 | 9 |
| topping, strawberry | 1 tbsp | 54 | 0 | 14 | 0 | 6 | 0 | 0 | 4 |

# EGGS

| FOOD ITEM | SERVING SIZE | CALORIES | PRO (g) | CARB (g) | FIBER (g) | SUGAR (g) | FAT (g) | SAT FAT (g) | SOD (mg) |
|---|---|---|---|---|---|---|---|---|---|
| egg, cooked, hard-boiled | 1 large | 78 | 6 | 1 | 0 | 1 | 5 | 2 | 62 |
| egg, cooked, poached | 1 large | 74 | 6 | 0 | 0 | 0 | 5 | 2 | 147 |
| egg, cooked, scrambled | 1 large | 100 | 7 | 1 | 0 | 1 | 8 | 3 | 105 |
| egg, deviled | ½ filled egg | 63 | 4 | 0 | 0 | 0 | 5 | 1 | 50 |
| egg, duck | 1 | 130 | 9 | 1 | 0 | 1 | 10 | 3 | 102 |
| egg, goose | 1 | 266 | 20 | 2 | 0 | 1 | 19 | 5 | 199 |
| egg, quail | 1 | 14 | 1 | 0 | 0 | 0 | 1 | 0 | 13 |
| egg, scrambled, cholesterol-free, frozen | ¼ cup | 61 | 4 | 2 | 0 | 2 | 4 | 1 | 109 |
| egg salad | ¼ cup | 146 | 4 | 1 | 0 | n/a | 14 | 3 | 116 |
| egg substitute, Better 'n Eggs | ¼ cup | 26 | 5 | 0 | 0 | 0 | 0 | 0 | 98 |
| egg substitute, frozen | ¼ cup | 96 | 7 | 2 | 0 | 2 | 7 | 1 | 119 |
| egg substitute, liquid | ¼ cup | 53 | 8 | 0 | 0 | 0 | 2 | 0 | 111 |
| egg substitute, Tofutti Egg Watchers | ¼ cup | 30 | 6 | 1 | 0 | 1 | 0 | 0 | 80 |
| egg white, cooked | 1 large | 17 | 4 | 0 | 0 | 0 | 0 | 0 | 55 |
| egg white, cooked, hard-boiled, chopped | ¼ cup | 53 | 4 | 0 | 0 | 0 | 4 | 1 | 43 |
| egg white, dried | 1 tbsp | 23 | 5 | 0 | 0 | 0 | 0 | 0 | 75 |
| egg white, dried, sifted | 1 tbsp | 26 | 5 | 1 | 0 | 0 | 0 | 0 | 86 |
| egg white, Egg Beaters | 3 tbsp | 25 | 5 | 0 | 0 | 0 | 0 | 0 | 75 |
| egg white, Egg Beaters | ¼ cup | 30 | 6 | 1 | 0 | 0 | 0 | 0 | 115 |
| egg white, Egg Beaters, Cheese & Chive | ¼ cup | 35 | 6 | 1 | 0 | 0 | 1 | 1 | 210 |
| egg white, Egg Beaters, Garden Vegetable | ¼ cup | 30 | 6 | 1 | 0 | 0 | 0 | 0 | 160 |
| egg white, Egg Beaters, Southwestern | ¼ cup | 30 | 6 | 1 | 0 | 0 | 0 | 0 | 180 |
| egg white, Eggology | ¼ cup | 30 | 7 | 0 | 0 | 0 | 0 | 0 | 100 |
| egg white, raw | 1 large | 17 | 4 | 0 | 0 | 0 | 0 | 0 | 55 |
| egg yolk, raw | 1 large | 53 | 3 | 1 | 0 | 0 | 4 | 2 | 8 |
| omelet, 1 egg with ham and cheese | 1 | 156 | 11 | 2 | 0 | n/a | 11 | 5 | 372 |
| quiche, cheese | ⅛ pie (4 oz) | 336 | 10 | 16 | 0 | n/a | 26 | 13 | 117 |

| FOOD ITEM | SERVING SIZE | CALORIES | PRO (g) | CARB (g) | FIBER (g) | SUGAR (g) | FAT (g) | SAT FAT (g) | SOD (mg) |
|---|---|---|---|---|---|---|---|---|---|
| quiche, spinach | ⅛ pie (4 oz) | 336 | 10 | 16 | 0 | n/a | 26 | 13 | 117 |
| quiche Lorraine | ⅛ pie (6 oz) | 526 | 15 | 25 | 1 | n/a | 41 | 19 | 220 |

# ENTRÉES AND SIDE DISHES

| FOOD ITEM | SERVING SIZE | CALORIES | PRO (g) | CARB (g) | FIBER (g) | SUGAR (g) | FAT (g) | SAT FAT (g) | SOD (mg) |
|---|---|---|---|---|---|---|---|---|---|
| beef goulash | ½ cup | 135 | 17 | 3 | 0 | 2 | 6 | 2 | 113 |
| beef goulash, with noodles | ½ cup | 180 | 15 | 13 | 1 | n/a | 7 | 2 | 65 |
| beef stew | 1 cup | 170 | 10 | 18 | 4 | 2 | 7 | 3 | 300 |
| black-eyed peas, with pork | ½ cup | 100 | 3 | 20 | 4 | n/a | 2 | 1 | 420 |
| breakfast burrito, ham and cheese | 4 oz | 210 | 9 | 30 | 0 | 2 | 6 | 2 | 500 |
| breakfast sandwich, bacon, egg, and cheese biscuit | 1 | 441 | 20 | 33 | 1 | 3 | 27 | 7 | 1250 |
| breakfast sandwich, sausage biscuit | 1 | 412 | 11 | 31 | 1 | 2 | 28 | 8 | 988 |
| broccoli in cheese sauce | ½ cup | 115 | 7 | 6 | 2 | n/a | 8 | 4 | 202 |
| burrito, bean | 4 oz | 224 | 7 | 36 | 4 | n/a | 7 | 3 | 493 |
| burrito, beef and bean | 4 oz | 256 | 8 | 34 | 3 | 3 | 10 | 4 | 672 |
| burrito, cheese and bean | 4 oz | 230 | 9 | 32 | 6 | 1 | 7 | 3 | 503 |
| cabbage, stuffed with rice and beef | 4 oz | 138 | 9 | 10 | 1 | n/a | 7 | 3 | 227 |
| cannelloni, beef | 4 oz | 261 | 13 | 19 | 1 | n/a | 14 | 5 | 448 |
| cannelloni, beef and pork | 4 oz | 100 | 8 | 10 | 1 | n/a | 3 | 1 | 252 |
| cannelloni, cheese | 4 oz | 96 | 9 | 12 | 1 | 4 | 2 | 1 | 241 |
| cannelloni, cheese and spinach | 4 oz | 182 | 8 | 20 | 1 | n/a | 8 | 3 | 92 |
| chicken, almond | 4 oz | 131 | 10 | 8 | 2 | 2 | 7 | 1 | 246 |
| chicken, barbecued, breast | 3 oz | 162 | 20 | 2 | 0 | n/a | 8 | 2 | 181 |
| chicken, barbecued, drumstick | 1 | 129 | 16 | 2 | 0 | n/a | 6 | 2 | 145 |
| chicken, barbecued, thigh | 1 | 141 | 17 | 2 | 0 | n/a | 7 | 2 | 157 |
| chicken ã la king | 4 oz | 129 | 7 | 16 | 1 | 2 | 4 | 1 | 452 |
| chicken à la king | 8 oz | 257 | 15 | 33 | 1 | 4 | 8 | 3 | 904 |

| FOOD ITEM | SERVING SIZE | CALORIES | PRO (g) | CARB (g) | FIBER (g) | SUGAR (g) | FAT (g) | SAT FAT (g) | SOD (mg) |
|---|---|---|---|---|---|---|---|---|---|
| chicken and bean tostado | 5.5 oz | 242 | 19 | 16 | 3 | 2 | 11 | 4 | 387 |
| chicken and dumplings | 8 oz | 272 | 17 | 28 | 2 | 7 | 10 | 4 | 800 |
| chicken buffalo wing, spicy | 3 oz | 261 | 22 | 0 | 0 | 0 | 19 | 5 | 68 |
| chicken burrito | 4 oz | 207 | 11 | 30 | 2 | n/a | 5 | 1 | 1756 |
| chicken burrito, Southwestern | 4 oz | 209 | 10 | 23 | 2 | 2 | 9 | 1 | 598 |
| chicken cacciatore | 4 oz | 213 | 20 | 6 | 1 | 2 | 12 | 3 | 115 |
| chicken cacciatore, breast | 4.5 oz | 241 | 22 | 7 | 1 | 2 | 13 | 3 | 130 |
| chicken cacciatore, thigh | 3 oz | 145 | 13 | 4 | 1 | 1 | 8 | 2 | 78 |
| chicken cashew | 4 oz | 302 | 20 | 8 | 2 | n/a | 21 | 4 | 635 |
| chicken chili cheese corn dog | 1 | 200 | 6 | 24 | 0 | 1 | 9 | n/a | 470 |
| chicken chow mein, without noodles | 1 cup | 193 | 20 | 10 | 2 | n/a | 8 | 2 | 651 |
| chicken chop suey, without noodles | 4 oz | 100 | 10 | 5 | 1 | n/a | 4 | 1 | 335 |
| chicken cordon bleu | 4 oz | 188 | 10 | 18 | 2 | 3 | 9 | 3 | 591 |
| chicken cordon bleu | 8 oz | 494 | 44 | 11 | 1 | n/a | 30 | 15 | 665 |
| chicken corn dog | 1 | 180 | 7 | 15 | 1 | 1 | 10 | n/a | 490 |
| chicken corn dog | 1 mini | 52 | 2 | 5 | 0 | n/a | 3 | n/a | 123 |
| chicken croquette | 3 oz | 218 | 14 | 11 | 0 | n/a | 13 | 3 | 176 |
| chicken curry | 8 oz | 294 | 27 | 10 | 2 | 1 | 16 | 3 | 620 |
| chicken divan | 4 oz | 156 | 20 | 4 | 1 | n/a | 7 | 3 | 214 |
| chicken dumpling shumai | 1 | 22 | 1 | 2 | 0 | 0 | 1 | 0 | 50 |
| chicken egg roll | 1 | 103 | 4 | 9 | 1 | n/a | 6 | 1 | 164 |
| chicken enchilada | 7 oz | 260 | 12 | 27 | n/a | n/a | 11 | n/a | 740 |
| chicken fajita | 8 oz | 363 | 20 | 44 | 5 | n/a | 12 | 2 | 343 |
| chicken flauta | 4 oz | 331 | 13 | 12 | 2 | n/a | 26 | 4 | 71 |
| chicken fricassee | 4 oz | 150 | 13 | 4 | 0 | n/a | 8 | 2 | 234 |
| chicken fried rice | 1 cup | 240 | 7 | 49 | 1 | 2 | 2 | 0 | 870 |
| chicken fried steak | 4 oz | 170 | 8 | 14 | 1 | 1 | 9 | 4 | 471 |
| chicken hash | 4 oz | 126 | 11 | 9 | 1 | n/a | 5 | 1 | 146 |
| chicken hot and spicy, drumstick | 1 | 150 | 13 | 4 | 0 | 0 | 9 | 3 | 380 |

| FOOD ITEM | SERVING SIZE | CALORIES | PRO (g) | CARB (g) | FIBER (g) | SUGAR (g) | FAT (g) | SAT FAT (g) | SOD (mg) |
|---|---|---|---|---|---|---|---|---|---|
| chicken Kiev | 4.5 oz | 321 | 37 | 5 | 0 | n/a | 16 | 8 | 227 |
| chicken kung pao | 4 oz | 302 | 20 | 8 | 2 | n/a | 21 | 4 | 635 |
| chicken Parmesan | 4 oz | 229 | 19 | 18 | 1 | 6 | 8 | 3 | 743 |
| chicken pot pie, frozen | 8 oz | 484 | 13 | 43 | 2 | 8 | 29 | 10 | 857 |
| chicken primavera, with pasta | 9.5 oz | 320 | 11 | 40 | 6 | 9 | 12 | 6 | 840 |
| chicken stew | 4 oz | 131 | 11 | 7 | 1 | n/a | 6 | 2 | 51 |
| chicken teriyaki, breast | 1 | 178 | 27 | 7 | 0 | n/a | 4 | 1 | 1683 |
| chicken teriyaki, drumstick | 1 | 95 | 14 | 4 | 0 | n/a | 2 | 1 | 894 |
| chicken teriyaki, thigh, no skin | 1 | 106 | 16 | 4 | 0 | n/a | 2 | 1 | 999 |
| chicken teriyaki, with vegetables and rice | 10 oz | 365 | 24 | 34 | 3 | n/a | 14 | 4 | 1976 |
| chicken tetrazzini | 4 oz | 169 | 9 | 13 | 1 | n/a | 9 | 3 | 325 |
| chicken turnover | 4 oz | 360 | 11 | 23 | 1 | n/a | 20 | 5 | 219 |
| chicken wrap | 4 oz | 184 | 15 | 25 | 1 | 3 | 3 | 1 | 529 |
| chili, vegetarian, with beans | 1 cup | 205 | 12 | 38 | 10 | 6 | 1 | 0 | 778 |
| chili, with beans | 1 cup | 287 | 15 | 30 | 11 | 3 | 14 | 6 | 1336 |
| chili, with beans and turkey | 1 cup | 203 | 19 | 26 | 6 | 6 | 3 | 1 | 876 |
| chili, without beans | 1 cup | 194 | 17 | 18 | 3 | 3 | 6 | 2 | 969 |
| chili con carne, with beans | 4 oz | 150 | 8 | 12 | 0 | 0 | 7 | 0 | 345 |
| chilies rellenos | 1 | 365 | 17 | 8 | 1 | n/a | 30 | 13 | 522 |
| chimichanga, beef and bean | 1 | 241 | 8 | 21 | 3 | n/a | 14 | 3 | 230 |
| chop suey, beef, with noodles | ½ cup | 211 | 11 | 16 | n/a | n/a | 12 | 2 | 475 |
| chop suey beef, without noodles | ½ cup | 136 | 11 | 6 | 1 | n/a | 8 | 2 | 462 |
| chop suey, chicken, without noodles | ½ cup | 97 | 10 | 5 | 1 | n/a | 4 | 1 | 325 |
| chop suey, pork, with noodles | ½ cup | 143 | 11 | 6 | 1 | n/a | 8 | 2 | 463 |
| chop suey, pork, without noodles | ½ cup | 224 | 11 | 16 | 2 | n/a | 14 | 2 | 424 |
| chop suey, shrimp, with noodles | ½ cup | 136 | 8 | 12 | 1 | n/a | 6 | 1 | 355 |
| chop suey, shrimp, without noodles | ½ cup | 77 | 8 | 5 | 1 | n/a | 3 | 0 | 337 |

| FOOD ITEM | SERVING SIZE | CALORIES | PRO (g) | CARB (g) | FIBER (g) | SUGAR (g) | FAT (g) | SAT FAT (g) | SOD (mg) |
|---|---|---|---|---|---|---|---|---|---|
| chow mein, beef, with noodles | ½ cup | 211 | 11 | 16 | n/a | n/a | 12 | 2 | 475 |
| chow mein, beef, without noodles | ½ cup | 136 | 11 | 6 | 1 | n/a | 8 | 2 | 462 |
| chow mein, chicken, without noodles | ½ cup | 97 | 10 | 5 | 1 | n/a | 4 | 1 | 325 |
| chow mein, pork, with noodles | ½ cup | 224 | 11 | 16 | 2 | n/a | 14 | 2 | 424 |
| chow mein, pork, without noodles | ½ cup | 143 | 11 | 6 | 1 | n/a | 8 | 2 | 463 |
| chow mein, shrimp, without noodles | 4 oz | 79 | 8 | 5 | 1 | n/a | 3 | 0 | 348 |
| coleslaw | ½ cup | 98 | 1 | 9 | 1 | 3 | 7 | 1 | 178 |
| collard greens, with pork | 1 cup | 78 | 6 | 7 | 3 | n/a | 4 | 1 | 522 |
| corn pudding | ½ cup | 164 | 5 | 21 | 2 | 9 | 6 | 3 | 351 |
| corned beef hash | 4 oz | 186 | 10 | 11 | 1 | 0 | 12 | 5 | 482 |
| crab cake | 1 | 160 | 11 | 5 | 0 | 0 | 10 | 2 | 491 |
| crab dumpling (shumai) | 1 | 23 | 1 | 2 | 0 | 0 | 1 | 0 | 67 |
| crab thermidor | 3 oz | 214 | 10 | 4 | 0 | 0 | 18 | 10 | 192 |
| creamed chipped beef | ½ cup | 164 | 9 | 9 | 0 | n/a | 10 | 3 | 735 |
| creamed spinach | 1 cup | 222 | 7 | 15 | 2 | 10 | 16 | 9 | 1130 |
| deviled crab | 3 oz | 168 | 11 | 11 | 1 | n/a | 9 | 2 | 460 |
| duck curry Thai | 4 oz | 130 | 7 | 2 | 0 | 0 | 10 | 3 | 247 |
| egg foo yung | 3 oz | 113 | 6 | 3 | 1 | n/a | 8 | 2 | 317 |
| egg foo yung, shrimp | 3 oz | 154 | 8 | 3 | 1 | n/a | 12 | 3 | 254 |
| eggplant caponata | ½ cup | 113 | 3 | 15 | 3 | 2 | 6 | 0 | 420 |
| eggplant moussaka | 1 cup | 238 | 17 | 13 | 4 | 7 | 13 | 5 | 460 |
| eggplant Parmesan, low-calorie | 4 oz | 104 | 8 | 7 | 2 | 0 | 5 | 3 | 384 |
| egg roll, shrimp | 1 | 104 | 4 | 10 | 1 | n/a | 6 | 1 | 293 |
| enchilada, cheese | 1 | 300 | 11 | 31 | n/a | n/a | 15 | 0 | 980 |
| fettuccine Alfredo | 8 oz | 280 | 13 | 40 | 2 | 7 | 7 | 4 | 690 |
| fettuccine Alfredo, with chicken | 9½ oz | 373 | 19 | 33 | 4 | n/a | 19 | 7 | 588 |
| fondue, cheese | ½ cup | 246 | 15 | 4 | 0 | n/a | 14 | 9 | 142 |
| French toast, prepared with 2% milk | 1 piece | 149 | 5 | 16 | 1 | n/a | 7 | 2 | 311 |

| FOOD ITEM | SERVING SIZE | CALORIES | PRO (g) | CARB (g) | FIBER (g) | SUGAR (g) | FAT (g) | SAT FAT (g) | SOD (mg) |
|---|---|---|---|---|---|---|---|---|---|
| fried chicken, with potatoes | 8 oz | 470 | 25 | 31 | 3 | n/a | 27 | 8 | 1247 |
| grape leaves, stuffed with meat and rice | 1 | 50 | 2 | 2 | 1 | 0 | 4 | 1 | 15 |
| ham and scalloped potatoes | ½ cup | 126 | 7 | 16 | 1 | n/a | 4 | 1 | 245 |
| ham salad | ½ cup | 270 | 9 | 6 | 2 | 3 | 24 | 5 | 1030 |
| hot dog, chicken, with bun | 1 | 235 | 9 | 24 | 1 | 6 | 11 | 3 | 819 |
| lamb and eggplant moussaka | ½ cup | 119 | 8 | 7 | 2 | 3 | 6 | 2 | 230 |
| lamb curry | ½ cup | 128 | 14 | 2 | 1 | 1 | 7 | 2 | 162 |
| lamb dolmas, grape leaves stuffed with lamb and rice | 1 | 56 | 2 | 3 | 1 | n/a | 4 | 1 | 14 |
| lamb goulash | ½ cup | 155 | 16 | 4 | 1 | n/a | 8 | 2 | 136 |
| lasagna, cheese | 5 oz | 160 | 9 | 19 | 2 | 3 | 6 | 3 | 331 |
| lasagna, vegetarian | 5 oz | 124 | 8 | 16 | 2 | 4 | 3 | 2 | 276 |
| lasagna, with Italian sausage | 5 oz | 188 | 9 | 19 | 2 | 3 | 9 | 4 | 534 |
| lasagna, with meat and sauce | 5 oz | 143 | 9 | 18 | 2 | 4 | 4 | 2 | 281 |
| lasagna, with veal, low-calorie | 10 oz | 271 | 22 | 30 | 4 | 0 | 7 | 3 | 947 |
| linguine, with clam sauce, low-calorie | 5 oz | 248 | 11 | 32 | 2 | n/a | 8 | 3 | 1768 |
| linguine with clam sauce, low-fat | 4 oz | 135 | 6 | 21 | 1 | 2 | 3 | 1 | 221 |
| lobster newburg | 4 oz | 284 | 14 | 5 | 0 | 3 | 23 | 14 | 301 |
| lobster thermidor | 4 oz | 284 | 14 | 5 | 0 | 3 | 23 | 14 | 301 |
| macaroni, with beef in tomato sauce | 5 oz | 125 | 8 | 20 | 3 | 5 | 1 | 0 | 262 |
| macaroni and cheese | 5 oz | 238 | 10 | 25 | 1 | 4 | 11 | 5 | 638 |
| macaroni and cheese, with beef | ½ cup | 170 | 14 | 11 | 1 | n/a | 8 | 4 | 368 |
| macaroni and cheese, with tuna | ½ cup | 208 | 13 | 15 | 1 | n/a | 10 | 4 | 437 |
| manicotti, cheese | 4 oz | 160 | 8 | 15 | 2 | 4 | 7 | 11 | 378 |
| manicotti, cheese, low-calorie, and sauce | 4 oz | 137 | 9 | 12 | n/a | n/a | 6 | 3 | 350 |
| manicotti, cheese with marinara sauce | 4 oz | 136 | 5 | 16 | 1 | 3 | 7 | 3 | 358 |
| manicotti, meat and tomato sauce | 4 oz | 148 | 10 | 10 | 1 | 3 | 8 | 4 | 214 |

| FOOD ITEM | SERVING SIZE | CALORIES | PRO (g) | CARB (g) | FIBER (g) | SUGAR (g) | FAT (g) | SAT FAT (g) | SOD (mg) |
|---|---|---|---|---|---|---|---|---|---|
| manicotti, three cheeses | 4 oz | 109 | 5 | 15 | 2 | 5 | 3 | 1 | 200 |
| okra curry | 3 oz | 220 | 2 | 6 | n/a | n/a | 21 | n/a | 817 |
| onions, creamed | ½ cup | 93 | 3 | 11 | 1 | 6 | 5 | 1 | 153 |
| onions, pickled, with beets | ¼ cup | 27 | 1 | 6 | 1 | 5 | 0 | 0 | 27 |
| pizza, cheese | 1 slice | 304 | 13 | 38 | 2 | 6 | 11 | 5 | 676 |
| pizza, pepperoni and cheese | 1 slice | 413 | 18 | 39 | n/a | n/a | 21 | 8 | 869 |
| pizza, sausage and cheese | 1 slice | 337 | 12 | 32 | n/a | n/a | 18 | 6 | 704 |
| pizza, vegetarian and cheese | 1 slice | 260 | 13 | 36 | 2 | 5 | 8 | 3 | 740 |
| poi | ¼ cup | 67 | 0 | 16 | 0 | 0 | 0 | 0 | 7 |
| pork and beans | ½ cup | 134 | 7 | 25 | 7 | n/a | 2 | 1 | 524 |
| pork dumpling shumai | 1 | 24 | 1 | 2 | 0 | 0 | 1 | 0 | 51 |
| pork lo mein | 4 oz | 160 | 11 | 12 | 2 | n/a | 8 | 1 | 80 |
| pork with black beans | 4 oz | 237 | 13 | 5 | n/a | n/a | 18 | n/a | n/a |
| pot pie, beef | 4 oz | 474 | 17 | 36 | 2 | n/a | 29 | 7 | 516 |
| pot pie, chicken | 4 oz | 253 | 7 | 22 | 1 | 4 | 15 | 5 | 448 |
| pot pie, turkey | 4 oz | 200 | 7 | 20 | 1 | n/a | 10 | 3 | 397 |
| potatoes, au gratin | ½ cup | 162 | 6 | 14 | 2 | n/a | 9 | 6 | 530 |
| potatoes, French fried | 1 cup | 185 | 3 | 28 | 3 | n/a | 7 | 3 | 239 |
| potatoes, hash browns | ½ cup | 103 | 1 | 14 | 1 | 1 | 5 | 1 | 133 |
| potatoes, mashed, with milk and butter | ½ cup | 119 | 2 | 18 | 2 | 2 | 4 | 2 | 333 |
| potatoes, O'Brien | ½ cup | 39 | 1 | 8 | 1 | n/a | 1 | 0 | 105 |
| potatoes, scalloped | ½ cup | 105 | 4 | 13 | 2 | n/a | 5 | 3 | 410 |
| potato, twice baked, with butter | 5 oz | 204 | 4 | 27 | 4 | 1 | 9 | 3 | 357 |
| radiatore, with Alfredo primavera | ½ cup | 175 | 6 | 24 | 1 | 4 | 6 | 3 | 420 |
| ravioli, beef in tomato and meat sauce | 4 oz | 107 | 4 | 17 | 2 | 2 | 3 | 1 | 545 |
| ravioli, cheese in tomato sauce | 4 oz | 170 | 7 | 21 | 2 | 2 | 6 | 3 | 290 |
| roast beef hash | ½ cup | 156 | 11 | 10 | 1 | n/a | 8 | 2 | 235 |
| salad, chicken | ½ cup | 250 | 10 | 9 | 2 | 4 | 20 | 4 | 600 |

| FOOD ITEM | SERVING SIZE | CALORIES | PRO (g) | CARB (g) | FIBER (g) | SUGAR (g) | FAT (g) | SAT FAT (g) | SOD (mg) |
|---|---|---|---|---|---|---|---|---|---|
| salad, corn | ½ cup | 102 | 4 | 23 | 4 | 2 | 2 | 0 | 327 |
| salad, crab | 3 oz | 115 | 11 | 5 | 0 | 0 | 6 | 1 | 286 |
| salad, crab and seafood, with light mayo | 3 oz | 54 | 2 | 5 | 1 | 0 | 3 | 1 | 263 |
| salad, cucumber, with vinegar | 1 cup | 48 | 1 | 12 | 2 | 11 | 0 | 0 | 3 |
| salad, lobster | ½ cup | 75 | 6 | 5 | 1 | n/a | 4 | 1 | 157 |
| salad, potato, German | ½ cup | 78 | 2 | 15 | 1 | n/a | 1 | 1 | 48 |
| salad, potato, mayonnaise | ½ cup | 151 | 2 | 19 | 2 | 8 | 8 | 1 | 553 |
| salad, potato, vinaigrette | ½ cup | 106 | 2 | 17 | 2 | 5 | 3 | 0 | 530 |
| salad, shrimp | 3 oz | 132 | 12 | 3 | 0 | n/a | 8 | 1 | 183 |
| salad, three-bean | ½ cup | 70 | 2 | 7 | 3 | 0 | 4 | 1 | 260 |
| Salisbury steak, with gravy | 4 oz | 192 | 14 | 6 | 0 | 0 | 12 | 5 | 385 |
| sandwich, barbecue, with bun | 6.5 oz | 322 | 23 | 34 | 2 | 0 | 10 | 3 | 948 |
| sandwich, chicken barbecue | 1 | 280 | 25 | 37 | 2 | 9 | 3 | 1 | 830 |
| sandwich, chicken pita | 1 | 311 | 22 | 28 | 2 | n/a | 12 | 5 | 784 |
| sandwich, chicken salad, on part wheat bread | 1 | 368 | 11 | 27 | 3 | 2 | 24 | 3 | 466 |
| sandwich, chicken salad, on whole wheat bread | 1 | 398 | 31 | 5 | 3 | 3 | 26 | 3 | 527 |
| sandwich, chicken salad, on white bread | 1 | 365 | 10 | 31 | 2 | 3 | 22 | 3 | 481 |
| sandwich, egg salad | 1 | 379 | 10 | 27 | 2 | 3 | 26 | 4 | 481 |
| sandwich, grilled cheese | 1 (4 oz) | 401 | 18 | 26 | 2 | 3 | 25 | 13 | 1194 |
| sandwich, grilled ham and cheese | 1 | 381 | 21 | 30 | 1 | n/a | 20 | 8 | 1465 |
| sandwich, ham and cheese | 1 | 352 | 21 | 33 | n/a | n/a | 15 | 6 | 771 |
| sandwich, sloppy joe on bun | 6 oz | 358 | 18 | 36 | 2 | n/a | 15 | 5 | 1008 |
| sandwich, tuna salad | 1 | 322 | 14 | 32 | 2 | 5 | 16 | 2 | 577 |
| sandwich, turkey | 1 | 337 | 25 | 2 | 2 | 15 | 2 | n/a | n/a |
| sandwich, turkey club | ½ (11 oz) | 325 | 20 | 32 | 2 | 8 | 13 | 4 | 795 |
| shell pasta, cooked, with American cheese | ½ cup | 140 | 6 | 18 | 1 | 4 | 5 | 2 | 405 |
| shepherd's pie | 4 oz | 130 | 8 | 15 | 1 | n/a | 4 | 1 | 146 |
| shrimp burger | 1 | 247 | 17 | 15 | 1 | n/a | 13 | 3 | 300 |

| FOOD ITEM | SERVING SIZE | CALORIES | PRO (g) | CARB (g) | FIBER (g) | SUGAR (g) | FAT (g) | SAT FAT (g) | SOD (mg) |
|---|---|---|---|---|---|---|---|---|---|
| shrimp cake | 1 | 247 | 17 | 15 | 1 | n/a | 13 | 3 | 300 |
| shrimp cocktail | 3 oz | 81 | 10 | 8 | 2 | 4 | 1 | 0 | 417 |
| shrimp Creole, with rice | ½ cup | 155 | 14 | 14 | 1 | n/a | 5 | 1 | 185 |
| shrimp curry | ½ cup | 149 | 14 | 7 | 0 | n/a | 7 | 2 | 171 |
| shrimp dumpling shumai | 1 | 23 | 1 | 2 | 0 | 0 | 1 | 0 | 56 |
| shrimp jambalaya | 4 oz | 145 | 13 | 13 | 1 | n/a | 4 | 1 | 173 |
| shrimp newburg | 4 oz | 247 | 6 | 23 | 3 | 2 | 15 | 5 | 487 |
| shrimp primavera | 4 oz | 95 | 6 | 14 | n/a | n/a | 2 | 0 | 174 |
| shrimp scampi | 3 oz | 194 | 16 | 1 | 0 | n/a | 14 | 8 | 245 |
| shrimp teriyaki | 4 oz | 140 | 22 | 7 | 0 | n/a | 2 | 0 | 1751 |
| spaghetti and meatballs | ½ cup | 181 | 9 | 14 | 1 | 2 | 9 | 2 | 566 |
| spinach dip | ¼ cup | 280 | 0 | 6 | 0 | 1 | 28 | 4 | 28 |
| spinach soufflé | 1 cup | 233 | 11 | 8 | 1 | 3 | 18 | 8 | 769 |
| stuffed crab | 3 oz | 128 | 13 | 3 | 0 | 0 | 7 | 2 | 221 |
| stuffed mushrooms | 1 | 69 | 3 | 8 | 0 | 1 | 4 | 1 | 149 |
| stuffed peppers | 1 | 210 | 16 | 21 | 5 | 2 | 7 | 3 | 250 |
| stuffed shrimp | 3 oz | 168 | 17 | 5 | 0 | n/a | 8 | 2 | 224 |
| Swedish meatballs, with pasta | 4 oz | 181 | 9 | 17 | 1 | 1 | 9 | 3 | 445 |
| sweet and sour beef | 4 oz | 168 | 8 | 14 | 1 | n/a | 9 | 3 | 465 |
| sweet and sour chicken, breast | 1 | 118 | 8 | 15 | 1 | n/a | 3 | 1 | 506 |
| sweet and sour chicken, drumstick | 1 | 65 | 4 | 8 | 1 | n/a | 2 | 0 | 278 |
| sweet and sour chicken, thigh | 1 | 70 | 5 | 9 | 1 | n/a | 2 | 0 | 301 |
| sweet and sour pork | 4 oz | 116 | 8 | 13 | 1 | 10 | 4 | 1 | 419 |
| sweet and sour shrimp | 4 oz | 310 | 8 | 30 | 1 | 25 | 19 | 2 | 1301 |
| taco, chicken, soft | 1 | 387 | 21 | 41 | 7 | n/a | 16 | 6 | 933 |
| tamale, with meat | 1 | 134 | 6 | 11 | 2 | n/a | 7 | 3 | 84 |
| tamale pie | 8 oz | 150 | 4 | 27 | 4 | 2 | 3 | 0 | 590 |
| turkey tetrazzini | 4 oz | 168 | 9 | 13 | 1 | n/a | 9 | 3 | 325 |
| tuna casserole | 4 oz | 128 | 6 | 15 | 0 | 2 | 4 | 2 | 319 |

| FOOD ITEM | SERVING SIZE | CALORIES | PRO (g) | CARB (g) | FIBER (g) | SUGAR (g) | FAT (g) | SAT FAT (g) | SOD (mg) |
|---|---|---|---|---|---|---|---|---|---|
| tuna salad | ½ cup | 260 | 12 | 9 | 2 | 4 | 19 | 3 | 580 |
| veal cordon bleu | 4 oz | 236 | 17 | 2 | 0 | n/a | 18 | 9 | 296 |
| veal Marsala | 4 oz | 315 | 14 | 7 | 0 | n/a | 23 | 10 | 170 |
| veal paprikash | 4 oz | 130 | 17 | 2 | 0 | n/a | 6 | 2 | 73 |
| veal parmigiana | 4 oz | 223 | 16 | 10 | 1 | n/a | 13 | 5 | 404 |
| veal parmigiana, low-calorie | 4 oz | 85 | 9 | 4 | 1 | n/a | 4 | 2 | 204 |
| veal pot stickers, Thai | 1 oz | 75 | 3 | 11 | 0 | 0 | 2 | 1 | 119 |
| veal scaloppini | 3 oz | 211 | 16 | 1 | 0 | 0 | 15 | 4 | 246 |
| veal schnitzel | 4 oz | 390 | 17 | 11 | 1 | 1 | 31 | n/a | 828 |
| veal stew | 3 oz | 64 | 5 | 6 | 1 | 0 | 2 | 1 | 56 |
| vegetable stir-fry | 4 oz | 96 | 4 | 17 | 1 | 6 | 1 | 0 | 753 |
| Welsh rarebit | 4 oz | 216 | 9 | 9 | 0 | 4 | 16 | 7 | 504 |

## FATS AND OILS

| FOOD ITEM | SERVING SIZE | CALORIES | PRO (g) | CARB (g) | FIBER (g) | SUGAR (g) | FAT (g) | SAT FAT (g) | SOD (mg) |
|---|---|---|---|---|---|---|---|---|---|
| bacon grease | 1 tsp | 39 | 0 | 0 | 0 | 0 | 4 | 2 | 6 |
| butter, light with salt | 1 tsp | 24 | 0 | 0 | 0 | 0 | 4 | 2 | 21 |
| butter, light without salt | 1 tsp | 24 | 0 | 0 | 0 | 0 | 3 | 2 | 2 |
| butter, with salt | 1 tsp | 33 | 0 | 0 | 0 | 0 | 4 | 2 | 27 |
| butter, without salt | 1 tsp | 33 | 0 | 0 | 0 | 0 | 4 | 2 | 0 |
| butter-margarine blend, stick, without salt | 1 tsp | 34 | 0 | 0 | 0 | 0 | 4 | 1 | 1 |
| butter replacement, powder | 1 tsp | 6 | 0 | 1 | 0 | 0 | 0 | 0 | 85 |
| buttery spread, Smart Balance 37% Light Buttery Spread | 1 tbsp | 45 | 0 | 0 | 0 | 0 | 5 | 2 | 85 |
| buttery spread, Smart Balance 67% Buttery Spread | 1 tbsp | 80 | 0 | 0 | 0 | 0 | 9 | 3 | 90 |
| buttery spread, Smart Balance Omega Plus Buttery Spread | 1 tbsp | 80 | 0 | 0 | 0 | 0 | 9 | 3 | 90 |
| buttery spread, Smart Balance buttery spread | 1 tsp | 7 | 0 | 0 | 0 | 0 | 1 | 0 | 35 |

| FOOD ITEM | SERVING SIZE | CALORIES | PRO (g) | CARB (g) | FIBER (g) | SUGAR (g) | FAT (g) | SAT FAT (g) | SOD (mg) |
|---|---|---|---|---|---|---|---|---|---|
| chicken fat | 1 tsp | 38 | 0 | 0 | 0 | 0 | 4 | 1 | 0 |
| cooking spray | ⅓ sec | 0 | 0 | 0 | 0 | 0 | 0 | 0 | 0 |
| cooking spray, baking | ⅓ sec | 0 | 0 | 0 | 0 | 0 | 0 | 0 | 0 |
| cooking spray, butter | ⅓ sec | 0 | 0 | 0 | 0 | 0 | 0 | 0 | 0 |
| cooking spray, butter | 1 sec | 10 | 0 | 0 | 0 | 0 | 2 | 0 | 0 |
| cooking spray, canola oil | ⅓ sec | 0 | 0 | 0 | 0 | 0 | 0 | 0 | 0 |
| cooking spray, canola oil, butter-flavored | ⅓ sec | 0 | 0 | 0 | 0 | 0 | 0 | 0 | 0 |
| cooking spray, canola oil, high heat | ⅓ sec | 0 | 0 | 0 | 0 | 0 | 0 | 0 | 0 |
| cooking spray, canola oil, nonaerosol | ⅓ sec | 0 | 0 | 0 | 0 | 0 | 0 | 0 | 0 |
| cooking spray, canola oil, roasted garlic | ⅓ sec | 0 | 0 | 0 | 0 | 0 | 0 | 0 | 0 |
| cooking spray, canola oil, water-based | ⅓ sec | 0 | 0 | 0 | 0 | 0 | 0 | 0 | 0 |
| cooking spray, canola oil, with butter | ⅓ sec | 0 | 0 | 0 | 0 | 0 | 0 | 0 | 0 |
| cooking spray, canola oil, with lemon | ⅓ sec | 0 | 0 | 0 | 0 | 0 | 0 | 0 | 0 |
| cooking spray, extra-virgin olive oil | ⅓ sec | 0 | 0 | 0 | 0 | 0 | 0 | 0 | 0 |
| cooking spray, flour and canola oil, baking | ⅓ sec | 0 | 0 | 0 | 0 | 0 | 0 | 0 | 0 |
| cooking spray, for the grill | ⅓ sec | 0 | 0 | 0 | 0 | 0 | 0 | 0 | 0 |
| cooking spray, for the grill, canola oil | ⅓ sec | 0 | 0 | 0 | 0 | 0 | 0 | 0 | 0 |
| cooking spray, grapeseed oil | ⅓ sec | 0 | 0 | 0 | 0 | 0 | 0 | 0 | 0 |
| cooking spray, I Can't Believe It's Not Butter | ⅓ sec | 0 | 0 | 0 | 0 | 0 | 0 | 0 | 0 |
| cooking spray, natural butter and soy oil | ⅓ sec | 0 | 0 | 0 | 0 | 0 | 0 | 0 | 0 |
| cooking spray, olive oil | ⅓ sec | 0 | 0 | 0 | 0 | 0 | 0 | 0 | 0 |
| cooking spray, original | ⅓ sec | 0 | 0 | 0 | 0 | 0 | 0 | 0 | 0 |
| cooking spray, Smart Balance Buttery Burst Cooking Spray with Organic Soy | 1 pump | 0 | 0 | 0 | 0 | 0 | 0 | 0 | 0 |
| cooking spray, soybean oil | ⅓ sec | 0 | 0 | 0 | 0 | 0 | 0 | 0 | 0 |
| cooking spray, Wescoat | ¼ sec | 0 | 0 | 0 | 0 | 0 | 0 | 0 | 0 |

| FOOD ITEM | SERVING SIZE | CALORIES | PRO (g) | CARB (g) | FIBER (g) | SUGAR (g) | FAT (g) | SAT FAT (g) | SOD (mg) |
|---|---|---|---|---|---|---|---|---|---|
| fish oil, cod | 1 tsp | 41 | 0 | 0 | 0 | 0 | 5 | 1 | 0 |
| fish oil, cod liver | 1 tsp | 41 | 0 | 0 | 0 | 0 | 5 | 1 | 0 |
| fish oil, salmon | 1 tsp | 41 | 0 | 0 | 0 | 0 | 5 | 1 | 0 |
| flaxseed oil | 1 tsp | 40 | 0 | 0 | 0 | 0 | 5 | 0 | 0 |
| ghee (clarified butter) | 1 tsp | 37 | 0 | 0 | 0 | 0 | 4 | 3 | 0 |
| lard | 1 tsp | 38 | 0 | 0 | 0 | 0 | 4 | 1 | 0 |
| margarine, hard, corn and soybean oils | 1 tsp | 34 | 0 | 0 | 0 | 0 | 4 | 1 | 44 |
| margarine, hard, corn oil | 1 tsp | 34 | 0 | 0 | 0 | 0 | 4 | 1 | 44 |
| margarine, hard, soybean oil | 1 tsp | 34 | 0 | 0 | 0 | 0 | 4 | 1 | 44 |
| margarine, regular, with salt | 1 tsp | 34 | 0 | 0 | 0 | 0 | 4 | 1 | 44 |
| margarine, regular, without salt | 1 tsp | 34 | 0 | 0 | 0 | 0 | 4 | 1 | 0 |
| margarine, spread, fat-free | 1 tsp | 2 | 0 | 0 | 0 | 0 | 0 | 0 | 28 |
| margarine, spread, 48% fat | 1 tsp | 20 | 0 | 0 | 0 | 0 | 2 | 0 | 30 |
| margarine, spread, 20% vegetable oil, with salt | 1 tsp | 9 | 0 | 0 | 0 | 0 | 1 | 0 | 37 |
| margarine, spread, 20% vegetable oil, without salt | 1 tsp | 7 | 0 | 0 | 0 | 0 | 1 | 0 | 0 |
| margarine, spread, 70% vegetable oil | 1 tsp | 29 | 0 | 0 | n/a | n/a | 3 | 1 | 33 |
| margarine, spread, 80% vegetable oil | 1 tsp | 33 | 0 | 0 | 0 | 0 | 4 | 1 | 31 |
| margarine, whipped | 1 tsp | 25 | 0 | 0 | 0 | 0 | 4 | 1 | 30 |
| margarine-like spread, liquid, with salt, fat-free | 1 tsp | 2 | 0 | 0 | 0 | 0 | 0 | 0 | 42 |
| oil, almond | 1 tsp | 40 | 0 | 0 | 0 | 0 | 5 | 0 | 0 |
| oil, apricot kernel | 1 tsp | 40 | 0 | 0 | 0 | 0 | 5 | 0 | 0 |
| oil, avocado | 1 tsp | 41 | 0 | 0 | 0 | 0 | 5 | 1 | 0 |
| oil, borage flaxseed | 1 tsp | 43 | 0 | 0 | 0 | 0 | 5 | 0 | 0 |
| oil, canola | 1 tsp | 41 | 0 | 0 | 0 | 0 | 5 | 0 | 0 |
| oil, canola and soybean | 1 tsp | 40 | 0 | 0 | 0 | 0 | 5 | 0 | 0 |
| oil, cashew nut, roasted, with salt | 1 tbsp | 47 | 1 | 2 | 0 | 0 | 4 | 1 | 25 |
| oil, cashew nut, roasted, without salt | 1 tbsp | 47 | 1 | 2 | 0 | 0 | 4 | 1 | 1 |

| FOOD ITEM | SERVING SIZE | CALORIES | PRO (g) | CARB (g) | FIBER (g) | SUGAR (g) | FAT (g) | SAT FAT (g) | SOD (mg) |
|---|---|---|---|---|---|---|---|---|---|
| oil, cocoa butter | 1 tsp | 40 | 0 | 0 | 0 | 0 | 5 | 3 | 0 |
| oil, coconut | 1 tsp | 39 | 0 | 0 | 0 | 0 | 5 | 4 | 0 |
| oil, corn and canola | 1 tsp | 41 | 0 | 0 | 0 | 0 | 5 | 0 | 0 |
| oil, corn, peanut, and olive | 1 tsp | 42 | 0 | 0 | 0 | 0 | 5 | 1 | 0 |
| oil, cottonseed | 1 tsp | 41 | 0 | 0 | 0 | 0 | 5 | 1 | 0 |
| oil, grapeseed | 1 tsp | 40 | 0 | 0 | 0 | 0 | 5 | 0 | 0 |
| oil, hazelnut | 1 tsp | 40 | 0 | 0 | 0 | 0 | 5 | 0 | 0 |
| oil, mustard | 1 tsp | 41 | 0 | 0 | 0 | 0 | 5 | 1 | 0 |
| oil, olive | 1 tsp | 40 | 0 | 0 | 0 | 0 | 5 | 1 | 0 |
| oil, palm | 1 tsp | 40 | 0 | 0 | 0 | 0 | 5 | 2 | 0 |
| oil, palm kernel | 1 tsp | 39 | 0 | 0 | 0 | 0 | 5 | 4 | 0 |
| oil, peanut | 1 tsp | 40 | 0 | 0 | 0 | 0 | 5 | 1 | 0 |
| oil, safflower | 1 tsp | 40 | 0 | 0 | 0 | 0 | 5 | 0 | 0 |
| oil, sesame | 1 tsp | 40 | 0 | 0 | 0 | 0 | 5 | 0 | 0 |
| oil, soybean | 1 tsp | 40 | 0 | 0 | 0 | 0 | 5 | 1 | 0 |
| oil, walnut | 1 tsp | 40 | 0 | 0 | 0 | 0 | 5 | 0 | 0 |
| oil, wheat germ | 1 tsp | 40 | 0 | 0 | 0 | 0 | 5 | 1 | 0 |

## FISH

| FOOD ITEM | SERVING SIZE | CALORIES | PRO (g) | CARB (g) | FIBER (g) | SUGAR (g) | FAT (g) | SAT FAT (g) | SOD (mg) |
|---|---|---|---|---|---|---|---|---|---|
| anchovies, raw | 3 oz | 111 | 17 | 0 | 0 | 0 | 4 | 1 | 88 |
| anchovies, with oil, drained | 3 oz | 179 | 25 | 0 | 0 | 0 | 8 | 2 | 3119 |
| bass, sea, baked | 3 oz | 105 | 20 | 0 | 0 | 0 | 2 | 1 | 74 |
| bass, sea, raw | 4 oz | 110 | 21 | 0 | 0 | 0 | 2 | 1 | 77 |
| bass, striped, baked | 3 oz | 105 | 19 | 0 | 0 | 0 | 3 | 1 | 75 |
| bass, striped, raw | 4 oz | 110 | 20 | 0 | 0 | 0 | 3 | 1 | 78 |
| brown trout, baked | 3 oz | 119 | 22 | 0 | 0 | 0 | 3 | 2 | 64 |
| burbot, baked | 3 oz | 98 | 21 | 0 | 0 | 0 | 1 | 0 | 105 |
| burbot, raw | 4 oz | 102 | 22 | 0 | 0 | 0 | 1 | 0 | 110 |

| FOOD ITEM | SERVING SIZE | CALORIES | PRO (g) | CARB (g) | FIBER (g) | SUGAR (g) | FAT (g) | SAT FAT (g) | SOD (mg) |
|---|---|---|---|---|---|---|---|---|---|
| butterfish, baked | 3 oz | 159 | 19 | 0 | 0 | 0 | 9 | 3 | 97 |
| butterfish, raw | 4 oz | 166 | 20 | 0 | 0 | 0 | 9 | 4 | 101 |
| carp, baked | 3 oz | 138 | 19 | 0 | 0 | 0 | 6 | 1 | 54 |
| carp, raw | 4 oz | 144 | 20 | 0 | 0 | 0 | 6 | 1 | 56 |
| catfish, farmed, raw | 4 oz | 153 | 18 | 0 | 0 | 0 | 9 | 2 | 60 |
| catfish, steamed | 3 oz | 144 | 17 | 0 | 0 | 0 | 8 | 2 | 51 |
| catfish, wild, baked | 3 oz | 89 | 16 | 0 | 0 | 0 | 2 | 1 | 43 |
| catfish, wild, raw | 4 oz | 108 | 19 | 0 | 0 | 0 | 3 | 1 | 49 |
| caviar, red/black | 1 tbsp | 40 | 4 | 1 | 0 | 0 | 3 | 1 | 240 |
| cisco, raw | 4 oz | 111 | 22 | 0 | 0 | 0 | 2 | 0 | 62 |
| cisco, smoked | 3 oz | 151 | 14 | 0 | 0 | 0 | n/a | 1 | 409 |
| cod, Atlantic, baked | 3 oz | 89 | 19 | 0 | 0 | 0 | 1 | 0 | 66 |
| cod, Atlantic, raw | 4 oz | 90 | 20 | 0 | 0 | 0 | 1 | 0 | 67 |
| cod, cooked | 3 oz | 91 | 20 | 0 | 0 | 0 | 1 | 0 | 56 |
| cod, Pacific, raw | 4 oz | 93 | 20 | 0 | 0 | 0 | 1 | 0 | 81 |
| cod, steamed | 4 oz | 116 | 25 | 0 | 0 | 0 | 1 | 0 | 91 |
| codfish ball | 1 | 125 | 9 | 8 | 1 | n/a | 7 | 1 | 175 |
| codfish cake | 1 | 237 | 16 | 15 | 1 | n/a | n/a | 3 | 334 |
| croaker, cooked | 3 oz | 242 | 18 | 12 | 0 | 1 | n/a | 3 | 203 |
| croaker, raw | 4 oz | 118 | 20 | 0 | 0 | 0 | 4 | 1 | 64 |
| cusk, baked | 3 oz | 95 | 21 | 0 | 0 | 0 | 1 | 0 | 34 |
| cusk , raw | 4 oz | 99 | 22 | 0 | 0 | 0 | 1 | 0 | 35 |
| cuttlefish, raw | 4 oz | 90 | 18 | 1 | 0 | n/a | 1 | 0 | 422 |
| cuttlefish, steamed | 3 oz | 134 | 28 | 1 | 0 | n/a | 1 | 0 | 633 |
| devilfish, Alaskan, raw | 4 oz | 110 | 13 | 1 | n/a | n/a | 6 | n/a | n/a |
| dolphin, baked | 3 oz | 93 | 20 | 0 | 0 | 0 | 1 | 0 | 96 |
| dolphin, raw | 4 oz | 96 | 21 | 0 | 0 | 0 | 1 | 0 | 100 |
| drumfish, baked | 3 oz | 130 | 19 | 0 | 0 | 0 | 5 | 1 | 82 |
| drumfish, raw | 4 oz | 135 | 20 | 0 | 0 | 0 | 6 | 1 | 85 |
| fish and chips | 4 oz | 196 | 8 | 24 | 2 | 7 | 8 | 2 | 411 |

| FOOD ITEM | SERVING SIZE | CALORIES | PRO (g) | CARB (g) | FIBER (g) | SUGAR (g) | FAT (g) | SAT FAT (g) | SOD (mg) |
|---|---|---|---|---|---|---|---|---|---|
| fish broth | 1 cup | 39 | 1 | 0 | 0 | 1 | 0 | 0 | 776 |
| fish cake | 2.5 oz | 149 | 13 | 6 | 0 | n/a | 8 | 2 | 127 |
| fish cake, Japanese | 0.5 oz | 19 | 2 | 2 | 0 | n/a | 0 | 0 | 10 |
| fish chowder | 1 cup | 194 | 24 | 12 | 1 | 4 | 5 | 2 | 180 |
| fish curry, Thai | 1 cup | 310 | 20 | 13 | 2 | 3 | n/a | 14 | 249 |
| fish paste, Japanese | 1 tbsp | 2 | 2 | 0 | n/a | n/a | n/a | 10 | n/a |
| fish roe | 1 tbsp | 40 | 4 | 1 | 0 | 0 | 3 | 1 | 240 |
| fish sandwich, with tartar sauce | 3 oz | 232 | 9 | 22 | 0 | n/a | n/a | 3 | 330 |
| fish sandwich, with tartar sauce and cheese | 3.5 oz | 284 | 11 | 26 | 0 | n/a | n/a | 4 | 508 |
| fish sandwich, without tartar sauce | 2 oz | 155 | 6 | 21 | 1 | n/a | 5 | n/a | 201 |
| fish sauce | 1 tbsp | 6 | 1 | 1 | 0 | 1 | 0 | 0 | 1390 |
| fish sticks | 2 oz | 112 | 4 | 13 | 1 | 2 | 4 | n/a | n/a |
| fish sticks, vegetarian | 1 piece | 81 | 6 | 3 | 2 | 0 | 5 | 1 | 137 |
| fish taco | 4 oz | 231 | 9 | 16 | 1 | 1 | n/a | 4 | 324 |
| fisherman's soup | 1 cup | 194 | 24 | 12 | 1 | 4 | 5 | 2 | 180 |
| flounder, baked | 3 oz | 100 | 21 | 0 | 0 | 0 | 1 | 0 | 89 |
| flounder, cooked | 3 oz | 101 | 19 | 0 | 0 | 0 | 2 | 0 | 101 |
| flounder, raw | 4 oz | 103 | 21 | 0 | 0 | 0 | 1 | 0 | 92 |
| flounder, stuffed | 3 oz | 135 | 17 | 5 | 0 | n/a | 4 | 1 | 190 |
| grouper, baked | 3 oz | 100 | 21 | 0 | 0 | 0 | 1 | 0 | 45 |
| grouper, raw | 4 oz | 104 | 22 | 0 | 0 | 0 | 1 | 0 | 60 |
| haddock , baked | 3 oz | 95 | 21 | 0 | 0 | 0 | 1 | 0 | 74 |
| haddock , raw | 4 oz | 99 | 21 | 0 | 0 | 0 | 1 | 0 | 77 |
| haddock, smoked | 3 oz | 99 | 21 | 0 | 0 | 0 | 1 | 0 | 649 |
| haddock, steamed | 3 oz | 94 | 21 | 0 | 0 | 0 | 1 | 0 | 66 |
| haddock cake | 4 oz | 237 | 16 | 15 | 1 | n/a | n/a | 3 | 334 |
| halibut, Atlantic, baked | 3 oz | 119 | 23 | 0 | 0 | 0 | 3 | 0 | 59 |
| halibut, Atlantic, raw | 4 oz | 125 | 24 | 0 | 0 | 0 | 3 | 0 | 61 |
| halibut, Greenland, baked | 3 oz | 203 | 16 | 0 | 0 | 0 | n/a | 3 | 88 |

FISH (cont.)

| FOOD ITEM | SERVING SIZE | CALORIES | PRO (g) | CARB (g) | FIBER (g) | SUGAR (g) | FAT (g) | SAT FAT (g) | SOD (mg) |
|---|---|---|---|---|---|---|---|---|---|
| halibut, Greenland, raw | 4 oz | 211 | 16 | 0 | 0 | 0 | n/a | 3 | 91 |
| halibut, smoked | 3 oz | 153 | 26 | 0 | 0 | 0 | 3 | 0 | n/a |
| herring, Atlantic, baked | 3 oz | 173 | 20 | 0 | 0 | 0 | 10 | 2 | 98 |
| herring, Atlantic, kippered, smoked | 1 small | 43 | 5 | 0 | 0 | 0 | 2 | 1 | 184 |
| herring, Atlantic, kippered, smoked | 1 medium | 87 | 10 | 0 | 0 | 0 | 5 | 1 | 367 |
| herring, Atlantic, kippered, smoked | 1 large | 141 | 16 | 0 | 0 | 0 | 8 | 2 | 597 |
| herring, Atlantic, pickled | 3 oz | 223 | 12 | 8 | 0 | 7 | 2 | n/a | n/a |
| herring, Pacific, cooked | 3 oz | 213 | 18 | 0 | 0 | 0 | n/a | 4 | 81 |
| herring, pickled | 1" cube | 52 | 3 | 2 | 0 | 2 | 4 | 0 | 174 |
| jellyfish, pickled | 3 oz | 10 | 2 | 0 | 0 | 0 | 0 | 0 | 2747 |
| ling, baked | 3 oz | 94 | 21 | 0 | 0 | 0 | 1 | n/a | 147 |
| ling, raw | 4 oz | 90 | 20 | 0 | 0 | 0 | 1 | n/a | 67 |
| lingcod, baked | 3 oz | 93 | 19 | 0 | 0 | 0 | 1 | 0 | 65 |
| lingcod, raw | 4 oz | 90 | 20 | 0 | 0 | 0 | 1 | n/a | 67 |
| mackerel, Atlantic, baked | 3 oz | 222 | 20 | 0 | 0 | 0 | n/a | 4 | 71 |
| mackerel, Atlantic, raw | 4 oz | 232 | 21 | 0 | 0 | 0 | n/a | 4 | 102 |
| mackerel, dried | 1 | 244 | 15 | 0 | 0 | 0 | n/a | 6 | 3560 |
| mackerel, king, baked | 3 oz | 114 | 22 | 0 | 0 | 0 | 2 | 0 | 173 |
| mackerel, king, raw | 4 oz | 119 | 23 | 0 | 0 | 0 | 2 | 0 | 179 |
| mackerel, Pacific, raw | 4 oz | 179 | 23 | 0 | 0 | 0 | 9 | 3 | 98 |
| mackerel, Spanish, baked | 3 oz | 134 | 20 | 0 | 0 | 0 | 5 | 2 | 56 |
| mackerel, Spanish, raw | 4 oz | 158 | 22 | 0 | 0 | 0 | 7 | 2 | 67 |
| mackerel cake | 4 oz | 297 | 19 | 15 | 1 | n/a | n/a | 4 | 479 |
| mahi mahi, baked | 3 oz | 93 | 20 | 0 | 0 | 0 | 1 | 0 | 96 |
| mahi mahi, raw | 4 oz | 96 | 21 | 0 | 0 | 0 | 1 | 0 | 100 |
| milkfish, baked | 3 oz | 162 | 22 | 0 | 0 | 0 | 7 | 2 | 78 |
| milkfish, raw | 4 oz | 168 | 23 | 0 | 0 | 0 | 8 | 2 | 82 |
| monkfish, baked | 3 oz | 83 | 16 | 0 | 0 | 0 | 2 | 0 | 20 |

| FOOD ITEM | SERVING SIZE | CALORIES | PRO (g) | CARB (g) | FIBER (g) | SUGAR (g) | FAT (g) | SAT FAT (g) | SOD (mg) |
|---|---|---|---|---|---|---|---|---|---|
| monkfish, raw | 4 oz | 86 | 16 | 0 | 0 | 0 | 2 | 0 | 20 |
| mullet, striped, baked | 3 oz | 128 | 21 | 0 | 0 | 0 | 4 | 1 | 60 |
| mullet, striped, raw | 4 oz | 133 | 22 | 0 | 0 | 0 | 4 | 1 | 74 |
| northern pike, baked | 3 oz | 96 | 21 | 0 | 0 | 0 | 1 | 0 | 42 |
| northern pike, raw | 4 oz | 100 | 22 | 0 | 0 | 0 | 1 | 0 | 44 |
| ocean perch, Atlantic, baked | 3 oz | 103 | 20 | 0 | 0 | 0 | 2 | 0 | 82 |
| ocean perch, Atlantic, cooked | 3 oz | 111 | 21 | 0 | 0 | 0 | 2 | 1 | 96 |
| ocean perch, Atlantic, raw | 4 oz | 107 | 21 | 0 | 0 | 0 | 2 | 0 | 85 |
| orange roughy, baked | 3 oz | 89 | 19 | 0 | 0 | 0 | 1 | 0 | 59 |
| orange roughy, cooked | 3 oz | 81 | 16 | 0 | 0 | 0 | 1 | 0 | 71 |
| orange roughy, raw | 4 oz | 86 | 19 | 0 | 0 | 0 | 1 | 0 | 82 |
| perch, baked | 3 oz | 103 | 20 | 0 | 0 | 0 | 2 | 0 | 82 |
| pike, walleye, baked | 3 oz | 101 | 21 | 0 | 0 | 0 | 1 | 0 | 55 |
| pike, walleye, raw | 4 oz | 105 | 22 | 0 | 0 | 0 | 1 | 0 | 58 |
| pollock, Atlantic, baked | 3 oz | 100 | 21 | 0 | 0 | 0 | 1 | 0 | 94 |
| pollock, Atlantic, raw | 4 oz | 104 | 22 | 0 | 0 | 0 | 1 | 0 | 98 |
| pollock, cooked | 3 oz | 101 | 20 | 0 | 0 | 0 | 1 | 0 | 11 |
| rockfish, cooked | 3 oz | 101 | 21 | 0 | 0 | 0 | 2 | 0 | 71 |
| rockfish, Pacific, raw | 4 oz | 107 | 21 | 0 | 0 | 0 | 2 | 0 | 68 |
| sablefish, baked | 3 oz | 213 | 15 | 0 | 0 | 0 | n/a | 3 | 61 |
| sablefish, raw | 4 oz | 221 | 15 | 0 | 0 | 0 | n/a | 4 | 64 |
| sablefish, smoked | 3 oz | 219 | 15 | 0 | 0 | 0 | n/a | 4 | 627 |
| salmon, Alaskan chinook, canned | 3 oz | 226 | 26 | 0 | 0 | 0 | n/a | n/a | n/a |
| salmon, Alaskan chinook, smoked | 3 oz | 128 | 20 | 1 | n/a | n/a | 5 | n/a | n/a |
| salmon, Atlantic, farmed, raw | 4 oz | 208 | 23 | 0 | 0 | 0 | n/a | 2 | 67 |
| salmon, Alaskan king, smoked, canned | 1 oz | 43 | 7 | 0 | n/a | n/a | 2 | n/a | n/a |
| salmon, Alaskan king, smoked, with brine | 3 oz | 375 | 34 | 2 | 2 | n/a | n/a | 6 | 589 |
| salmon, Alaskan, smoked | 1 oz | 43 | 7 | 0 | n/a | n/a | 2 | n/a | n/a |

| FOOD ITEM | SERVING SIZE | CALORIES | PRO (g) | CARB (g) | FIBER (g) | SUGAR (g) | FAT (g) | SAT FAT (g) | SOD (mg) |
|---|---|---|---|---|---|---|---|---|---|
| salmon, Atlantic, wild, baked | 3 oz | 155 | 22 | 0 | 0 | 0 | 7 | 1 | 48 |
| salmon, Atlantic, wild, raw | 4 oz | 161 | 23 | 0 | 0 | 0 | 7 | 1 | 50 |
| salmon, chinook, raw | 4 oz | 203 | 23 | 0 | 0 | 0 | n/a | 4 | 53 |
| salmon, chinook, lox | 3 oz | 100 | 16 | 0 | 0 | 0 | 4 | 1 | 1701 |
| salmon, chinook, smoked | 3 oz | 100 | 16 | 0 | 0 | 0 | 4 | 1 | 667 |
| salmon, chinook, smoked lox | 1 oz | 33 | 5 | 0 | 0 | 0 | 1 | 0 | 567 |
| salmon, chum, baked | 3 oz | 131 | 22 | 0 | 0 | 0 | 4 | 1 | 54 |
| salmon, chum, canned, drained | 3 oz | 120 | 18 | 0 | 0 | 0 | 5 | 1 | 414 |
| salmon, chum, raw | 4 oz | 136 | 23 | 0 | 0 | 0 | 4 | 1 | 57 |
| salmon, coho, cooked | 4 oz | 192 | 24 | 0 | 0 | 0 | n/a | 2 | 66 |
| salmon, coho, farmed, baked | 3 oz | 151 | 21 | 0 | 0 | 0 | 7 | 2 | 44 |
| salmon, coho, wild, baked | 3 oz | 118 | 20 | 0 | 0 | 0 | 4 | 1 | 49 |
| salmon, coho, wild, raw | 4 oz | 166 | 25 | 0 | 0 | 0 | 7 | 1 | 52 |
| salmon, coho, wild, steamed | 3 oz | 156 | 23 | 0 | 0 | 0 | 6 | 1 | 45 |
| salmon, pink, canned, drained | 3 oz | 116 | 20 | 0 | 0 | 0 | 4 | 1 | 339 |
| salmon, pink, raw | 4 oz | 132 | 23 | 0 | 0 | 0 | 4 | 1 | 76 |
| salmon, pink chum, baked | 3 oz | 131 | 22 | 0 | 0 | 0 | 4 | 1 | 54 |
| salmon, sockeye, baked | 3 oz | 184 | 23 | 0 | 0 | 0 | 9 | 2 | 56 |
| salmon, sockeye, cooked | 3 oz | 192 | 24 | 0 | 0 | 0 | n/a | 2 | 66 |
| salmon, sockeye, raw | 4 oz | 191 | 24 | 0 | 0 | 0 | n/a | 2 | 53 |
| salmon cake | 3 oz | 185 | 12 | 10 | 1 | n/a | n/a | 3 | 359 |
| salmon jerky | 1 oz | 81 | 13 | 4 | 0 | 4 | 1 | 0 | 456 |
| sardine, Atlantic | 1 oz | 59 | 7 | 0 | 0 | 0 | 3 | 0 | 143 |
| sardine, Atlantic, with bone and oil, drained | 1 piece | 33 | 4 | 0 | 0 | 0 | 2 | 0 | 81 |
| sardine, with mustard, canned | 1 oz | 51 | 5 | 0 | 0 | n/a | 3 | 1 | 118 |
| sardine, without skin and bone, water packed | 3 oz | 185 | 21 | 0 | 0 | 0 | n/a | 2 | 781 |
| shad, baked | 3 oz | 214 | 18 | 0 | 0 | 0 | n/a | 4 | 55 |
| shad, raw | 4 oz | 223 | 19 | 0 | 0 | 0 | n/a | 4 | 58 |

| FOOD ITEM | SERVING SIZE | CALORIES | PRO (g) | CARB (g) | FIBER (g) | SUGAR (g) | FAT (g) | SAT FAT (g) | SOD (mg) |
|---|---|---|---|---|---|---|---|---|---|
| shark, baked | 3 oz | 153 | 21 | 0 | 0 | n/a | 7 | 1 | 108 |
| shark, hammerhead, raw | 4 oz | 120 | 27 | 0 | 0 | 0 | 0 | 0 | n/a |
| shark, raw | 4 oz | 147 | 24 | 0 | 0 | 0 | 5 | 1 | 90 |
| smelt, rainbow, baked | 3 oz | 105 | 19 | 0 | 0 | 0 | 3 | 0 | 65 |
| smelt, rainbow, raw | 4 oz | 110 | 20 | 0 | 0 | 0 | 3 | 1 | 68 |
| smelt, rainbow, smoked | 3 oz | 145 | 26 | 0 | 0 | 0 | 4 | 1 | n/a |
| snapper, baked | 3 oz | 109 | 22 | 0 | 0 | 0 | 1 | 0 | 48 |
| snapper, raw | 4 oz | 113 | 23 | 0 | 0 | 0 | 2 | 0 | 73 |
| sole, baked | 3 oz | 100 | 21 | 0 | 0 | 0 | 1 | 0 | 89 |
| sole, cooked | 3 oz | 101 | 19 | 0 | 0 | 2 | 0 | 0 | 101 |
| sole, raw | 4 oz | 103 | 21 | 0 | 0 | 0 | 1 | 0 | 92 |
| sole, steamed | 3 oz | 98 | 20 | 0 | 0 | 0 | 1 | 0 | 78 |
| sturgeon, baked | 3 oz | 115 | 18 | 0 | 0 | 0 | 4 | 1 | 59 |
| sturgeon, raw | 4 oz | 119 | 18 | 0 | 0 | 0 | 5 | 1 | 61 |
| sturgeon, smoked | 3 oz | 147 | 27 | 0 | 0 | 0 | 4 | 1 | 629 |
| surimi fish | 3 oz | 84 | 13 | 6 | 0 | 0 | 1 | 0 | 122 |
| swordfish, baked | 3 oz | 131 | 22 | 0 | 0 | 0 | 4 | 1 | 98 |
| swordfish, cooked | 3 oz | 122 | 16 | 0 | 0 | 0 | 6 | 2 | 101 |
| swordfish, raw | 4 oz | 137 | 22 | 0 | 0 | 0 | 5 | 1 | 102 |
| swordfish, steamed | 3 oz | 130 | 21 | 0 | 0 | 0 | 4 | 1 | 87 |
| tarpon, raw | 4 oz | 105 | 24 | 0 | 0 | 0 | 1 | 0 | n/a |
| tilapia, baked | 3 oz | 109 | 22 | 0 | 0 | 0 | 2 | 1 | 48 |
| tilapia, cooked | 3 oz | 110 | 22 | 0 | 0 | 0 | 3 | 1 | 30 |
| tilapia, raw | 4 oz | 109 | 23 | 0 | 0 | 0 | 2 | 1 | 59 |
| tilefish, baked | 3 oz | 125 | 21 | 0 | 0 | 0 | 4 | 1 | 50 |
| tilefish, raw | 4 oz | 109 | 20 | 0 | 0 | 0 | 3 | 1 | 60 |
| trout, rainbow, farmed, baked | 3 oz | 144 | 21 | 0 | 0 | 0 | 6 | 2 | 36 |
| trout, rainbow, farmed, raw | 4 oz | 156 | 24 | 0 | 0 | 0 | 6 | 2 | 40 |
| trout, rainbow, wild, baked | 3 oz | 128 | 19 | 0 | 0 | 0 | 5 | 1 | 48 |
| trout, rainbow, wild, raw | 4 oz | 135 | 23 | 0 | 0 | 0 | 4 | 1 | 35 |
| trout, sea, baked | 3 oz | 113 | 18 | 0 | 0 | 0 | 4 | 1 | 63 |

| FOOD ITEM | SERVING SIZE | CALORIES | PRO (g) | CARB (g) | FIBER (g) | SUGAR (g) | FAT (g) | SAT FAT (g) | SOD (mg) |
|---|---|---|---|---|---|---|---|---|---|
| trout, sea, raw | 4 oz | 118 | 19 | 0 | 0 | 0 | 4 | 1 | 66 |
| trout, sea, smoked | 1 oz | 50 | 8 | 0 | 0 | 0 | 2 | 0 | n/a |
| tuna, bluefin, baked | 3 oz | 156 | 25 | 0 | 0 | 0 | 5 | 1 | 43 |
| tuna, bluefin, raw | 4 oz | 163 | 26 | 0 | 0 | 0 | 6 | 1 | 44 |
| tuna, chunk light, canned in water, drained | 3 oz | 105 | 23 | 0 | 0 | 0 | 0 | 0 | 345 |
| tuna, cooked | 3 oz | 130 | 26 | 0 | 0 | 0 | 2 | 0 | 40 |
| tuna, dried | 1 oz | 51 | 8 | 0 | 0 | 0 | 2 | 0 | 14 |
| tuna, skipjack, baked | 3 oz | 112 | 24 | 0 | 0 | 0 | 1 | 0 | 40 |
| tuna, skipjack, raw | 4 oz | 117 | 25 | 0 | 0 | 0 | 1 | 0 | 42 |
| tuna, smoked | 3 oz | 171 | 22 | 0 | 0 | 0 | 9 | 2 | 94 |
| tuna, StarKist Light | 3 oz | 99 | 22 | 0 | 0 | 0 | 1 | 0 | 43 |
| tuna, white, canned in water, drained | 3 oz | 109 | 20 | 0 | 0 | 0 | 3 | 1 | 321 |
| tuna, yellowfin, baked | 3 oz | 118 | 25 | 0 | 0 | 0 | 1 | 0 | 40 |
| tuna, yellowfin, raw | 4 oz | 122 | 27 | 0 | 0 | 0 | 1 | 0 | 42 |
| tuna jerky | 1 oz | 81 | 16 | 4 | 0 | 4 | 0 | 0 | 456 |
| tuna patty | 3 oz | 212 | 16 | 10 | 1 | n/a | n/a | 3 | 299 |
| turbot, baked | 3 oz | 104 | 18 | 0 | 0 | 0 | 3 | n/a | 163 |
| turbot, raw | 4 oz | 108 | 18 | 0 | 0 | 0 | 3 | 1 | 170 |
| whitefish, Alaskan, raw | 4 oz | 149 | 21 | 0 | 0 | 0 | 7 | 2 | 58 |
| whiting, baked | 3 oz | 176 | 7 | 0 | 0 | 8 | 2 | 0 | 224 |
| whiting, raw | 4 oz | 102 | 21 | 0 | 0 | 0 | 1 | 0 | 82 |
| wolffish, Atlantic, baked | 3 oz | 105 | 19 | 0 | 0 | 0 | 3 | 0 | 93 |
| wolffish, Atlantic, raw | 4 oz | 109 | 20 | 0 | 0 | 0 | 3 | 0 | 96 |

## FRUIT

| FOOD ITEM | SERVING SIZE | CALORIES | PRO (g) | CARB (g) | FIBER (g) | SUGAR (g) | FAT (g) | SAT FAT (g) | SOD (mg) |
|---|---|---|---|---|---|---|---|---|---|
| apricot | 1 | 17 | 0 | 4 | 1 | 3 | 0 | 0 | 0 |
| apple | 1 | 72 | 0 | 19 | 3 | 14 | 0 | 0 | 0 |
| apple, crab | 1 (1 oz) | 20 | 0 | 5 | 0 | n/a | 0 | 0 | 0 |
| apple, crab, sliced | ½ cup | 42 | 0 | 11 | 1 | n/a | 0 | 0 | 0 |

| FOOD ITEM | SERVING SIZE | CALORIES | PRO (g) | CARB (g) | FIBER (g) | SUGAR (g) | FAT (g) | SAT FAT (g) | SOD (mg) |
|---|---|---|---|---|---|---|---|---|---|
| apple, Mammy (Jamaican), peeled | 3 oz | 26 | 0 | 6 | 2 | n/a | 0 | 0 | 8 |
| apple, peeled | 1 | 61 | 0 | 16 | 2 | 13 | 0 | 0 | 0 |
| apple, Rose | 1 (4 oz) | 28 | 1 | 6 | n/a | n/a | 0 | n/a | 0 |
| apple, sugar (sweetsop), peeled | 4 oz | 107 | 2 | 27 | 5 | n/a | 0 | 0 | 10 |
| apples, dried, stewed, with added sugar | ⅓ cup | 77 | 0 | 19 | 2 | 17 | 0 | 0 | 18 |
| apples, dried, stewed, without added sugar | ⅓ cup | 48 | 0 | 13 | 2 | 11 | 0 | 0 | 17 |
| applesauce, canned sweetened, with salt | ⅓ cup | 65 | 0 | 17 | 1 | n/a | 0 | 0 | 24 |
| applesauce, canned, sweetened, without salt | ⅓ cup | 64 | 0 | 17 | 1 | 14 | 0 | 0 | 3 |
| applesauce, Gravenstein, canned, unsweetened | ⅓ cup | 33 | 0 | 9 | 1 | 7 | 0 | 0 | 3 |
| apricot | 1 | 17 | 0 | 4 | 1 | 3 | 0 | 0 | 0 |
| apricot, halved | ½ cup | 25 | 1 | 6 | 1 | 0 | 0 | 0 | 0 |
| apricot, sliced | ½ cup | 40 | 1 | 9 | 2 | 8 | 0 | 0 | 1 |
| apricots, canned in water | ½ cup | 33 | 1 | 8 | 2 | 6 | 0 | 0 | 4 |
| apricots, canned in water, peeled | ½ cup | 25 | 1 | 6 | 1 | n/a | 0 | 0 | 12 |
| apricots, dried | 1 | 18 | 0 | 4 | 0 | n/a | 0 | 0 | 0 |
| apricots, dried, chopped | 2 tbsp | 42 | 0 | 11 | 1 | 8 | 0 | 0 | 0 |
| apricots, dried, stewed | ⅓ cup | 70 | 1 | 18 | 2 | 16 | 0 | 0 | 8 |
| avocado | ¼ cup | 58 | 1 | 3 | 2 | 0 | 5 | 1 | 3 |
| avocado, California | ⅕ of medium | 13 | 0 | 1 | 1 | 0 | 1 | 0 | 0 |
| avocado, cubed | 2 tbsp | 30 | 0 | 2 | 1 | 0 | 3 | 0 | 1 |
| avocado, Florida | ¼ of medium | 91 | 2 | 6 | 4 | 2 | 8 | 1 | 2 |
| avocado, pureed | 2 tbsp | 46 | 1 | 2 | 2 | 0 | 4 | 1 | 2 |
| avocado, sliced | 1 tbsp | 15 | 0 | 1 | 1 | 0 | 1 | 0 | 1 |
| avocado salsa | 1 oz | 12 | 0 | 1 | 0 | 0 | 1 | 0 | 204 |
| banana | 1 large (8") | 121 | 1 | 31 | 4 | 17 | 0 | 0 | 1 |
| banana | 1 extra large (9") | 135 | 2 | 35 | 4 | 19 | 1 | 0 | 2 |
| banana, dried | 1 | 181 | 1 | 24 | 2 | 19 | 10 | 2 | 116 |
| banana, dried, powdered | 1 tbsp | 21 | 0 | 5 | 1 | 3 | 0 | 0 | 0 |

| FOOD ITEM | SERVING SIZE | CALORIES | PRO (g) | CARB (g) | FIBER (g) | SUGAR (g) | FAT (g) | SAT FAT (g) | SOD (mg) |
|---|---|---|---|---|---|---|---|---|---|
| banana, green, fried | 1 | 155 | 1 | 22 | 2 | 14 | 8 | 1 | 1 |
| banana, mashed | ⅓ cup | 66 | 1 | 17 | 2 | 9 | 0 | 0 | 1 |
| banana, pureed | 2 oz | 54 | 0 | 12 | 1 | 11 | 0 | 0 | 5 |
| banana, red | 3 oz | 79 | 1 | 20 | 1 | 13 | 0 | 0 | 0 |
| banana, sliced | ⅓ cup | 44 | 1 | 11 | 1 | 6 | 0 | 0 | 1 |
| banana, yellow | 1 extra small (6") | 72 | 1 | 19 | 2 | 10 | 0 | 0 | 1 |
| banana, yellow | ½ of medium (7") | 55 | 1 | 15 | 2 | 11 | 0 | 0 | 0 |
| banana, yellow | 1 medium (7") | 105 | 1 | 27 | 3 | 14 | 0 | 0 | 1 |
| banana chips, dried, Melissa's | 0.5 oz | 75 | 0 | 10 | 1 | 3 | 4 | 3 | n/a |
| banana flakes | 1 tbsp | 22 | 0 | 6 | 1 | 4 | 0 | 0 | 0 |
| banana melon | 3 oz | 18 | 1 | 3 | 0 | 3 | 0 | 0 | 9 |
| blackberries | 1 cup | 62 | 2 | 14 | 7 | 6 | 1 | 0 | 1 |
| blackberries, frozen, unsweetened | ½ cup | 45 | 1 | 11 | 4 | 8 | 0 | 0 | 0 |
| blueberries | ½ cup | 41 | 1 | 11 | 2 | 7 | 0 | 0 | 1 |
| blueberries, frozen | 4 oz | 50 | 1 | 12 | n/a | n/a | 0 | 0 | n/a |
| breadfruit | ¼ cup | 57 | 1 | 15 | 3 | 6 | 0 | 0 | 1 |
| breadfruit, seeds, cooked | 1 oz | 54 | 2 | 8 | 1 | n/a | 2 | 0 | 7 |
| breadfruit, seeds, raw | 1 oz | 48 | 2 | 9 | 1 | n/a | 1 | 0 | 7 |
| cantaloupe, balled | 1 cup | 60 | 1 | 14 | n/a | n/a | 0 | 0 | 28 |
| cantaloupe, cubed | 1 cup | 54 | 1 | 13 | n/a | n/a | 0 | 0 | 26 |
| cantaloupe, diced | 1 cup | 53 | 1 | 13 | n/a | n/a | 0 | 0 | 25 |
| cantaloupe, wedged | ⅛ of small | 19 | 0 | 4 | n/a | n/a | 0 | 0 | 9 |
| cantaloupe, wedged | ⅛ of medium | 23 | 1 | 6 | n/a | n/a | 0 | 0 | 11 |
| cantaloupe, wedged | ⅛ of large | 35 | 1 | 8 | n/a | n/a | 0 | 0 | 16 |
| casaba, cubed | 1 cup | 48 | 2 | 11 | 2 | 10 | 0 | 0 | 15 |
| casaba, wedged | 1/10 of melon | 46 | 2 | 11 | 1 | 9 | 0 | 0 | 15 |
| cherimoya, whole, without skin and seeds | ⅛ | 52 | 1 | 12 | 2 | n/a | 0 | n/a | 3 |
| cherries, Barbados | ½ cup | 16 | 0 | 4 | 1 | n/a | 0 | 0 | 3 |

| FOOD ITEM | SERVING SIZE | CALORIES | PRO (g) | CARB (g) | FIBER (g) | SUGAR (g) | FAT (g) | SAT FAT (g) | SOD (mg) |
|---|---|---|---|---|---|---|---|---|---|
| cherries, Barbados | 1 cup | 31 | 0 | 8 | 1 | n/a | 0 | 0 | 7 |
| cherries, Bing, dried | 2 tsp | 60 | 1 | 13 | 1 | 8 | 0 | 0 | 3 |
| cherries, black, canned, drained | ¼ cup | 44 | 1 | 11 | 1 | 10 | 0 | 0 | 3 |
| cherries, dark, sweet, pitted | 1 oz | 0 | 6 | 0 | 6 | 0 | 0 | 0 | n/a |
| cherries, groundcherries | ½ cup | 37 | 1 | 8 | 2 | n/a | 0 | 0 | 1 |
| cherries, Maraschino, green, canned | 1 | 10 | 0 | 3 | 0 | 3 | 0 | 0 | 0 |
| cherries, Maraschino, red, with stems | 1 | 10 | 0 | 3 | 0 | 3 | 0 | 0 | 0 |
| cherries, red, sour, canned in water | ½ cup | 44 | 1 | 11 | 1 | 9 | 0 | 0 | 9 |
| cherries, red, sour, freeze-dried | 0.5 oz | 60 | 1 | 12 | 0 | n/a | 0 | n/a | 2 |
| cherries, red, sour, frozen, unsweetened | ½ cup | 36 | 1 | 9 | 1 | 7 | 0 | 0 | 1 |
| cherries, sour | ½ cup | 39 | 1 | 9 | 1 | 7 | 0 | 0 | 2 |
| cherries, Surinam (pitanga) | ½ cup | 29 | 1 | 6 | n/a | n/a | 0 | n/a | 6 |
| cherries, Surinam (pitanga) | 1 cup | 57 | 1 | 13 | n/a | n/a | 1 | 0 | 5 |
| cherries, sweet | ¼ cup | 23 | 0 | 6 | 1 | 5 | 0 | 0 | 0 |
| cherries, sweet | 10 | 43 | 1 | 10 | 1 | 9 | 0 | n/a | 0 |
| cherries, sweet | ½ cup | 46 | 1 | 12 | 2 | 9 | 0 | 0 | 0 |
| cherries, sweet, canned in water | ½ cup | 57 | 1 | 15 | 2 | 13 | 0 | 0 | 1 |
| cherries, sweet, frozen | ½ cup | 45 | 1 | 11 | 2 | 10 | 0 | 0 | 0 |
| cherries, sweet, Montmorency | 3 oz | 44 | 1 | 10 | 1 | n/a | 0 | 0 | 12 |
| cherries, tart, dried | 2 tbsp | 53 | 0 | 13 | 4 | 7 | 0 | 0 | 0 |
| cherries, tart, dried, pitted | 2 tbsp | 62 | 1 | 22 | 1 | n/a | 0 | 0 | 0 |
| cherries, tart, Montmorency | 2 tbsp | 51 | 0 | 12 | 0 | 10 | 0 | 0 | 1 |
| cherries, tart, red, dried, pitted | 2 tbsp | 62 | 1 | 22 | 1 | n/a | 0 | 0 | 0 |
| cherries, West Indian | ½ cup | 16 | 0 | 4 | 1 | n/a | 0 | 0 | 3 |
| cherries, West Indian | 1 cup | 31 | 0 | 8 | 1 | n/a | 0 | 0 | 7 |
| clementine, mandarin orange | 1 | 40 | 1 | 9 | 2 | 6 | 0 | 0 | 1 |
| coconut, dried, Melissa's | 2 tsp | 55 | 0 | 2 | 0 | 1 | 5 | 5 | 2 |
| cranberries | 1 cup | 44 | 0 | 12 | 4 | 4 | 0 | 0 | 2 |

| FOOD ITEM | SERVING SIZE | CALORIES | PRO (g) | CARB (g) | FIBER (g) | SUGAR (g) | FAT (g) | SAT FAT (g) | SOD (mg) |
|---|---|---|---|---|---|---|---|---|---|
| cranberries, chopped | ½ cup | 25 | 0 | 7 | 3 | 2 | 0 | 0 | 1 |
| cranberries, dried | 2 tbsp | 45 | 0 | 11 | 1 | 10 | 0 | 0 | 0 |
| cranberries, dried, with orange bits | 2 tbsp | 45 | 0 | 12 | 1 | 9 | 0 | 0 | 0 |
| cranberries, frozen | 1 cup | 44 | 0 | 12 | 4 | 4 | 0 | 0 | 2 |
| cranberry bits, dried | 2 tbsp | 53 | 0 | 13 | 1 | 11 | 0 | 0 | 0 |
| cranberry-orange relish | 2 tbsp | 61 | 0 | 16 | 0 | n/a | 0 | 0 | 11 |
| cranberry sauce, canned, sweetened | ½ slice | 86 | 0 | 22 | 1 | 22 | 0 | 0 | 17 |
| currants, black, dried | 2 tbsp | 50 | 1 | 14 | 1 | 12 | 0 | 0 | 0 |
| currants, black, European | ½ cup | 35 | 1 | 9 | 4 | n/a | 0 | 0 | 1 |
| currants, dried, Melissa's | 2 tsp | 65 | 1 | 15 | 1 | 10 | 0 | 0 | 5 |
| currants, dried, zante | 2 tbsp | 51 | 1 | 13 | 1 | 12 | 0 | 0 | 1 |
| currants, red | ½ cup | 31 | 1 | 8 | 2 | 4 | 0 | 0 | 1 |
| currants, stewed, with sugar | ¼ cup | 43 | 0 | 10 | n/a | n/a | 0 | 0 | 1 |
| currants, stewed, without sugar | ½ cup | 36 | 1 | 17 | 10 | 7 | 1 | 0 | 4 |
| currants, white | ½ cup | 31 | 1 | 8 | 2 | 4 | 0 | 0 | 1 |
| date, Chinese | 1 oz | 22 | 0 | 6 | n/a | n/a | 0 | n/a | 1 |
| date, chopped | 1 tbsp | 30 | 0 | 8 | 1 | 7 | 0 | 0 | 0 |
| date, deglet noor | 1 | 23 | 0 | 6 | 1 | 5 | 0 | 0 | 0 |
| date, deglet noor, pitted, chopped | 1 tbsp | 31 | 0 | 8 | 1 | 7 | 0 | 0 | 0 |
| date, Indian | 1 | 5 | 0 | 1 | 0 | 1 | 0 | 0 | 1 |
| date, medjool, pitted | 1 | 66 | 0 | 18 | 2 | 16 | 0 | 0 | 0 |
| date pulp, Indian | 1 tbsp | 18 | 0 | 5 | 1 | 4 | 0 | 0 | 2 |
| durian | 1 oz | 42 | 0 | 8 | 1 | n/a | 2 | n/a | 1 |
| durian, chopped | 2 tbsp | 45 | 0 | 8 | 1 | n/a | 2 | n/a | 1 |
| durian, frozen | 1 oz | 42 | 0 | 8 | 1 | n/a | 2 | n/a | 1 |
| elderberries | ¼ cup | 26 | 0 | 7 | 3 | n/a | 0 | 0 | 2 |
| elderberries, canned | 2 tbsp | 38 | 0 | 10 | 2 | 8 | 0 | 0 | 2 |
| elderberries, cooked | 2 tbsp | 38 | 0 | 10 | 2 | 8 | 0 | 0 | 2 |
| feijoa | 1 | 25 | 1 | 5 | 2 | n/a | 0 | 0 | 2 |
| feijoa, pureed | ¼ cup | 30 | 1 | 6 | 3 | n/a | 0 | 0 | 2 |

| FOOD ITEM | SERVING SIZE | CALORIES | PRO (g) | CARB (g) | FIBER (g) | SUGAR (g) | FAT (g) | SAT FAT (g) | SOD (mg) |
|---|---|---|---|---|---|---|---|---|---|
| fig | 1 small | 30 | 0 | 8 | 1 | 7 | 0 | 0 | 0 |
| fig | 1 medium | 37 | 0 | 10 | 1 | 8 | 0 | 0 | 1 |
| fig | 1 large | 47 | 0 | 12 | 2 | 10 | 0 | 0 | 1 |
| fig, Barbary | 2 oz | 23 | 0 | 5 | 2 | n/a | 0 | 0 | 3 |
| fig, dried | 2 tbsp | 62 | 1 | 16 | 2 | 12 | 0 | 0 | 2 |
| fig, dried | 1 oz | 71 | 1 | 18 | 3 | 14 | 0 | 0 | 3 |
| fig, dried, Calimyrna, Melissa's | 2 tsp | 55 | 1 | 13 | 2 | 10 | 0 | 0 | 0 |
| figs, canned, Kadota | 1 | 28 | 0 | 6 | 1 | 4 | 0 | 0 | 1 |
| figs, canned, undrained | ¼ cup | 33 | 0 | 9 | 1 | 7 | 0 | 0 | 1 |
| fruit cocktail, canned, natural style | ¼ cup | 40 | 0 | 10 | 1 | 6 | 0 | 0 | 10 |
| fruit cocktail, canned, with juice | ½ cup | 55 | 1 | 14 | 1 | 13 | 0 | 0 | 5 |
| fruit cocktail, canned, with water | ½ cup | 38 | 1 | 10 | 1 | 0 | 0 | 0 | 5 |
| fruit mix, dried | 1 oz | 1 | 18 | 2 | n/a | 0 | 0 | 5 | n/a |
| fruit salad, canned, with water | ½ cup | 37 | 0 | 10 | 1 | n/a | 0 | 0 | 4 |
| fruit salad, fresh, with citrus | ½ cup | 50 | 0 | 13 | 2 | n/a | 0 | 0 | 0 |
| fruit salad, fresh, without citrus | ½ cup | 51 | 1 | 13 | 2 | 11 | 0 | 0 | 0 |
| fruit salad, with walnuts | 0.5 oz | 50 | 1 | 7 | n/a | 5 | 2 | 0 | 13 |
| gooseberries | 1 cup | 66 | 1 | 15 | 6 | n/a | 1 | 0 | 2 |
| gooseberries, Cape (groundcherries) | 1 cup | 74 | 3 | 16 | 4 | n/a | 1 | n/a | 1 |
| grapefruit | ½ of medium | 60 | 1 | 16 | 6 | 10 | 0 | 0 | 0 |
| grapefruit, pink | ½ of small | 32 | 1 | 8 | 1 | 7 | 0 | 0 | 0 |
| grapefruit, pink | ½ of medium | 41 | 1 | 10 | 1 | 9 | 0 | 0 | 0 |
| grapefruit, pink | ½ of large | 53 | 1 | 13 | 2 | 12 | 0 | 0 | 0 |
| grapefruit, pink, sections | ½ cup | 48 | 1 | 12 | 2 | 8 | 0 | 0 | 0 |
| grapefruit, pink, sections, canned in water | ½ cup | 44 | 1 | 11 | 0 | 11 | 0 | 0 | 2 |
| grapefruit, pink California, sections | 4 oz | 42 | 1 | 11 | 1 | n/a | 0 | 0 | 1 |
| grapefruit, red | ½ of small | 32 | 1 | 8 | 1 | 7 | 0 | 0 | 0 |
| grapefruit, red | ½ of medium | 41 | 1 | 10 | 1 | 9 | 0 | 0 | 0 |

| FOOD ITEM | SERVING SIZE | CALORIES | PRO (g) | CARB (g) | FIBER (g) | SUGAR (g) | FAT (g) | SAT FAT (g) | SOD (mg) |
|---|---|---|---|---|---|---|---|---|---|
| grapefruit, red | ½ of large | 53 | 1 | 13 | 2 | 12 | 0 | 0 | 0 |
| grapefruit, red, sections | ½ of medium | 48 | 1 | 12 | 2 | 8 | 0 | 0 | 0 |
| grapefruit, red, sections | ½ cup | 37 | 1 | 9 | 1 | 8 | 0 | 0 | 0 |
| grapefruit, red, sections, canned in water | ½ cup | 44 | 1 | 11 | 0 | 11 | 0 | 0 | 2 |
| grapefruit, white | ½ of medium | 41 | 1 | 10 | 1 | 9 | 0 | 0 | 0 |
| grapefruit, white | ½ of large | 53 | 1 | 13 | 2 | 12 | 0 | 0 | 0 |
| grapefruit, white, sections | ½ cup | 37 | 1 | 9 | 1 | 8 | 0 | 0 | 0 |
| grapes, black | ½ cup | 50 | 1 | 13 | 1 | 12 | 0 | 0 | 3 |
| grapes, champagne | ½ cup | 50 | 1 | 15 | 1 | 14 | 0 | 0 | 0 |
| grapes, concord | 1 cup | 61 | 1 | 16 | 1 | 15 | 0 | 0 | 2 |
| grapes, European, green | ½ cup | 55 | 1 | 14 | 1 | 12 | 0 | 0 | 2 |
| grapes, European, red | ½ cup | 55 | 1 | 14 | 1 | 12 | 0 | 0 | 2 |
| grapes, green | ½ cup | 55 | 1 | 14 | 1 | 12 | 0 | 0 | 2 |
| grapes, red | ½ cup | 55 | 1 | 14 | 1 | 12 | 0 | 0 | 2 |
| grapes, slip skin | ½ cup | 31 | 0 | 8 | 0 | 7 | 0 | 0 | 1 |
| grapes, Thompson, seedless | ½ cup | 55 | 1 | 14 | 1 | 12 | 0 | 0 | 2 |
| grapes, Thompson, seedless, canned in water | ½ cup | 49 | 1 | 13 | 1 | 12 | 0 | 0 | 7 |
| grapes, Tokay | ½ cup | 55 | 1 | 14 | 1 | 12 | 0 | 0 | 2 |
| guava | 1 | 61 | 2 | 13 | 5 | 8 | 1 | 0 | 2 |
| guava, Brazilian | 1 | 25 | 1 | 5 | 2 | n/a | 0 | 0 | 2 |
| guava, Brazilian, pureed | ¼ cup | 30 | 1 | 6 | 3 | n/a | 0 | 0 | 2 |
| guava, pineapple | 1 | 25 | 1 | 5 | 2 | n/a | 0 | 0 | 2 |
| guava, pineapple, pureed | ¼ cup | 30 | 1 | 6 | 3 | n/a | 0 | 0 | 2 |
| guava, pink, pureed | 2 oz | 29 | 0 | 7 | n/a | n/a | 0 | 0 | 2 |
| guava, strawberry | 5 ea | 21 | 0 | 5 | 2 | n/a | 0 | 0 | 11 |
| guava, strawberry, pureed | ¼ cup | 42 | 0 | 11 | 3 | n/a | 0 | 0 | 23 |
| guava paste | 0.5 oz | 40 | 0 | 10 | 0 | 0 | 0 | 0 | 0 |
| guavasteen | 1 | 25 | 1 | 5 | 2 | n/a | 0 | 0 | 2 |
| guavasteen, pureed | ¼ cup | 30 | 1 | 6 | 3 | n/a | 0 | 0 | 2 |
| honeydew, balled | 1 cup | 64 | 1 | 16 | 1 | 14 | 0 | 0 | 32 |

| FOOD ITEM | SERVING SIZE | CALORIES | PRO (g) | CARB (g) | FIBER (g) | SUGAR (g) | FAT (g) | SAT FAT (g) | SOD (mg) |
|---|---|---|---|---|---|---|---|---|---|
| honeydew, diced | 1 cup | 61 | 1 | 15 | 1 | 14 | 0 | 0 | 31 |
| honeydew, wedged | ⅛ of small | 45 | 1 | 11 | 1 | 10 | 0 | 0 | 23 |
| honeydew, wedged | ⅛ of medium | 58 | 1 | 15 | 1 | 14 | 0 | 0 | 29 |
| jackfruit, dried | ¼ cup | 19 | 0 | 5 | 0 | 4 | 0 | 0 | 0 |
| jackfruit, sliced | ⅓ cup | 47 | 1 | 12 | 1 | n/a | 0 | 0 | 1 |
| jujube | 1 oz | 22 | 0 | 6 | n/a | n/a | 0 | 0 | 1 |
| jujube, dried | 0.5 oz | 41 | 1 | 10 | n/a | n/a | 0 | n/a | 1 |
| kiwifruit (Chinese gooseberry), dried | 0.5 oz | 15 | 0 | 4 | 1 | 2 | 0 | 0 | 1 |
| kiwifruit (Chinese gooseberry), peeled | 1 small | 35 | 1 | 8 | 2 | 5 | 0 | 0 | 2 |
| kiwifruit (Chinese gooseberry), peeled | 1 medium | 46 | 1 | 11 | 2 | 7 | 0 | 0 | 2 |
| kiwifruit (Chinese gooseberry), peeled | 1 large | 56 | 1 | 13 | 3 | 8 | 0 | 0 | 3 |
| kumquat | 3 oz | 60 | 2 | 14 | 6 | 7 | 1 | 0 | 9 |
| kumquats, canned | 1 oz | 39 | 0 | 10 | n/a | n/a | 0 | 0 | 31 |
| lemon | 1 medium | 15 | 0 | 5 | 1 | 1 | 0 | 0 | 5 |
| lemon peel | 1 tbsp | 3 | 0 | 1 | 1 | 0 | 0 | 0 | 0 |
| lemon peel, dried, Melissa's | 1½ tsp | 45 | 0 | 12 | 6 | 6 | 0 | 0 | 0 |
| lime | 1 | 20 | 0 | 7 | 2 | 1 | 0 | 0 | 1 |
| lime peel | 1 tsp | 3 | 0 | 1 | 1 | 0 | 0 | 0 | 0 |
| loganberries | 1 cup | 62 | 2 | 14 | 7 | 7 | 1 | 0 | 1 |
| loquat | 6 small | 38 | 0 | 10 | 1 | n/a | 0 | 0 | 1 |
| loquat | 5 medium | 38 | 0 | 10 | 1 | 0 | 0 | 0 | 1 |
| loquat | 3 large | 28 | 0 | 7 | 1 | 0 | 0 | 0 | 1 |
| loquat, canned | 2 oz | 48 | 0 | 13 | n/a | n/a | 0 | n/a | n/a |
| loquat, cubed | ½ cup | 35 | 9 | 1 | n/a | n/a | 0 | 0 | 1 |
| lychee (litchi) | 6 | 38 | 0 | 10 | 1 | 9 | 0 | 0 | 1 |
| lychee (litchi) | ½ cup | 63 | 1 | 16 | 1 | 14 | 0 | 0 | 1 |
| lychee (litchi), dried | 5 | 35 | 0 | 9 | 1 | 8 | 0 | 0 | 0 |
| mango | ½ | 67 | 1 | 18 | 2 | 15 | 0 | 0 | 2 |
| mango, dried, chips | 0.5 oz | 46 | 0 | 12 | n/a | n/a | n/a | n/a | n/a |
| mango, dried, slices | 0.5 oz | 52 | 0 | 13 | 1 | 10 | 0 | 0 | 8 |

| FOOD ITEM | SERVING SIZE | CALORIES | PRO (g) | CARB (g) | FIBER (g) | SUGAR (g) | FAT (g) | SAT FAT (g) | SOD (mg) |
|---|---|---|---|---|---|---|---|---|---|
| mango, freeze-dried | 0.5 oz | 50 | 1 | 13 | 1 | n/a | 0 | 0 | 5 |
| mangosteen | 2 oz | 40 | 0 | 10 | n/a | n/a | 0 | n/a | n/a |
| mulberries | 4 oz | 49 | 2 | 11 | 2 | 9 | 0 | 0 | 11 |
| mulberries | 1 cup | 60 | 2 | 14 | 2 | 11 | 1 | 0 | 14 |
| muskmelon, balled | 1 cup | 60 | 1 | 14 | n/a | n/a | 0 | 0 | 28 |
| nectarine | 1 medium | 70 | 1 | 17 | 1 | 13 | 0 | 0 | 0 |
| nectarine, sliced | ½ cup | 30 | 1 | 7 | 1 | 5 | 0 | 0 | 0 |
| oheloberries | 3 oz | 24 | 0 | 6 | 1 | 0 | 0 | 0 | 1 |
| oheloberries | 1 cup | 39 | 1 | 10 | 2 | n/a | 0 | 0 | 1 |
| orange | 1 small (2⅜") | 45 | 1 | 11 | 2 | 9 | 0 | 0 | 0 |
| orange | 1 large (3¹⁄₁₆") | 86 | 2 | 22 | 4 | 17 | 0 | 0 | 0 |
| orange, blood | 1 medium | 70 | 1 | 16 | 3 | 12 | 0 | 0 | 0 |
| orange, California navel | 1 medium | 69 | 1 | 18 | 3 | 12 | 0 | 0 | 1 |
| orange, California navel, without membranes | 1 medium | 69 | 1 | 18 | 3 | 12 | 0 | 0 | 1 |
| orange, California Valencia | 1 (2⅝") | 59 | 1 | 14 | 3 | 11 | 0 | 0 | 0 |
| orange, California Valencia, without membrane | 1 | 56 | 1 | 13 | 3 | 10 | 0 | 0 | 0 |
| orange, cara cara | 1 medium | 80 | 1 | 21 | 7 | 14 | 0 | 0 | 0 |
| orange, mandarin | 1 small | 37 | 1 | 9 | 1 | 7 | 0 | 0 | 1 |
| orange, mandarin | 1 large | 50 | 1 | 15 | 3 | 12 | 1 | 0 | 0 |
| orange, mandarin, sectioned | ½ cup | 52 | 1 | 13 | 2 | 10 | 0 | 0 | 2 |
| oranges, mandarin, canned with juice | ½ cup | 46 | 1 | 12 | 1 | 11 | 0 | 0 | 6 |
| orange, moro | 1 medium | 70 | 1 | 16 | 3 | 12 | 0 | 0 | 0 |
| orange peel | 1 tbsp | 6 | 0 | 2 | 1 | n/a | 0 | 0 | 0 |
| orange peel, candied | 0.5 oz | 38 | 0 | 11 | 1 | 9 | 0 | 0 | 17 |
| orange peel, dehydrated | 0.5 oz | 47 | 1 | 12 | 5 | 0 | 0 | 0 | 1 |
| oroblanco | ¼ | 50 | 1 | 11 | 2 | 8 | 0 | 0 | 0 |
| papaya | 1 small | 59 | 1 | 15 | 3 | 9 | 0 | 0 | 5 |
| papaya | ½ of medium | 59 | 1 | 15 | 3 | 9 | 0 | 0 | 5 |
| papaya | ½ of large | 74 | 1 | 19 | 3 | 11 | 0 | 0 | 6 |

| FOOD ITEM | SERVING SIZE | CALORIES | PRO (g) | CARB (g) | FIBER (g) | SUGAR (g) | FAT (g) | SAT FAT (g) | SOD (mg) |
|---|---|---|---|---|---|---|---|---|---|
| papaya, cubed | ½ cup | 27 | 0 | 7 | 1 | 4 | 0 | 0 | 2 |
| papaya, dried | 1 piece | 59 | 1 | 15 | 3 | 9 | 0 | 0 | 5 |
| papaya, mashed | ½ cup | 45 | 1 | 11 | 2 | 7 | 0 | 0 | 3 |
| passion fruit, purple | 1 | 17 | 0 | 4 | 2 | 2 | 0 | 0 | 5 |
| passion fruit, purple, cubed | ½ cup | 57 | 1 | 14 | 6 | 7 | 0 | 0 | 17 |
| peach | 1 small | 31 | 1 | 8 | 1 | 6 | 0 | 0 | 0 |
| peach | 1 medium | 38 | 1 | 9 | 1 | 8 | 0 | 0 | 0 |
| peach | 1 large | 61 | 1 | 15 | 2 | 13 | 0 | 0 | 0 |
| peaches, canned, in water, undrained | 1 cup | 59 | 1 | 15 | 3 | 12 | 0 | 0 | 7 |
| peaches, canned, light with extra light syrup | ½ cup | 60 | 0 | 14 | 1 | 13 | 0 | 0 | 10 |
| peaches, dehydrated | 2 tbsp | 47 | 1 | 12 | 2 | 10 | 0 | 0 | 1 |
| peaches, dehydrated, stewed | 2 tbsp | 40 | 1 | 10 | 1 | 9 | 0 | 0 | 1 |
| peaches, halved, dried | 2 tbsp | 48 | 1 | 12 | 2 | 8 | 0 | 0 | 1 |
| peaches, sliced, frozen, unsweetened | 1 cup | 60 | 1 | 14 | 1 | 12 | 0 | 0 | 0 |
| peaches, sliced, frozen, with puree | 3 oz | 66 | 1 | 16 | 1 | 15 | 0 | 0 | 0 |
| peaches, sliced, peeled | ½ cup | 33 | 1 | 8 | 1 | 7 | 0 | 0 | 0 |
| pear | ½ | 50 | 1 | 13 | 2 | 9 | 1 | 0 | 0 |
| pear, Asian | 1 (2.25") | 51 | 1 | 13 | 4 | 9 | 0 | 0 | 0 |
| pear, Bartlett | ½ of medium | 48 | 0 | 13 | 3 | 8 | 0 | 0 | 1 |
| pear, Bosc | ½ of small | 40 | 0 | 11 | 2 | 7 | 0 | 0 | 1 |
| pear, halved, dried | 2 tbsp | 59 | 0 | 16 | 2 | 14 | 0 | 0 | 1 |
| pear, prickly | 1 | 42 | 1 | 10 | 4 | n/a | 1 | 0 | 5 |
| pear, prickly, cubed | ½ cup | 31 | 1 | 7 | 3 | n/a | 0 | 0 | 4 |
| persimmon, Fuyu, dried | 2 tbsp | 53 | 0 | 13 | 1 | 10 | 0 | 0 | 4 |
| persimmon, Japanese | ½ | 59 | 0 | 16 | 3 | 11 | 0 | 0 | 1 |
| persimmon, Japanese, dried | ½ | 47 | 0 | 12 | 2 | 10 | 0 | 0 | 1 |
| persimmon, native | 1 | 32 | 0 | 8 | 0 | n/a | 0 | n/a | 0 |
| pineapple | ¼ | 57 | 1 | 15 | 2 | 11 | 0 | 0 | 1 |
| pineapple, diced | ½ cup | 37 | 0 | 10 | 1 | 7 | 0 | 0 | 1 |
| pineapple, extra sweet, sliced | 4 oz | 58 | 1 | 15 | 2 | 12 | 0 | 0 | 0 |

| FOOD ITEM | SERVING SIZE | CALORIES | PRO (g) | CARB (g) | FIBER (g) | SUGAR (g) | FAT (g) | SAT FAT (g) | SOD (mg) |
|---|---|---|---|---|---|---|---|---|---|
| pineapple, freeze-dried | 0.5 oz | 49 | 0 | 13 | 0 | n/a | 0 | n/a | 1 |
| pineapple, sliced | 2 slices (3.5 oz) | 54 | 1 | 14 | 2 | 10 | 0 | 0 | 1 |
| pineapple, South African | 1 baby (4 oz) | 57 | 1 | 14 | n/a | n/a | 0 | 0 | 0 |
| plantain | ¼ of medium | 55 | 1 | 14 | 1 | 7 | 0 | 0 | 2 |
| plantain, cooked, mashed | ¼ cup | 58 | 0 | 16 | 1 | 7 | 0 | 0 | 3 |
| plantain, fried | 2 tbsp | 53 | 0 | 8 | 1 | 0 | 3 | 0 | 1 |
| plantain, green, fried (tostones) | ¼ cup | 67 | 0 | 10 | 1 | n/a | 3 | 0 | 2 |
| plantain, sliced, cooked | ¼ cup | 45 | 0 | 12 | 1 | 5 | 0 | 0 | 2 |
| plantain chips | 0.5 oz | 74 | 0 | 8 | 1 | n/a | 5 | 4 | 1 |
| plum | 1 (2⅛") | 30 | 0 | 8 | 1 | 7 | 0 | 0 | 0 |
| plum, Caribbean June | 1 (2 oz) | 45 | 1 | 11 | n/a | n/a | 0 | n/a | 2 |
| plum, date | ½ (6 oz) | 59 | 0 | 16 | 3 | 11 | 0 | 0 | 1 |
| plum, java (jambolan) | 1 (4 oz) | 55 | 1 | 14 | n/a | n/a | 0 | n/a | 13 |
| plum, Indian | 1 (2 oz) | 45 | 1 | 11 | n/a | n/a | 0 | n/a | 2 |
| plum, sliced | ½ cup | 47 | 0 | 10 | n/a | n/a | 1 | 0 | 2 |
| plum, yellow | 1 | 20 | 0 | 5 | 1 | 4 | 0 | 0 | 1 |
| plums, purple, canned in water | ½ cup | 51 | 0 | 14 | 1 | 13 | 0 | 0 | 1 |
| plums, purple, canned, whole | ¼ cup | 65 | 0 | 16 | 1 | 13 | 0 | 0 | 8 |
| pomegranate | ½ of 3⅜" | 53 | 0 | 13 | 0 | 13 | 0 | 0 | 2 |
| prunes | 0.5 oz | 39 | 0 | 10 | 2 | 8 | 0 | 0 | 0 |
| prunes | 3 medium | 50 | 1 | 13 | 2 | 6 | 0 | 0 | 3 |
| prunes | 2 large | 40 | 0 | 10 | 1 | 4 | 0 | 0 | 2 |
| prunes, Caribbean June | 0.5 oz | 41 | 1 | 10 | n/a | n/a | 0 | n/a | 1 |
| prunes, dried with rock salt | 2 tbsp | 52 | 1 | 14 | 1 | n/a | 0 | 0 | 506 |
| prunes, Japanese, dried with rock salt | 2 tbsp | 52 | 1 | 14 | 1 | n/a | 0 | 0 | 506 |
| prunes, pitted | ¼ cup | 68 | 1 | 18 | 2 | 10 | 0 | 0 | 4 |
| prunes, pitted, bite-size | 1 oz | 71 | 1 | 18 | 2 | 8 | 0 | 0 | 4 |
| prunes, powdered | 0.5 oz | 46 | 1 | 12 | 1 | n/a | n/a | n/a | 1 |
| prunes, pureed | 0.5 oz | 45 | 0 | 11 | 1 | 5 | 0 | 0 | 5 |

| FOOD ITEM | SERVING SIZE | CALORIES | PRO (g) | CARB (g) | FIBER (g) | SUGAR (g) | FAT (g) | SAT FAT (g) | SOD (mg) |
|---|---|---|---|---|---|---|---|---|---|
| pummelo | ¼ | 58 | 1 | 15 | 2 | n/a | 0 | n/a | 2 |
| pummelo, sectioned | ½ cup | 36 | 1 | 9 | 1 | n/a | 0 | n/a | 1 |
| quince | 1 | 52 | 0 | 14 | 2 | n/a | 0 | 0 | 4 |
| raisins, golden, seedless | 0.5 oz | 46 | 0 | 11 | 1 | 10 | 0 | 0 | 4 |
| raisins, golden, seedless, packed | 2 tbsp | 65 | 1 | 16 | 1 | 15 | 0 | 0 | 5 |
| raisins, purple | 1 mini box | 42 | 0 | 11 | 1 | 8 | 0 | 0 | 2 |
| raisins, purple, cooked | 1 oz | 62 | 0 | 16 | 1 | n/a | 0 | 0 | 2 |
| raisins, purple, plumped, seedless | 2 tbsp | 52 | 1 | 14 | 1 | n/a | 0 | 0 | 2 |
| raisins, purple, seedless | 0.5 oz | 42 | 0 | 11 | 1 | 8 | 0 | 0 | 2 |
| raisins, purple, seedless, packed | 2 tbsp | 61 | 1 | 16 | 1 | n/a | 0 | 0 | 6 |
| raisins, purple, seedless, unpacked | 2 tbsp | 54 | 0 | 14 | 1 | n/a | 0 | 0 | 5 |
| raisins, purple, unsulfured | 2 tbsp | 49 | 0 | 12 | 1 | 10 | 0 | 0 | 2 |
| rambutan, canned with syrup, drained | ½ cup | 62 | 0 | 16 | 1 | 0 | 0 | 0 | 8 |
| raspberries, black | 3 oz | 61 | 1 | 14 | 1 | 4 | 0 | 0 | 0 |
| raspberries, dried flakes | 0.5 oz | 37 | 1 | 12 | 4 | 3 | 0 | 0 | 1 |
| raspberries, freeze-dried | 0.5 oz | 57 | 1 | 12 | 4 | 6 | 0 | 0 | 0 |
| raspberries, red | 3 oz | 44 | 1 | 10 | 6 | 4 | 1 | 0 | 1 |
| raspberries, red | 1 cup | 64 | 1 | 15 | 8 | 5 | 1 | 0 | 1 |
| raspberries, red, frozen, unsweetened | 4 oz | 46 | 1 | 10 | 2 | 6 | 0 | 0 | 1 |
| rhubarb | 1 stalk | 11 | 0 | 2 | 1 | 1 | 0 | 0 | 2 |
| rhubarb, diced | 1 cup | 26 | 1 | 6 | 2 | 1 | 0 | 0 | 5 |
| rhubarb, flash-frozen, with sugar, cooked | ¼ cup | 70 | 0 | 19 | 1 | 17 | 0 | 0 | 1 |
| roselle | 5 oz | 42 | 1 | 10 | n/a | n/a | 1 | n/a | 5 |
| rowal | ¼ cup | 63 | 1 | 14 | 4 | 8 | 1 | 0 | 2 |
| sapodilla | ½ | 71 | 0 | 17 | 5 | n/a | 1 | 0 | 10 |
| sapodilla pulp | ¼ cup | 50 | 0 | 12 | 3 | n/a | 1 | 0 | 7 |
| satsuma, mandarin | 1 | 50 | 1 | 11 | 2 | 9 | 0 | 0 | 0 |
| soursop | ⅛ | 53 | 1 | 13 | 3 | 11 | 0 | 0 | 11 |
| soursop pulp | ¼ cup | 37 | 1 | 9 | 2 | 8 | 0 | 0 | 8 |

| FOOD ITEM | SERVING SIZE | CALORIES | PRO (g) | CARB (g) | FIBER (g) | SUGAR (g) | FAT (g) | SAT FAT (g) | SOD (mg) |
|---|---|---|---|---|---|---|---|---|---|
| starfruit (carambola) | 1 medium | 28 | 1 | 6 | 3 | 4 | 0 | 0 | 2 |
| starfruit (carambola) | 1 large | 39 | 1 | 9 | 4 | 5 | 0 | 0 | 3 |
| starfruit (carambola), cubed | 1 cup | 42 | 1 | 9 | 4 | 5 | 0 | 0 | 3 |
| starfruit (carambola), dried | 0.5 oz | 43 | 1 | 10 | 0 | 9 | 0 | 0 | 2 |
| starfruit (carambola), sliced | 1 cup | 33 | 1 | 7 | 3 | 4 | 0 | 0 | 2 |
| strawberry | 1 small | 2 | 0 | 1 | 0 | 0 | 0 | 0 | 0 |
| strawberry | 1 medium | 4 | 0 | 1 | 0 | 1 | 0 | 0 | 0 |
| strawberry | 1 large | 6 | 0 | 1 | 0 | 1 | 0 | 0 | 0 |
| strawberry | 1 extra large | 9 | 0 | 2 | 1 | 1 | 0 | 0 | 0 |
| strawberries, dried | ¼ cup | 75 | 1 | 17 | 2 | 15 | 0 | 0 | 0 |
| strawberries, flash-frozen, cooked | 1 cup | 49 | 1 | 11 | 4 | 7 | 1 | 0 | 4 |
| strawberries, freeze-dried, diced | 0.5 oz | 48 | 1 | 13 | 3 | 8 | 0 | 0 | 0 |
| strawberries, frozen, unsweetened | 1 | 4 | 0 | 1 | 0 | 0 | 0 | 0 | 0 |
| strawberries, frozen, unsweetened | 5 oz | 50 | 1 | 13 | 3 | 6 | 0 | 0 | 3 |
| strawberries, sliced | 1 cup | 53 | 1 | 13 | 3 | 8 | 1 | 0 | 2 |
| tamarind, Spanish, pulp | 2 tbsp | 36 | 0 | 9 | 1 | 9 | 0 | 0 | 4 |
| tamarind pulp | 2 tbsp | 36 | 0 | 9 | 1 | 9 | 0 | 0 | 4 |
| tamarind pulp, dried, sweetened | 2 tbsp | 70 | 1 | 18 | 1 | n/a | 0 | 0 | 7 |
| tangelo minneola | 1 | 70 | 1 | 13 | 2 | 11 | 1 | 0 | 0 |
| tangerine | 1 small | 37 | 1 | 9 | 1 | 7 | 0 | 0 | 1 |
| tangerine | 1 medium | 50 | 1 | 13 | 3 | 8 | 1 | 0 | 0 |
| tangerine, Ojai Pixies, sectioned | ½ cup | 52 | 1 | 13 | 2 | 10 | 1 | 0 | 2 |
| tangerine, sectioned | 2 oz | 30 | 1 | 8 | 1 | 6 | 0 | 0 | 1 |
| tangerines, canned with juice | ½ cup | 46 | 1 | 12 | 1 | 11 | 0 | 0 | 6 |
| watermelon, balled | 4 oz | 34 | 1 | 9 | 0 | 7 | 0 | 0 | 1 |
| watermelon, balled | 1 cup | 46 | 1 | 12 | 1 | 10 | 0 | 0 | 2 |
| watermelon, diced | 1 cup | 45 | 1 | 11 | 1 | 9 | 0 | 0 | 2 |
| watermelon, sliced | 10 oz | 86 | 2 | 22 | 1 | 18 | 0 | 0 | 3 |

## GELATINS AND PUDDINGS

| FOOD ITEM | SERVING SIZE | CALORIES | PRO (g) | CARB (g) | FIBER (g) | SUGAR (g) | FAT (g) | SAT FAT (g) | SOD (mg) |
|---|---|---|---|---|---|---|---|---|---|
| custard, apple | 2 oz | 57 | 1 | 14 | 1 | n/a | 0 | 0 | 2 |
| flan | ½ cup | 150 | 4 | 25 | 0 | n/a | 4 | 2 | 149 |
| gelatin, black cherry, sugar-free | 1 cup | 20 | 2 | 0 | 0 | 0 | 0 | 0 | 140 |
| gelatin, cranberry, sugar-free | 1 cup | 20 | 2 | 0 | 0 | 0 | 0 | 0 | 140 |
| gelatin, fruit-flavored | ½ cup | 80 | 2 | 19 | 0 | 19 | 0 | 0 | 80 |
| gelatin, fruit-flavored, sugar-free | ½ cup | 23 | 1 | 5 | 0 | 0 | 0 | 0 | 56 |
| gelatin, lemon, sugar-free | 1 cup | 20 | 2 | 0 | 0 | 0 | 0 | 0 | 110 |
| gelatin, orange, sugar-free | 1 cup | 20 | 2 | 0 | 0 | 0 | 0 | 0 | 130 |
| gelatin, mixed fruit, sugar-free | 1 cup | 20 | 2 | 0 | 0 | 0 | 0 | 0 | 100 |
| gelatin, raspberry, sugar-free | 1 cup | 20 | 2 | 0 | 0 | 0 | 0 | 0 | 110 |
| gelatin, strawberry, sugar-free | 1 cup | 20 | 2 | 0 | 0 | 0 | 0 | 0 | 110 |
| gelatin, strawberry-banana, sugar-free | 1 cup | 20 | 2 | 0 | 0 | 0 | 0 | 0 | 100 |
| gelatin, strawberry-kiwi, sugar-free | 1 cup | 20 | 2 | 0 | 0 | 0 | 0 | 0 | 140 |
| gelatin, tropical berry, sugar-free | 1 snack cup | 10 | 1 | 0 | 0 | 0 | 0 | 0 | 45 |
| gelatin, watermelon, sugar-free | 1 cup | 20 | 2 | 0 | 0 | 0 | 0 | 0 | 110 |
| pudding, banana cream, fat-free, sugar-free | 1 snack cup | 25 | 0 | 6 | 0 | 0 | 0 | 0 | 320 |
| pudding, bread | ½ cup | 237 | 7 | 33 | 1 | 20 | 8 | 4 | 333 |
| pudding, butterscotch | 1 snack cup | 120 | 1 | 22 | 0 | 17 | 4 | 1 | 150 |
| pudding, cheesecake | 1 serving | 100 | 0 | 24 | 0 | 20 | 0 | 0 | 360 |
| pudding, chocolate, fat-free | 1 snack cup | 102 | 3 | 23 | 1 | 17 | 0 | 0 | 192 |
| pudding, chocolate, fat-free, sugar-free | 1 serving | 35 | 1 | 8 | 1 | 0 | 0 | 0 | 300 |
| pudding, chocolate, reduced-calorie, sugar-free | ½ cup | 80 | 5 | 14 | 1 | 0 | 0 | 0 | 390 |
| pudding, chocolate, sugar-free | 1 snack cup | 60 | 2 | 14 | 1 | 0 | 2 | 1 | 180 |
| pudding, chocolate, with whole milk | ½ cup | 169 | 5 | 28 | 1 | 17 | 4 | 3 | 139 |
| pudding, chocolate-cherry | 1 serving | 100 | 1 | 25 | 1 | 19 | 0 | 0 | 420 |
| pudding, chocolate chip | 1 serving | 120 | 2 | 22 | 1 | 16 | 4 | 1 | 160 |

| FOOD ITEM | SERVING SIZE | CALORIES | PRO (g) | CARB (g) | FIBER (g) | SUGAR (g) | FAT (g) | SAT FAT (g) | SOD (mg) |
|---|---|---|---|---|---|---|---|---|---|
| pudding, chocolate-mint | 1 serving | 100 | 1 | 25 | 1 | 17 | 0 | 0 | 380 |
| pudding, chocolate-vanilla swirl, fat-free | 1 snack cup | 100 | 3 | 23 | 1 | 17 | 0 | 0 | 190 |
| pudding, coconut cream | ½ cup | 160 | 4 | 25 | 0 | n/a | 5 | 4 | 227 |
| pudding, date | ½ cup | 176 | 2 | 26 | 1 | 18 | 8 | 4 | 88 |
| pudding, devil's food, fat-free | 1 snack cup | 100 | 2 | 22 | 1 | 16 | 0 | 0 | 190 |
| pudding, egg custard | 1 serving | 140 | 4 | 19 | 0 | 16 | 5 | 2 | 150 |
| pudding, instant, banana cream, fat-free, sugar-free | 1 serving | 25 | 0 | 6 | 0 | 0 | 0 | 0 | 320 |
| pudding, instant, butterscotch, fat-free, sugar-free | 1 serving | 25 | 0 | 6 | 0 | 0 | 0 | 0 | 320 |
| pudding, instant, chocolate, fat-free, sugar-free | 1 serving | 35 | 1 | 8 | 1 | 0 | 0 | 0 | 300 |
| pudding, instant, chocolate fudge | 1 serving | 100 | 1 | 25 | 1 | 17 | 0 | 0 | 380 |
| pudding, instant, lemon | 1 serving | 95 | 0 | 24 | 0 | n/a | 0 | 0 | 333 |
| pudding, instant, white chocolate, fat-free, sugar-free | 1 serving | 25 | 0 | 6 | 0 | 0 | 0 | 0 | 320 |
| pudding, plum | 3 oz | 235 | 4 | 42 | 2 | 30 | 6 | n/a | 293 |
| pudding, rice, fat-free | ½ cup | 140 | 5 | 29 | 0 | 19 | 0 | 0 | 160 |
| pudding, tapioca, fat-free | 1 snack cup | 80 | 2 | 19 | 0 | 13 | 0 | 0 | 150 |
| pudding, tapioca, fat-free | ½ cup | 111 | 2 | 26 | 0 | 20 | 0 | 0 | 265 |
| pudding, tapioca, with whole milk | ½ cup | 162 | 4 | 27 | 0 | n/a | 4 | 2 | 169 |
| pudding, vanilla | ½ cup | 116 | 3 | 28 | 0 | 20 | 0 | 0 | 266 |
| pudding, vanilla, fat-free | 1 snack cup | 80 | 1 | 18 | 0 | 13 | 0 | 0 | 140 |

## GRAINS AND RICES

| FOOD ITEM | SERVING SIZE | CALORIES | PRO (g) | CARB (g) | FIBER (g) | SUGAR (g) | FAT (g) | SAT FAT (g) | SOD (mg) |
|---|---|---|---|---|---|---|---|---|---|
| amaranth, uncooked | 2 tbsp | 91 | 4 | 16 | 2 | 0 | 2 | 0 | 5 |
| arrowroot flour | 2 tbsp | 57 | 0 | 14 | 1 | 0 | 0 | 0 | n/a |
| barley, pearled, cooked | ¼ cup | 48 | 1 | 11 | 1 | 0 | 0 | 0 | 1 |
| barley, pearled, raw | 2 tbsp | 81 | 3 | 17 | 4 | 0 | 1 | 0 | 3 |

| FOOD ITEM | SERVING SIZE | CALORIES | PRO (g) | CARB (g) | FIBER (g) | SUGAR (g) | FAT (g) | SAT FAT (g) | SOD (mg) |
|---|---|---|---|---|---|---|---|---|---|
| barley, whole, cooked | ¼ cup | 68 | 2 | 15 | 3 | n/a | 1 | 0 | 0 |
| barley grits, uncooked | 2 tbsp | 70 | 3 | 15 | 3 | 0 | 1 | 0 | 3 |
| barley groats | 2 tbsp | 63 | 2 | 16 | n/a | n/a | 0 | n/a | 1 |
| barley malt flour | 2 tbsp | 73 | 2 | 16 | 1 | 0 | 0 | 0 | 2 |
| basmati rice, Melissa's, uncooked | ¼ cup | 150 | 2 | 32 | 1 | 1 | 0 | n/a | 230 |
| buckwheat, dry | 1½ tbsp | 55 | 2 | 11 | 2 | n/a | 1 | 0 | 0 |
| buckwheat flour, whole-groat | 2 tbsp | 50 | 2 | 11 | 2 | 0 | 0 | 0 | 2 |
| buckwheat groats (kasha), roasted, cooked | ⅓ cup | 51 | 2 | 11 | 2 | 1 | 0 | 0 | 2 |
| buckwheat groats (kasha), roasted, dry | 2 tbsp | 71 | 2 | 15 | 2 | n/a | 1 | 0 | 2 |
| bulgur, cooked | ⅓ cup | 50 | 2 | 11 | 3 | 0 | 0 | 0 | 3 |
| bulgur, dry | 2 tbsp | 60 | 2 | 13 | 3 | 0 | 0 | 0 | 3 |
| bulgur, hard wheat | 2 tbsp | 70 | 3 | 15 | 4 | 0 | 0 | 0 | 3 |
| bulgur, soft wheat | 2 tbsp | 75 | 2 | 16 | 2 | 0 | 0 | 0 | 0 |
| corn bran, crude | ¼ cup | 43 | 2 | 16 | 15 | 0 | 0 | 0 | 1 |
| corn flour, degermed, unenriched, yellow | 2 tbsp | 59 | 1 | 13 | 0 | 0 | 0 | 0 | 0 |
| corn flour, masa, enriched, yellow | 2 tbsp | 52 | 1 | 11 | 2 | n/a | 1 | 0 | 1 |
| corn flour, whole grain, white | 2 tbsp | 53 | 1 | 11 | 1 | 0 | 1 | 0 | 1 |
| corn flour, whole grain, yellow | 2 tbsp | 53 | 1 | 11 | 2 | 0 | 1 | 0 | 1 |
| corn grits, white, quick, cooked | ⅓ cup | 48 | 1 | 10 | 0 | 0 | 0 | 0 | 2 |
| corn grits, white, quick, dry | 2 tbsp | 72 | 2 | 16 | 0 | 0 | 0 | 0 | 0 |
| corn grits, white, regular, cooked | ⅓ cup | 48 | 1 | 10 | 1 | 0 | 0 | 0 | 2 |
| corn grits, white, regular, dry | 2 tbsp | 72 | 2 | 16 | 0 | 0 | 0 | 0 | 0 |
| corn grits, yellow, quick, cooked | ⅓ cup | 47 | 1 | 10 | 0 | 0 | 0 | 0 | 2 |
| corn grits, yellow, quick, dry | 2 tbsp | 72 | 2 | 16 | 0 | 0 | 0 | 0 | 0 |
| corn grits, yellow, regular, cooked | ⅓ cup | 47 | 1 | 10 | 1 | 0 | 0 | 0 | 2 |
| corn grits, yellow, regular, dry | 2 tbsp | 72 | 2 | 16 | 0 | 0 | 0 | 0 | 0 |

| FOOD ITEM | SERVING SIZE | CALORIES | PRO (g) | CARB (g) | FIBER (g) | SUGAR (g) | FAT (g) | SAT FAT (g) | SOD (mg) |
|---|---|---|---|---|---|---|---|---|---|
| cornmeal, degermed, enriched, white, dry | 2 tbsp | 63 | 1 | 13 | 1 | 0 | 0 | 0 | 1 |
| cornmeal, degermed, enriched, yellow, dry | 2 tbsp | 61 | 1 | 14 | 1 | 0 | 0 | 0 | 1 |
| cornmeal, whole grain, white, dry | 2 tbsp | 55 | 1 | 12 | 1 | 0 | 1 | 0 | 5 |
| cornmeal, whole grain, yellow, dry | 2 tbsp | 55 | 1 | 12 | 1 | 0 | 1 | 0 | 5 |
| cornstarch | 1 tbsp | 30 | 0 | 7 | 0 | 0 | 0 | 0 | 1 |
| couscous, cooked | ⅓ cup | 59 | 2 | 12 | 1 | 0 | 0 | 0 | 3 |
| couscous, dry | 2 tbsp | 81 | 3 | 17 | 1 | n/a | 0 | 0 | 2 |
| hominy, canned, white | ½ cup | 59 | 1 | 12 | 2 | 2 | 1 | 0 | 173 |
| hominy, canned, yellow | ½ cup | 58 | 1 | 11 | 2 | n/a | 1 | 0 | 168 |
| hominy, cooked | ½ cup | 69 | 1 | 12 | 2 | n/a | 1 | 0 | 173 |
| millet, cooked | ¼ cup | 52 | 2 | 10 | 1 | 0 | 0 | 0 | 1 |
| millet, dry | 1½ tbsp | 71 | 2 | 14 | 2 | 0 | 1 | 0 | 1 |
| millet, puffed | ½ cup | 37 | 1 | 8 | 0 | 0 | 0 | 0 | 1 |
| millet, whole grain, dry | 0.5 oz | 47 | 2 | 10 | 0 | n/a | 1 | 0 | 0 |
| millet grits, dry | 1 tbsp | 55 | 2 | 11 | 2 | 0 | 1 | 0 | 0 |
| oat bran, cooked | ⅓ cup | 29 | 2 | 8 | 2 | n/a | 1 | 0 | 1 |
| oat bran, raw | 2 tbsp | 29 | 2 | 8 | 2 | 0 | 1 | 0 | 0 |
| oat flour, partially debranned | 0.5 oz | 57 | 2 | 9 | 1 | 0 | 1 | 0 | 3 |
| oats, rolled, dry | 2 tbsp | 38 | 2 | 7 | 1 | 0 | 1 | 0 | 0 |
| oats, unprocessed whole grain | 2 tbsp | 76 | 3 | 13 | 2 | n/a | 1 | 0 | 0 |
| pilaf, Kashi 7 Grain Whole Pilaf, cooked | ¼ cup | 85 | 3 | 15 | 3 | 0 | 2 | 0 | 8 |
| quinoa, cooked | ¼ cup | 81 | 3 | 15 | 1 | n/a | 1 | 0 | 4 |
| quinoa, dry | 2 tbsp | 79 | 3 | 15 | 1 | n/a | 1 | 0 | 4 |
| quinoa, Melissa's, dry | 1 tbsp | 54 | 2 | 10 | 2 | n/a | 1 | n/a | 16 |
| quinoa flour | 2 tbsp | 60 | 2 | 11 | 2 | 0 | 1 | 0 | 4 |
| rice, brown, glutinous, dry | 1½ tbsp | 62 | 1 | 13 | 0 | n/a | 0 | n/a | 2 |
| rice, brown, long grain, cooked | ¼ cup | 54 | 1 | 11 | 1 | 0 | 0 | 0 | 2 |
| rice, brown, long grain, dry | 1½ tbsp | 64 | 1 | 13 | 1 | 0 | 1 | 0 | 1 |

| FOOD ITEM | SERVING SIZE | CALORIES | PRO (g) | CARB (g) | FIBER (g) | SUGAR (g) | FAT (g) | SAT FAT (g) | SOD (mg) |
|---|---|---|---|---|---|---|---|---|---|
| rice, brown, long grain basmati, dry | 1½ tbsp | 53 | 1 | 12 | 1 | 0 | 1 | 0 | 0 |
| rice, brown, medium grain, cooked | ¼ cup | 55 | 1 | 11 | 1 | n/a | 0 | 0 | 0 |
| rice, brown, medium grain, dry | 1½ tbsp | 64 | 1 | 14 | 1 | 0 | 0 | 0 | 1 |
| rice, brown, short grain, dry | 1½ tbsp | 66 | 1 | 15 | 1 | 0 | 1 | 0 | 2 |
| rice, brown, Uncle Ben's 10-minute, cooked | ¼ cup | 48 | 1 | 11 | 1 | 0 | 0 | 0 | 5 |
| rice, white, glutinous, cooked | ¼ cup | 42 | 1 | 9 | 0 | 0 | 0 | 0 | 2 |
| rice, white, glutinous, raw | 2 tbsp | 86 | 2 | 19 | 1 | n/a | 0 | 0 | 2 |
| rice, white, long-grain, cooked | ¼ cup | 51 | 1 | 11 | 0 | 0 | 0 | 0 | 0 |
| rice, white, long-grain, enriched, cooked, with salt | ¼ cup | 51 | 1 | 11 | 0 | 0 | 0 | 0 | 151 |
| rice, white, long-grain, enriched, cooked, without salt | ½ cup | 51 | 1 | 11 | 0 | 0 | 0 | 0 | 0 |
| rice, white, long-grain, regular, raw, enriched | 2 tbsp | 84 | 2 | 18 | 0 | 0 | 0 | 0 | 1 |
| rice, white, medium-grain, cooked | ¼ cup | 60 | 1 | 13 | 0 | 0 | 0 | 0 | 0 |
| rice, white, medium-grain, raw, enriched | 2 tbsp | 88 | 2 | 19 | 0 | 0 | 0 | 0 | 0 |
| rice, white, short-grain, cooked | ¼ cup | 60 | 1 | 13 | 0 | n/a | 0 | 0 | 0 |
| rice, white, short-grain, raw | 2 tbsp | 90 | 2 | 20 | 1 | 0 | 0 | 0 | 0 |
| rice, wild, cooked | ⅓ cup | 55 | 2 | 12 | 1 | 0 | 0 | 0 | 2 |
| rice, wild, raw | 2 tbsp | 71 | 15 | 1 | 1 | 0 | 0 | 1 | n/a |
| rice bran, crude | 2 tbsp | 47 | 2 | 7 | 3 | 0 | 3 | 1 | 1 |
| rice flour, brown | 2 tbsp | 72 | 1 | 15 | 1 | 0 | 1 | 0 | 2 |
| rice flour, white | 2 tbsp | 72 | 1 | 16 | 0 | 0 | 0 | 0 | 0 |
| risotto, Melissa's | 2 tbsp | 75 | 1 | 16 | 0 | 0 | 0 | 0 | 130 |
| risotto, rice, arborio, dry | 2 tbsp | 85 | 2 | 19 | 1 | 0 | 0 | 0 | 0 |
| risotto, rice, dry | 2 tbsp | 48 | 1 | 10 | 0 | 0 | 0 | 0 | 272 |
| rye flour, dark | 2 tbsp | 52 | 2 | 11 | 4 | 0 | 0 | 0 | 0 |
| rye flour, light | 2 tbsp | 47 | 1 | 10 | 2 | 0 | 0 | 0 | 0 |
| rye flour, medium | 2 tbsp | 45 | 1 | 10 | 2 | 0 | 0 | 0 | 0 |

| FOOD ITEM | SERVING SIZE | CALORIES | PRO (g) | CARB (g) | FIBER (g) | SUGAR (g) | FAT (g) | SAT FAT (g) | SOD (mg) |
|---|---|---|---|---|---|---|---|---|---|
| semolina, enriched | 2 tbsp | 75 | 3 | 15 | 1 | 0 | 0 | 0 | 0 |
| semolina, unenriched | 2 tbsp | 75 | 3 | 15 | 1 | 0 | 0 | 0 | 0 |
| sorghum flour | 2 tbsp | 60 | 2 | 13 | 2 | 0 | 1 | 0 | 0 |
| tabbouleh, Melissa's | 1½ tbsp | 60 | 2 | 12 | 1 | n/a | 0 | n/a | 205 |
| tapioca, pearl, dry | 2 tbsp | 68 | 0 | 17 | 0 | 1 | 0 | 0 | 0 |
| triticale flour, whole grain | 2 tbsp | 55 | 2 | 12 | 2 | 1 | 0 | 0 | 0 |
| triticale grain, whole berries | 2 tbsp | 38 | 2 | 8 | 2 | 0 | 0 | 0 | 0 |
| vital wheat gluten | 0.5 oz | 52 | 11 | 2 | 0 | 0 | 0 | 0 | 4 |
| wheat, durum | 2 tbsp | 81 | 3 | 17 | 3 | n/a | 1 | 0 | 0 |
| wheat, hard red bulgur | 2 tbsp | 70 | 3 | 15 | 4 | 0 | 0 | 0 | 3 |
| wheat, hard red spring whole grain, dry | 2 tbsp | 79 | 4 | 16 | 3 | 3 | 0 | 0 | 0 |
| wheat, hard white wheat berries, raw | 2 tbsp | 80 | 3 | 17 | 3 | 0 | 0 | 0 | 0 |
| wheat, soft red white whole grain, raw | 2 tbsp | 70 | 2 | 16 | 3 | 0 | 0 | 0 | 0 |
| wheat, soft red white whole grain, raw | 2 tbsp | 70 | 2 | 16 | 3 | 0 | 0 | 0 | 0 |
| wheat, sprouted | 2 tbsp | 27 | 1 | 6 | 0 | 0 | 0 | 2 | n/a |
| wheat bran, crude | 2 tbsp | 16 | 1 | 5 | 3 | 0 | 0 | 0 | 0 |
| wheat flour, white, all-purpose, enriched, bleached | 2 tbsp | 57 | 2 | 12 | 0 | 0 | 0 | 0 | 0 |
| wheat flour, white, all-purpose, enriched, self-rising | 2 tbsp | 55 | 2 | 12 | 0 | 0 | 0 | 0 | 198 |
| wheat flour, white, all-purpose, unenriched | 2 tbsp | 57 | 2 | 12 | 0 | 0 | 0 | 0 | 0 |
| wheat flour, white, all-purpose, unenriched, unbleached, organic | 2 tbsp | 62 | 2 | 13 | 1 | 1 | 0 | 1 | n/a |
| wheat flour, white, bread, enriched | 2 tbsp | 50 | 2 | 11 | 1 | 0 | 0 | 0 | 0 |
| wheat flour, white, cake, enriched | 2 tbsp | 49 | 1 | 11 | 0 | 0 | 0 | 0 | 0 |
| wheat flour, white, tortilla mix, enriched | 2 tbsp | 56 | 1 | 9 | 0 | 0 | 1 | 1 | 93 |
| wheat flour, whole grain | 2 tbsp | 51 | 2 | 11 | 2 | 0 | 0 | 0 | 1 |
| wheat germ, crude | 2 tbsp | 52 | 3 | 7 | 2 | n/a | 1 | 0 | 2 |

# HERBS AND SPICES

| FOOD ITEM | SERVING SIZE | CALORIES | PRO (g) | CARB (g) | FIBER (g) | SUGAR (g) | FAT (g) | SAT FAT (g) | SOD (mg) |
|---|---|---|---|---|---|---|---|---|---|
| allspice, ground | 1 tsp | 7 | 0 | 1 | 1 | 0 | 0 | 0 | 1 |
| almond extract | 1 tsp | 12 | 0 | 0 | 0 | 0 | 0 | 0 | 0 |
| anise seed | 1 tsp | 7 | 0 | 1 | 0 | 0 | 0 | 0 | 0 |
| annatto | 1 tsp | 7 | 0 | 1 | 1 | 0 | 0 | 0 | 0 |
| asafetida | 1 g | 3 | 0 | 0 | 0 | 0 | 0 | 0 | 0 |
| basil, dried | 1 tsp | 6 | 1 | 1 | 1 | 0 | 0 | 1 | n/a |
| basil, fresh | 1 tbsp | 2 | 0 | 0 | 0 | 0 | 0 | 0 | 0 |
| basil, fresh, chopped | 1 tbsp | 2 | 0 | 0 | 0 | 0 | 0 | 0 | 0 |
| bay leaves, crumbled | 1 tsp | 2 | 0 | 0 | 0 | 0 | 0 | 0 | 0 |
| bay leaves, ground | 1 tsp | 2 | 0 | 0 | 0 | 0 | 0 | 0 | 0 |
| borage, fresh | 1 tbsp | 1 | 0 | 0 | 0 | 0 | 0 | 0 | 4 |
| caraway seed | 1 tsp | 7 | 0 | 1 | 1 | 0 | 0 | 0 | 0 |
| caraway seed, ground | 1 tsp | 9 | 0 | 1 | 1 | 0 | 0 | 0 | 0 |
| cardamom seed | 1 tsp | 7 | 0 | 1 | 1 | 0 | 0 | 0 | 0 |
| cardamom seed, ground | 1 tsp | 6 | 0 | 1 | 1 | 0 | 0 | 0 | 0 |
| celery salt | 1 tsp | 3 | 0 | 0 | 0 | 0 | 0 | 0 | 1485 |
| celery seed | 1 tsp | 8 | 0 | 1 | 0 | 0 | 1 | 0 | 3 |
| celery seed, ground | 1 tsp | 9 | 0 | 1 | 1 | 0 | 0 | 0 | 3 |
| chervil, dried | 1 tsp | 1 | 0 | 0 | 0 | 0 | 0 | 0 | 1 |
| chervil, fresh, Melissa's | 1½ tsp | 0 | 0 | 0 | 0 | 0 | 0 | 0 | n/a |
| chicory, fresh, chopped | 1 tbsp | 3 | 0 | 1 | 0 | 0 | 0 | 0 | 5 |
| chili powder | 1 tsp | 12 | 0 | 2 | 0 | 0 | 0 | 0 | 59 |
| chives, freeze-dried | 1 tbsp | 1 | 0 | 0 | 0 | 0 | 0 | 0 | 0 |
| chives, fresh | 1 tbsp | 1 | 0 | 0 | 0 | 0 | 0 | 0 | 0 |
| cilantro, fresh | ¼ cup | 1 | 0 | 0 | 0 | 0 | 0 | 0 | 2 |
| cinnamon, ground | 1 tsp | 6 | 0 | 2 | 1 | 0 | 0 | 0 | 1 |
| cloves, ground | 1 tsp | 7 | 0 | 1 | 1 | 0 | 0 | 0 | 5 |
| cocoa powder, unsweetened | 1 tsp | 4 | 0 | 1 | 1 | 0 | 0 | 0 | 0 |
| coriander, dried | 1 tsp | 2 | 0 | 0 | 0 | 0 | 0 | 0 | 1 |
| coriander, fresh (cilantro) | ¼ cup | 1 | 0 | 0 | 0 | 0 | 0 | 0 | 2 |

| FOOD ITEM | SERVING SIZE | CALORIES | PRO (g) | CARB (g) | FIBER (g) | SUGAR (g) | FAT (g) | SAT FAT (g) | SOD (mg) |
|---|---|---|---|---|---|---|---|---|---|
| coriander seed | 1 tsp | 5 | 0 | 1 | 1 | 0 | 0 | 0 | 1 |
| cumin seed | 1 tsp | 8 | 0 | 1 | 0 | 0 | 0 | 0 | 4 |
| cumin seed, ground | 1 tsp | 9 | 0 | 1 | 1 | 0 | 0 | 0 | 4 |
| curry, fresh | 1 tbsp | 3 | 0 | 0 | 0 | 0 | 0 | 0 | n/a |
| curry powder | 1 tsp | 7 | 0 | 1 | 1 | 0 | 0 | 0 | 1 |
| dill seed | 1 tsp | 6 | 0 | 1 | 0 | 0 | 0 | 0 | 0 |
| dill seed, ground | 1 tsp | 9 | 0 | 1 | 1 | 0 | 0 | 0 | 0 |
| dill weed, dried | 1 tsp | 3 | 0 | 1 | 0 | 0 | 0 | 0 | 2 |
| dill weed, fresh | ¼ cup | 1 | 0 | 0 | 0 | 0 | 0 | 0 | 1 |
| epazote, fresh | ¼ cup | 1 | 0 | 0 | 0 | 0 | 0 | 0 | 1 |
| fennel seed | 1 tsp | 7 | 0 | 1 | 1 | 0 | 0 | 0 | 2 |
| fennel seed, ground | 1 tsp | 9 | 0 | 1 | 1 | 0 | 0 | 0 | 2 |
| fenugreek leaves, fresh | 1 tbsp | 2 | 0 | 0 | 0 | 0 | 0 | 0 | 5 |
| fenugreek seed | 1 tsp | 12 | 1 | 2 | 1 | 0 | 0 | 0 | 2 |
| fenugreek seed, ground | 1 tsp | 15 | 1 | 2 | 2 | 0 | 0 | 0 | 2 |
| five-spice powder, Chinese | 1 tsp | 9 | 0 | 2 | 0 | 0 | 0 | 0 | n/a |
| galangal, Thai ginger | 1 tsp | 2 | 0 | 0 | 0 | 0 | 0 | 0 | 0 |
| garlic powder | 1 tsp | 9 | 0 | 2 | 0 | 1 | 0 | 0 | 1 |
| garlic salt | 1 tsp | 0 | 0 | 0 | 0 | 0 | 0 | 0 | 968 |
| ginger, ground | 1 tsp | 6 | 0 | 1 | 0 | 0 | 0 | 0 | 1 |
| gingerroot | 1 slice | 2 | 0 | 0 | 0 | 0 | 0 | 0 | 0 |
| Italian seasoning | 1 tsp | 8 | 0 | 1 | 0 | 0 | 1 | 0 | 62 |
| jerk seasoning | 1 tsp | 0 | 0 | 0 | 0 | 0 | 0 | 0 | 280 |
| lemongrass | 1 tbsp | 4 | 0 | 1 | 0 | 0 | 0 | 0 | 0 |
| lemongrass, fresh | 1 tbsp | 4 | 0 | 1 | 0 | 0 | 0 | 0 | 0 |
| lemon-pepper seasoning | 1 tsp | 8 | 0 | 1 | 0 | 0 | 1 | 0 | 75 |
| lemon-pepper, with seasoned salt | 1 tsp | 0 | 0 | 0 | 0 | 0 | 0 | 0 | 520 |
| mace, ground | 1 tsp | 9 | 0 | 1 | 0 | 0 | 0 | 0 | 2 |
| marjoram, dried | 1 tsp | 2 | 0 | 0 | 0 | 0 | 0 | 0 | 0 |
| marjoram, fresh, Melissa's | 1½ tsp | 0 | 0 | 0 | 0 | 0 | 0 | 0 | 0 |

## HERBS AND SPICES (cont.)

| FOOD ITEM | SERVING SIZE | CALORIES | PRO (g) | CARB (g) | FIBER (g) | SUGAR (g) | FAT (g) | SAT FAT (g) | SOD (mg) |
|---|---|---|---|---|---|---|---|---|---|
| Mexican seasoning blend | 1 tsp | 0 | 0 | 0 | 0 | 0 | 0 | 0 | 200 |
| mustard seed | 1 tsp | 15 | 1 | 1 | 0 | 0 | 1 | 0 | 0 |
| mustard seed, ground | 1 tsp | 15 | 1 | 1 | 0 | 0 | 1 | 0 | 0 |
| nutmeg, ground | 1 tsp | 10 | 0 | 1 | 0 | 0 | 1 | 0 | 0 |
| onion powder | 1 tsp | 7 | 0 | 2 | 0 | 1 | 0 | 0 | 1 |
| oregano, dried | 1 tsp | 5 | 0 | 1 | 1 | 0 | 0 | 0 | 1 |
| oregano, fresh | 1 tbsp | 4 | 0 | 1 | 0 | 0 | 0 | 0 | 0 |
| paprika, ground | 1 tsp | 7 | 0 | 1 | 1 | 0 | 0 | 0 | 2 |
| parsley, fresh | 3 sprigs | 1 | 0 | 0 | 0 | 0 | 0 | 0 | 2 |
| parsley, fresh, chopped | 1 tbsp | 1 | 0 | 0 | 0 | 0 | 0 | 0 | 2 |
| pepper, black, ground | 1 tsp | 7 | 0 | 1 | 1 | 0 | 0 | 0 | 0 |
| pepper, black, ground, with seasoned salt | 1 tsp | 0 | 0 | 0 | 0 | 0 | 0 | 0 | 640 |
| pepper, cayenne, ground | 1 tsp | 6 | 0 | 1 | 0 | 0 | 0 | 0 | 1 |
| pepper, chili flakes | 1 tsp | 6 | 0 | 1 | 0 | 0 | 0 | 0 | 1 |
| pepper, white, ground | 1 tsp | 7 | 0 | 1 | 0 | 0 | 0 | 0 | 0 |
| peppermint, dried | 1 tsp | 2 | 0 | 0 | 0 | 0 | 0 | 0 | 2 |
| peppermint, fresh | 1 tbsp | 4 | 0 | 1 | 0 | 0 | 0 | 0 | 2 |
| poppy seed | 1 tsp | 15 | 1 | 1 | 0 | 0 | 1 | 0 | 1 |
| poppy seed, ground | 1 tsp | 17 | 1 | 1 | 1 | 0 | 1 | 0 | 0 |
| poultry seasoning | 1 tsp | 5 | 0 | 1 | 0 | 0 | 0 | 0 | 0 |
| pumpkin pie spice | 1 tsp | 6 | 0 | 1 | 0 | 0 | 0 | 0 | 1 |
| rosemary, dried | 1 tsp | 4 | 0 | 1 | 1 | 0 | 0 | 0 | 1 |
| rosemary, fresh | 1 tsp | 1 | 0 | 0 | 0 | 0 | 0 | 0 | 0 |
| rosemary, ground | 1 tsp | 4 | 0 | 1 | 1 | 0 | 0 | 0 | 1 |
| saffron | 1 tsp | 2 | 0 | 0 | 0 | 0 | 0 | 0 | 1 |
| sage, ground | 1 tsp | 1 | 0 | 0 | 0 | 0 | 0 | 0 | 0 |
| salt, hickory smoked | 1 tsp | 0 | 0 | 0 | 0 | 0 | 0 | 0 | 1820 |
| salt substitute, Mrs. Dash Extra Spicy | 1 tsp | 0 | 0 | 0 | 0 | 0 | 0 | 0 | 0 |
| salt substitute, Mrs. Dash Garlic & Herb | 1 tsp | 0 | 0 | 0 | 0 | 0 | 0 | 0 | 0 |

| FOOD ITEM | SERVING SIZE | CALORIES | PRO (g) | CARB (g) | FIBER (g) | SUGAR (g) | FAT (g) | SAT FAT (g) | SOD (mg) |
|---|---|---|---|---|---|---|---|---|---|
| salt, table | 1 tsp | 0 | 0 | 0 | 0 | 0 | 0 | 0 | 2325 |
| salt, table, iodized | 1 tsp | 0 | 0 | 0 | 0 | 0 | 0 | 0 | 2360 |
| salt, table, noniodized | 1 tsp | 0 | 0 | 0 | 0 | 0 | 0 | 0 | 2360 |
| savory, ground | 1 tsp | 4 | 0 | 1 | 1 | 0 | 0 | 0 | 0 |
| seasoning mix, bean soup | 1 tsp | 4 | 0 | 0 | 0 | 0 | 0 | 0 | 56 |
| seasoning mix, beef stew | 1 tsp | 8 | 0 | 2 | 0 | 0 | 0 | 0 | 205 |
| seasoning mix, beef stroganoff | 1 tsp | 7 | 0 | 2 | 0 | 0 | 0 | 0 | 167 |
| seasoning mix, buffalo wings | 1 tsp | 10 | 0 | 2 | 0 | 0 | 0 | 0 | 237 |
| seasoning mix, burrito | 1 tsp | 8 | 0 | 2 | 0 | 0 | 0 | 0 | 205 |
| seasoning mix, chicken herb | 1 tsp | 0 | 0 | 0 | 0 | 0 | 0 | 0 | 340 |
| seasoning mix, chicken taco | 1 tsp | 13 | 0 | 2 | 0 | 0 | 0 | 0 | 225 |
| seasoning mix, chili | 1 tsp | 5 | 0 | 1 | 0 | 0 | 0 | 0 | 190 |
| seasoning mix, chili, hot | 1 tsp | 9 | 0 | 1 | 0 | 0 | 0 | 0 | 85 |
| seasoning mix, chili, mild | 1 tsp | 8 | 0 | 1 | 0 | 0 | 0 | 0 | 100 |
| seasoning mix, chili, vegetarian | 1 tsp | 4 | 0 | 1 | 0 | 0 | 0 | 0 | 20 |
| seasoning mix, country chicken | 1 tsp | 13 | 0 | 2 | 0 | 0 | 1 | 0 | 440 |
| seasoning mix, crab cake | 1 tsp | 10 | 0 | 1 | 0 | 0 | 0 | 0 | 97 |
| seasoning mix, guacamole | 1 tsp | 10 | 0 | 2 | 0 | 0 | 0 | 0 | 260 |
| seasoning mix, fajita | 1 tsp | 8 | 0 | 1 | 0 | 0 | 0 | 0 | 145 |
| seasoning mix, fajita marinade | 1 tsp | 10 | 0 | 3 | 0 | 0 | 0 | 0 | 280 |
| seasoning mix, meat loaf | 1 tsp | 15 | 0 | 2 | 0 | 0 | 0 | 0 | 350 |
| seasoning mix, Mexican rice | 1 tsp | 7 | 0 | 1 | 0 | 0 | 0 | 0 | 218 |
| seasoning mix, pork chops | 1 tsp | 8 | 0 | 2 | 0 | 0 | 0 | 0 | 295 |
| seasoning mix, pot roast | 1 tsp | 10 | 0 | 1 | 0 | 0 | 0 | 0 | 390 |
| seasoning mix, salsa | 1 tsp | 10 | 0 | 2 | 0 | 0 | 0 | 0 | 180 |
| seasoning mix, sloppy joe | 1 tsp | 20 | 0 | 3 | 0 | 0 | 0 | 0 | 300 |
| seasoning mix, split pea soup | 1 tsp | 3 | 0 | 1 | 0 | 0 | 0 | 0 | 21 |

| FOOD ITEM | SERVING SIZE | CALORIES | PRO (g) | CARB (g) | FIBER (g) | SUGAR (g) | FAT (g) | SAT FAT (g) | SOD (mg) |
|---|---|---|---|---|---|---|---|---|---|
| seasoning mix, stir-fry | 1 tsp | 10 | 0 | 2 | 0 | 0 | 0 | 0 | 260 |
| seasoning mix, stir-fry, chicken | 1 tsp | 10 | 0 | 2 | 0 | 0 | 0 | 0 | 260 |
| seasoning mix, Swiss steak | 1 tsp | 15 | 0 | 2 | 0 | 0 | 0 | 0 | 430 |
| seasoning mix, taco | 1 tsp | 15 | 0 | 3 | 0 | 0 | 0 | 0 | 200 |
| seasoning mix, taco, 30% less salt | 1 tsp | 10 | 0 | 2 | 0 | 0 | 0 | 0 | 165 |
| seasoning mix, taco, 40% less salt | 1 tsp | 8 | 0 | 0 | 0 | 0 | 2 | 0 | 150 |
| seasoning mix, taco, cheesy | 1 tsp | 5 | 0 | 1 | 0 | 0 | 0 | 0 | 120 |
| seasoning mix, taco, spicy | 1 tsp | 7 | 0 | 1 | 0 | 0 | 0 | 0 | 117 |
| seasoning mix, taco salad | 1 tsp | 15 | 0 | 3 | 0 | 0 | 0 | 0 | 200 |
| seasoning mix, tofu burger | 1 tsp | 9 | 0 | 1 | 0 | 0 | 0 | 0 | 44 |
| seasoning mix, tofu scrambler | 1 tsp | 12 | 0 | 2 | 0 | 0 | 0 | 0 | 87 |
| seasoning mix, tuna, classic | 1 tsp | 10 | 0 | 1 | 0 | 0 | 0 | 0 | 40 |
| sesame seed | 1 tsp | 20 | 1 | 0 | 0 | 0 | 2 | 0 | 1 |
| sesame seed, ground | 1 tsp | 17 | 1 | 0 | 0 | 0 | 2 | 0 | 6 |
| spearmint, dried | 1 tsp | 2 | 0 | 0 | 0 | 0 | 0 | 0 | 2 |
| spearmint, fresh | 1 tbsp | 3 | 0 | 0 | 0 | 0 | 0 | 0 | 2 |
| spice blend, Mrs. Dash Onion & Herb | ¼ tsp | 0 | 0 | 0 | 0 | 0 | 0 | 0 | 0 |
| spice blend, Mrs. Dash Original Blend | 1 tsp | 0 | 0 | 0 | 0 | 0 | 0 | 0 | 0 |
| spice blend, Mrs. Dash Table Blend | 1 tsp | 0 | 0 | 0 | 0 | 0 | 0 | 0 | 0 |
| spice blend, Mrs. Dash Tomato Basil Garlic | ¼ tsp | 0 | 0 | 0 | 0 | 0 | 0 | 0 | 0 |
| tarragon, dried | 1 tsp | 6 | 0 | 1 | 0 | 0 | 0 | 0 | 1 |
| tarragon, fresh | 1 tbsp | 3 | 0 | 0 | 0 | 0 | 0 | 0 | 1 |
| tarragon, ground | 1 tsp | 5 | 0 | 1 | 0 | 0 | 0 | 0 | 1 |
| turmeric powder | 1 tsp | 8 | 0 | 1 | 0 | 0 | 0 | 0 | 1 |
| vanilla extract, imitation | 1 tsp | 10 | 0 | 0 | 0 | 0 | 0 | 0 | 0 |
| vanilla extract, pure | 1 tsp | 12 | 0 | 1 | 0 | 1 | 0 | 0 | 0 |

## MEATS

| FOOD ITEM | SERVING SIZE | CALORIES | PRO (g) | CARB (g) | FIBER (g) | SUGAR (g) | FAT (g) | SAT FAT (g) | SOD (mg) |
|---|---|---|---|---|---|---|---|---|---|
| **Beef** | | | | | | | | | |
| bottom round, all lean, cooked | 3 oz | 139 | 24 | 0 | 0 | 0 | 5 | 2 | 31 |
| bottom round, all lean, roasted, boneless | 3 oz | 112 | 18 | 0 | 0 | 0 | 4 | 1 | 23 |
| bottom round, raw | 4 oz | 145 | 25 | 0 | 0 | 0 | 5 | 2 | 67 |
| bottom round, trimmed, boneless, braised | 3 oz | 108 | 17 | 0 | 0 | 0 | 4 | 1 | 27 |
| brisket flat, lean, braised | 3 oz | 174 | 28 | 0 | 0 | 0 | 6 | 2 | 46 |
| brisket flat, lean, raw | 4 oz | 176 | 24 | 0 | 0 | 0 | 8 | 3 | 90 |
| chuck arm, lean, raw | 4 oz | 150 | 25 | 0 | 0 | 0 | 5 | 2 | 84 |
| chuck blade roast, lean, braised | 3 oz | 216 | 26 | 0 | 0 | 0 | 11 | 4 | 60 |
| chuck roast, lean, braised | 3 oz | 179 | 28 | 0 | 0 | 0 | 6 | 2 | 56 |
| corned beef, canned | 3 oz | 164 | 7 | 10 | 1 | 1 | 11 | 4 | 604 |
| corned beef, cooked | 3 oz | 213 | 15 | 0 | 0 | 0 | 16 | 5 | 964 |
| corned beef lunch meat, sliced | 3 oz | 98 | 16 | 2 | 0 | 0 | 2 | 2 | 736 |
| cotto salami, beef | 1 oz | 58 | 4 | 1 | 0 | 0 | 4 | 2 | 371 |
| eye round, lean, raw | 4 oz | 184 | 33 | 0 | 0 | 0 | 5 | 2 | 43 |
| eye round, lean, roasted | 3 oz | 138 | 25 | 0 | 0 | 0 | 3 | 1 | 32 |
| filet mignon, extra lean, raw | 4 oz | 120 | 22 | 0 | 0 | 0 | 4 | 2 | 55 |
| filet mignon, lean, broiled | 3 oz | 179 | 24 | 0 | 0 | 0 | 9 | 3 | 54 |
| flank steak, lean, braised | 3 oz | 224 | 23 | 0 | 0 | 0 | 14 | 6 | 60 |
| flank steak, lean, broiled | 3 oz | 158 | 24 | 0 | 0 | 0 | 6 | 3 | 48 |
| flank steak, lean, raw | 4 oz | 160 | 24 | 0 | 0 | 0 | 6 | 2 | 62 |
| ground, 10% fat, raw | 4 oz | 200 | 23 | 0 | 0 | 0 | 11 | 5 | 75 |
| ground, 20% fat, pan broiled | 3 oz | 230 | 22 | 0 | 0 | 0 | 15 | 6 | 64 |
| ground, 20% fat, raw | 4 oz | 288 | 19 | 0 | 0 | 0 | 23 | 9 | 76 |
| ground, 30% fat, pan broiled | 3 oz | 202 | 19 | 0 | 0 | 0 | 13 | 5 | 78 |
| ground, 30% fat, raw | 4 oz | 376 | 16 | 0 | 0 | 0 | 34 | 13 | 76 |
| ground, extra lean, raw | 4 oz | 130 | 22 | 0 | 0 | 0 | 5 | 2 | 65 |
| hot dog, beef, 97% fat-free | 1.7 oz | 45 | 6 | 3 | 0 | 0 | 1 | 1 | 400 |

| FOOD ITEM | SERVING SIZE | CALORIES | PRO (g) | CARB (g) | FIBER (g) | SUGAR (g) | FAT (g) | SAT FAT (g) | SOD (mg) |
|---|---|---|---|---|---|---|---|---|---|
| **Beef (cont.)** | | | | | | | | | |
| jerky, beef | 0.7 oz | 81 | 7 | 2 | 0 | 2 | 5 | 2 | 438 |
| jerky, beef, California-style, hot and spicy | 1 oz | 81 | 13 | 3 | 0 | 2 | 1 | 0 | 486 |
| jerky, beef, California-style, original | 1 oz | 81 | 14 | 3 | 0 | 3 | 1 | 0 | 597 |
| jerky, beef, California-style, teriyaki | 1 oz | 81 | 13 | 5 | 0 | 1 | 1 | 0 | 648 |
| pastrami, beef, 98% fat-free | 1 oz | 27 | 6 | 0 | 0 | 0 | 0 | 0 | 286 |
| pastrami, beef, deli | 1 oz | 33 | 6 | 0 | 0 | 0 | 1 | 0 | 242 |
| rib pot roast, lean, with bone, raw | 4 oz | 131 | 15 | 0 | 0 | 0 | 7 | 3 | 40 |
| rib pot roast, lean, with bone, roasted | 3 oz | 131 | 15 | 0 | 0 | 0 | 7 | 3 | 40 |
| rib steak, lean, with bone, broiled | 3 oz | 81 | 12 | 0 | 0 | 0 | 3 | 1 | 25 |
| rib steak, lean, with bone, raw | 4 oz | 108 | 16 | 0 | 0 | 0 | 4 | 2 | 34 |
| rib steak, select lean, with bone, roasted | 3 oz | 81 | 11 | 0 | 0 | 0 | 4 | 2 | 28 |
| roast, lean, roasted | 3 oz | 169 | 24 | 0 | 0 | 0 | 7 | 3 | 57 |
| roast beef, lunch meat, 97% fat-free, 25% less salt | 1 oz | 35 | 7 | 1 | 0 | 0 | 1 | 0 | 100 |
| roast beef, lunch meat, deli sliced, Cajun | 1 oz | 30 | 6 | 1 | 0 | 0 | 1 | 0 | 180 |
| roast beef, lunch meat, deli sliced, Italian-style | 1 oz | 30 | 6 | 1 | 0 | 0 | 1 | 0 | 180 |
| roast beef, lunch meat, medium rare | 1 oz | 30 | 6 | 1 | 0 | 1 | 1 | 1 | 235 |
| round tip roast, lean, raw | 4 oz | 143 | 24 | 0 | 0 | 0 | 4 | 2 | 61 |
| salami, beef, beerwurst | 1 oz | 79 | 4 | 1 | 0 | 0 | 6 | 2 | 208 |
| salami, beef, cooked | 1 oz | 73 | 4 | 1 | 0 | 0 | 6 | 3 | 323 |
| salami, beef, lean, sliced | 1 oz | 45 | 4 | 1 | 0 | 0 | 2 | 1 | 239 |
| sausage, beef, precooked | 1 oz | 115 | 4 | 0 | 0 | 0 | 11 | 4 | 258 |
| shank, lean, with bone, raw | 4 oz | 88 | 15 | 0 | 0 | 0 | 3 | 1 | 43 |
| short ribs, lean, with bone, braised | 3 oz | 65 | 7 | 0 | 0 | 0 | 4 | 2 | 13 |
| short ribs, lean, with bone, raw | 4 oz | 80 | 9 | 0 | 0 | 0 | 5 | 2 | 30 |

| FOOD ITEM | SERVING SIZE | CALORIES | PRO (g) | CARB (g) | FIBER (g) | SUGAR (g) | FAT (g) | SAT FAT (g) | SOD (mg) |
|---|---|---|---|---|---|---|---|---|---|
| steak, sirloin strip, ⅛ trim, broiled | 3 oz | 236 | 22 | 0 | 0 | 0 | 16 | 6 | 44 |
| steak, sirloin strip, ⅛ trim, raw | 4 oz | 254 | 23 | 0 | 0 | 0 | 17 | 7 | 59 |
| steak, top sirloin, lean, broiled | 3 oz | 166 | 26 | 0 | 0 | 0 | 6 | 2 | 56 |
| stew meat, lean, cooked | 3 oz | 201 | 27 | 0 | 0 | 0 | 10 | 4 | 57 |
| stew meat, lean, raw | 4 oz | 163 | 22 | 0 | 0 | 0 | 8 | 3 | 46 |
| T-bone, lean, broiled | 3 oz | 168 | 22 | 0 | 0 | 0 | 8 | 3 | 60 |
| T-bone, raw | 4 oz | 148 | 20 | 0 | 0 | 0 | 7 | 2 | 56 |
| tenderloin, lean, boneless, raw | 4 oz | 163 | 24 | 0 | 0 | 0 | 7 | 3 | 50 |
| tenderloin, select lean, boneless, roasted | 3 oz | 152 | 24 | 0 | 0 | 0 | 6 | 2 | 50 |
| top round steak, braised | 3 oz | 178 | 30 | 0 | 0 | 0 | 5 | 2 | 38 |
| top round steak, lean, raw | 4 oz | 177 | 24 | 0 | 0 | 0 | 8 | 3 | 32 |
| trip tip sirloin, lean, raw | 4 oz | 171 | 23 | 0 | 0 | 0 | 8 | 3 | 62 |
| trip tip sirloin, lean, roasted | 3 oz | 152 | 23 | 0 | 0 | 0 | 6 | 2 | 49 |
| **Game** | | | | | | | | | |
| alligator meat | 3 oz | 197 | 39 | 0 | 0 | 0 | 4 | 0 | n/a |
| bison, ground, pan broiled | 3 oz | 202 | 20 | 0 | 0 | 0 | 13 | 6 | 62 |
| bison, ground, raw | 4 oz | 253 | 21 | 0 | 0 | 0 | 18 | 8 | 75 |
| bison, meat, raw | 4 oz | 124 | 25 | 0 | 0 | 0 | 2 | 1 | 61 |
| bison, meat, roasted | 3 oz | 123 | 24 | 0 | 0 | 0 | 2 | 1 | 48 |
| bison, rib eye steak, lean, braised | 3 oz | 151 | 25 | 0 | 0 | 0 | 5 | 2 | 44 |
| bison, rib eye steak, lean, raw | 4 oz | 132 | 25 | 0 | 0 | 0 | 3 | 1 | 54 |
| boar, wild, cooked | 3 oz | 136 | 24 | 0 | 0 | 0 | 4 | 1 | 51 |
| boar, wild, raw | 4 oz | 138 | 24 | 0 | 0 | 0 | 4 | 1 | 52 |
| goat, baked | 3 oz | 122 | 12 | 0 | 0 | 0 | 3 | 1 | 73 |
| goat, broiled | 3 oz | 122 | 12 | 0 | 0 | 0 | 3 | 1 | 73 |
| goat, raw | 4 oz | 124 | 24 | 0 | 0 | 0 | 3 | 1 | 93 |
| goat, roasted | 3 oz | 122 | 23 | 0 | 0 | 0 | 3 | 1 | 73 |
| venison (deer), chop, cooked | 3 oz | 177 | 25 | 0 | 0 | 0 | 8 | 2 | 47 |

| FOOD ITEM | SERVING SIZE | CALORIES | PRO (g) | CARB (g) | FIBER (g) | SUGAR (g) | FAT (g) | SAT FAT (g) | SOD (mg) |
|---|---|---|---|---|---|---|---|---|---|
| **Game (cont.)** | | | | | | | | | |
| venison (deer), stewed | 3 oz | 145 | 28 | 0 | 0 | 0 | 3 | 1 | 34 |
| venison jerky | 1 oz | 97 | 10 | 4 | 0 | n/a | 4 | 2 | 830 |
| venison meat loaf | 3.8-oz slice | 148 | 22 | 6 | 0 | 0 | 3 | 1 | 111 |
| venison stew | 4 oz | 72 | 8 | 8 | 1 | n/a | 1 | 0 | 110 |
| **Lamb** | | | | | | | | | |
| Australian, center slice, broiled | 3 oz | 183 | 22 | 0 | 0 | 0 | 10 | 5 | 55 |
| Australian, center slice, lean, raw | 4 oz | 162 | 23 | 0 | 0 | 0 | 7 | 3 | 73 |
| Australian, leg, whole, lean, raw | 4 oz | 153 | 23 | 0 | 0 | 0 | 6 | 2 | 92 |
| Australian, leg, whole, lean, roasted | 3 oz | 162 | 23 | 0 | 0 | 0 | 7 | 3 | 61 |
| Australian, loin, lean, broiled | 3 oz | 163 | 23 | 0 | 0 | 0 | 7 | 3 | 68 |
| Australian, loin, lean, raw | 4 oz | 166 | 24 | 0 | 0 | 0 | 7 | 3 | 85 |
| Australian, ribs, lean, raw | 4 oz | 181 | 23 | 0 | 0 | 0 | 9 | 4 | 92 |
| Australian, ribs, lean, roasted | 3 oz | 179 | 21 | 0 | 0 | 0 | 10 | 4 | 70 |
| Australian, shank, braised | 3 oz | 200 | 21 | 0 | 0 | 0 | 12 | 6 | 79 |
| Australian, shank, raw | 4 oz | 221 | 21 | 0 | 0 | 0 | 14 | 7 | 109 |
| Australian, sirloin chop, lean, raw | 4 oz | 150 | 23 | 0 | 0 | 0 | 6 | 2 | 73 |
| Australian, sirloin chop, lean, broiled | 3 oz | 160 | 24 | 0 | 0 | 0 | 7 | 3 | 56 |
| ground, 20% fat, broiled | 3 oz | 241 | 21 | 0 | 0 | 0 | 17 | 7 | 69 |
| ground, 20% fat, raw | 4 oz | 218 | 19 | 0 | 0 | 0 | 15 | 6 | 62 |
| kebab, lean, braised | 3 oz | 190 | 29 | 0 | 0 | 0 | 7 | 3 | 60 |
| kebab, lean, raw | 4 oz | 152 | 23 | 0 | 0 | 0 | 6 | 2 | 74 |
| loin, lean, roasted | 3 oz | 172 | 23 | 0 | 0 | 0 | 8 | 3 | 56 |
| loin chop, lean, broiled | 3 oz | 184 | 26 | 0 | 0 | 0 | 8 | 3 | 71 |
| loin chop, lean, raw | 4 oz | 162 | 24 | 0 | 0 | 0 | 7 | 2 | 77 |
| meat loaf | 3.8-oz slice | 196 | 15 | 9 | 0 | 0 | 11 | 5 | 200 |
| New Zealand, leg, whole, raw | 4 oz | 228 | 21 | 0 | 0 | 0 | 15 | 8 | 46 |

| FOOD ITEM | SERVING SIZE | CALORIES | PRO (g) | CARB (g) | FIBER (g) | SUGAR (g) | FAT (g) | SAT FAT (g) | SOD (mg) |
|---|---|---|---|---|---|---|---|---|---|
| New Zealand, leg, whole, roasted | 3 oz | 199 | 22 | 0 | 0 | 0 | 12 | 6 | 37 |
| New Zealand, loin chop, broiled | 3 oz | 252 | 21 | 0 | 0 | 0 | 18 | 9 | 43 |
| New Zealand, loin chop, raw | 4 oz | 310 | 19 | 0 | 0 | 0 | 25 | 13 | 44 |
| stew meat, lean, braised | 3 oz | 190 | 29 | 0 | 0 | 0 | 7 | 3 | 60 |
| stew meat, lean, raw | 4 oz | 152 | 23 | 0 | 0 | 0 | 6 | 2 | 74 |
| **Pork** | | | | | | | | | |
| bacon, medium slice, cooked | 0.2 oz | 34 | 2 | 0 | 0 | 0 | 3 | 1 | 146 |
| bacon, medium slice, raw | 0.8 oz | 104 | 3 | 0 | 0 | 0 | 10 | 3 | 189 |
| breakfast strip, cooked | 0.4 oz | 52 | 3 | 0 | 0 | 0 | 4 | 1 | 238 |
| breakfast strip, raw | 0.8 oz | 88 | 3 | 0 | 0 | 0 | 8 | 3 | 224 |
| Canadian bacon, grilled | 1 oz | 52 | 7 | 0 | 0 | 0 | 2 | 1 | 439 |
| Canadian bacon, raw | 2 oz | 89 | 12 | 1 | 0 | 0 | 4 | 1 | 799 |
| chitins, cooked | 1 oz | 66 | 4 | 0 | 0 | 0 | 6 | 3 | 5 |
| chitins, raw | 2 oz | 103 | 4 | 0 | 0 | 0 | 9 | 4 | 14 |
| chop, center lean, with bone, braised | 2.6 oz | 149 | 22 | 0 | 0 | 0 | 6 | 2 | 46 |
| chop, lean, smoked, cooked | 2.4 oz | 114 | 17 | 0 | 0 | 0 | 5 | 2 | 825 |
| chop, stuffed | 5.5 oz | 287 | 26 | 24 | 1 | 0 | 9 | 3 | 1261 |
| chop, with barbecue sauce | 4 oz | 209 | 21 | 3 | 0 | 0 | 11 | 4 | 860 |
| chop sirloin, lean, raw | 3.3 oz | 133 | 20 | 0 | 0 | 0 | 5 | 2 | 48 |
| chop sirloin, lean, with bone, braised | 2.5 oz | 142 | 19 | 0 | 0 | 0 | 6 | 2 | 38 |
| dehydrated, Oriental-style pork | 1 oz | 174 | 3 | 0 | 0 | 0 | 18 | 7 | 194 |
| ground, cooked | 3 oz | 253 | 22 | 0 | 0 | 0 | 18 | 7 | 62 |
| ground, raw | 4 oz | 298 | 19 | 0 | 0 | 0 | 24 | 9 | n/a |
| ham, low-sodium, 96% fat-free | 1 oz | 31 | 5 | 1 | 0 | 1 | 1 | 0 | 235 |
| ham, rump, lean, raw | 4 oz | 155 | 24 | 0 | 0 | 0 | 6 | 2 | 78 |
| hot dog, pork | 2.7 oz | 204 | 10 | 0 | 0 | 0 | 18 | 7 | 620 |
| hot dog, pork, beef, and turkey, fat-free | 1.8 oz | 50 | 6 | 6 | 0 | 2 | 0 | 0 | 490 |

| FOOD ITEM | SERVING SIZE | CALORIES | PRO (g) | CARB (g) | FIBER (g) | SUGAR (g) | FAT (g) | SAT FAT (g) | SOD (mg) |
|---|---|---|---|---|---|---|---|---|---|
| **Pork (cont.)** | | | | | | | | | |
| hot dog, pork and turkey, fat-free | 2 oz | 62 | 7 | 6 | 0 | 0 | 1 | 0 | 452 |
| meatballs | 1 oz | 54 | 6 | 2 | 0 | 0 | 2 | 1 | 259 |
| prosciutto, sliced | 0.5 oz | 50 | 4 | 0 | 0 | 0 | 2 | 1 | 375 |
| prosciutto, pork Parmesan, without skin | 1 oz | 61 | 8 | 0 | 0 | 0 | 4 | 1 | 545 |
| prosciutto, pork primissimo, with skin | 1 oz | 106 | 6 | 0 | 0 | 0 | 9 | 4 | 556 |
| pulled pork, with sauce | 3 oz | 147 | 13 | 8 | 0 | n/a | 7 | 2 | 626 |
| ribs, country-style, lean, braised | 3 oz | 199 | 22 | 0 | 0 | 0 | 12 | 4 | 54 |
| ribs, country-style, lean, raw | 4 oz | 178 | 22 | 0 | 0 | 0 | 9 | 3 | 76 |
| ribs, with barbecue sauce | 4 oz | 178 | 22 | 0 | 0 | 0 | 9 | 3 | 76 |
| roast, center loin, lean, raw | 4 oz | 159 | 25 | 0 | 0 | 0 | 6 | 2 | 75 |
| roast, center loin, lean, roasted | 3 oz | 169 | 23 | 0 | 0 | 0 | 8 | 3 | 56 |
| salami, Italian pork | 1 oz | 120 | 6 | 0 | 0 | 0 | 10 | 4 | 536 |
| salami, Italian pork, reduced-sodium | 1 oz | 99 | 6 | 2 | 0 | 0 | 7 | 3 | 265 |
| sausage, Chinese | 1 oz | 100 | 6 | 2 | 0 | 0 | 8 | n/a | 249 |
| sausage, cooked | 0.5 oz | 44 | 3 | 0 | 0 | 0 | 4 | 1 | 97 |
| sausage, frozen | 1 oz | 65 | 4 | 0 | 0 | 0 | 5 | 1 | 144 |
| sausage link, frozen | 1 oz | 65 | 4 | 0 | 0 | 0 | 5 | 1 | 144 |
| scrapple | 2 oz | 119 | 5 | 8 | 0 | 0 | 8 | 3 | 369 |
| skins | 1 oz | 155 | 17 | 0 | 0 | 0 | 9 | 3 | 521 |
| tenderloin, raw | 4 oz | 136 | 24 | 0 | 0 | 0 | 4 | 1 | 57 |
| tenderloin, roasted | 3 oz | 139 | 24 | 0 | 0 | 0 | 4 | 1 | 48 |
| tenderloin, teriyaki | 3 oz | 101 | 15 | 4 | 0 | 3 | 3 | 1 | 351 |
| tenderloin chop, lean, broiled | 3 oz | 159 | 26 | 0 | 0 | 0 | 5 | 2 | 55 |
| **Veal** | | | | | | | | | |
| breast, braised | 3 oz | 226 | 23 | 0 | 0 | 0 | 14 | 6 | 55 |
| breast, raw | 4 oz | 236 | 20 | 0 | 0 | 0 | 17 | 7 | 81 |
| cube steak, frozen | 3 oz | 220 | 14 | 0 | 0 | 0 | 18 | 8 | 58 |

| FOOD ITEM | SERVING SIZE | CALORIES | PRO (g) | CARB (g) | FIBER (g) | SUGAR (g) | FAT (g) | SAT FAT (g) | SOD (mg) |
|---|---|---|---|---|---|---|---|---|---|
| ground, 7% fat, raw | 4 oz | 163 | 22 | 0 | 0 | 0 | 8 | 3 | 93 |
| ground, 8% fat, broiled | 3 oz | 146 | 21 | 0 | 0 | 0 | 6 | 3 | 71 |
| ground, 8% fat, raw | 4 oz | 115 | 16 | 0 | 0 | 0 | 5 | 2 | 56 |
| leg, lean, cubed, braised | 3 oz | 160 | 30 | 0 | 0 | 0 | 4 | 1 | 79 |
| leg, lean, cubed, raw | 4 oz | 124 | 23 | 0 | 0 | 0 | 3 | 1 | 94 |
| leg, top round steak, lean, roasted | 3 oz | 128 | 24 | 0 | 0 | 0 | 3 | 1 | 58 |
| liver, braised | 3 oz | 163 | 24 | 3 | 0 | 0 | 5 | 2 | 66 |
| liver, raw | 4 oz | 159 | 23 | 3 | 0 | 0 | 6 | 2 | 87 |
| loin, roasted | 3 oz | 185 | 21 | 0 | 0 | 0 | 10 | 4 | 79 |
| loin chop, lean, braised | 3 oz | 192 | 29 | 0 | 0 | 0 | 8 | 2 | 71 |
| loin chop, lean, raw | 4 oz | 141 | 21 | 0 | 0 | 0 | 6 | 2 | 52 |
| loin chop cutlet, braised | 3 oz | 242 | 26 | 0 | 0 | 0 | 15 | 6 | 68 |
| loin chop cutlet, raw | 4 oz | 177 | 19 | 0 | 0 | 0 | 11 | 4 | 50 |
| shank roast, braised | 3 oz | 151 | 27 | 0 | 0 | 0 | 4 | 1 | 80 |
| shank roast, lean, raw | 4 oz | 110 | 20 | 0 | 0 | 0 | 3 | 1 | 59 |
| short rib, lean, raw | 4 oz | 151 | 22 | 0 | 0 | 0 | 6 | 2 | 83 |
| short rib, lean, roasted | 3 oz | 143 | 21 | 0 | 0 | 0 | 6 | 2 | 78 |
| shoulder arm steak, braised | 3 oz | 171 | 30 | 0 | 0 | 0 | 5 | 1 | 77 |
| shoulder arm steak, raw | 4 oz | 167 | 30 | 0 | 0 | 0 | 4 | 1 | 75 |
| shoulder blade roast, braised | 3 oz | 168 | 28 | 0 | 0 | 0 | 6 | 2 | 86 |
| shoulder blade roast, raw | 4 oz | 123 | 20 | 0 | 0 | 0 | 4 | 1 | 63 |
| sirloin roast, lean, raw | 4 oz | 127 | 21 | 0 | 0 | 0 | 4 | 1 | 51 |
| top round steak, lean, raw | 4 oz | 121 | 24 | 0 | 0 | 0 | 2 | 1 | 73 |
| veal, with gravy | 3 oz | 131 | 16 | 2 | 0 | 0 | 6 | 2 | 249 |
| **Vegetarian "meats"** | | | | | | | | | |
| bacon bits | 1 tbsp | 33 | 2 | 2 | 1 | 0 | 2 | 0 | 124 |
| bacon strip | 1 oz | 88 | 3 | 2 | 1 | 0 | 8 | 1 | 415 |
| breakfast link, soy | 0.9 oz | 30 | 6 | 2 | 1 | 1 | 0 | 0 | 195 |
| breakfast patty, Morning Star Farms Veggie Breakfast Sausage Patties | 1 patty | 10 | 4 | 2 | 1 | 3 | 1 | 0 | 259 |

## MEATS (cont.)

| FOOD ITEM | SERVING SIZE | CALORIES | PRO (g) | CARB (g) | FIBER (g) | SUGAR (g) | FAT (g) | SAT FAT (g) | SOD (mg) |
|---|---|---|---|---|---|---|---|---|---|
| **Vegetarian "meats" (cont.)** | | | | | | | | | |
| burger, Morning Star Farms Garden Veggie Patties | 1 patty | 119 | 11 | 10 | 4 | 1 | 4 | 1 | 382 |
| burger, Morning Star Farms Spicy Black Bean Veggie Burgers | 1 patty | 115 | 12 | 15 | 5 | 1 | 1 | 0 | 499 |
| burger, soy | 2.5 oz | 125 | 13 | 9 | 3 | 1 | 4 | 1 | 385 |
| burger, soy, with cheese | 4.75 oz | 308 | 20 | 30 | 4 | 0 | 12 | 4 | 921 |
| burger crumbles, Morning Star Farms Recipe Crumbles | 1 oz | 59 | 6 | 2 | 1 | 0 | 3 | 1 | 122 |
| Canadian bacon, soy, sliced | 0.7 oz | 27 | 6 | 1 | 0 | 0 | 0 | 0 | 160 |
| chicken soy filet | 3 oz | 90 | 15 | 8 | 4 | 2 | 2 | 0 | 170 |
| ground beef, GimmeLean! | 3 oz | 105 | 14 | 12 | 2 | 2 | 0 | 0 | 360 |
| hot dog, Morning Star Farms America's Original Veggie Dog | 1 | 112 | 10 | 4 | 3 | 1 | 6 | 1 | 431 |
| meatballs | 3 oz | 168 | 18 | 7 | 4 | 1 | 8 | 1 | 468 |
| pepperoni, soy, sliced | 1 oz | 41 | 8 | 2 | 2 | 0 | 0 | 0 | 230 |
| sausage, GimmeLean | 1 oz | 35 | 5 | 4 | 1 | 1 | 0 | 0 | 145 |
| soy, ground, Melissa's | 2 oz | 70 | 11 | 4 | 3 | 0 | 3 | 0 | 250 |
| soyrizo meat, Melissa's | 2 oz | 120 | 7 | 5 | 3 | 2 | 9 | 1 | 440 |
| soyrizo sausage | 3 oz | 186 | 11 | 8 | 5 | 3 | 14 | 1 | 680 |
| taco meat, soy, Melissa's | 1 oz | 50 | 4 | 3 | 2 | 0 | 3 | 0 | 180 |

## NUTS, SEEDS, AND BUTTERS

| FOOD ITEM | SERVING SIZE | CALORIES | PRO (g) | CARB (g) | FIBER (g) | SUGAR (g) | FAT (g) | SAT FAT (g) | SOD (mg) |
|---|---|---|---|---|---|---|---|---|---|
| acorns, dried | 6 | 36 | 1 | 4 | n/a | n/a | 2 | 0 | 0 |
| acorns, raw | 6 | 27 | 0 | 3 | n/a | n/a | 2 | 0 | 0 |
| almond butter, natural, chocolate-flavored | 1 tbsp | 90 | 3 | 5 | 2 | 2 | 8 | 1 | 0 |
| almond butter, plain, with salt | 1 tbsp | 99 | 2 | 3 | 1 | 1 | 9 | 1 | 70 |
| almond butter, plain, without salt | 1 tbsp | 101 | 2 | 3 | 1 | n/a | 9 | 1 | 2 |

| FOOD ITEM | SERVING SIZE | CALORIES | PRO (g) | CARB (g) | FIBER (g) | SUGAR (g) | FAT (g) | SAT FAT (g) | SOD (mg) |
|---|---|---|---|---|---|---|---|---|---|
| almond paste | 1 tbsp | 65 | 1 | 7 | 1 | 5 | 4 | 0 | 1 |
| almonds, blanched | 1 tbsp | 53 | 2 | 2 | 1 | 0 | 5 | 0 | 3 |
| almonds, dried, sliced | 1 tbsp | 34 | 1 | 1 | 1 | 0 | 3 | 0 | 0 |
| almonds, dry-roasted, blanched | 1 tbsp | 52 | 2 | 1 | n/a | 0 | 5 | 0 | 0 |
| almonds, dry-roasted, with salt | 1 tbsp | 51 | 2 | 2 | 1 | 0 | 5 | 0 | 29 |
| almonds, dry-roasted, without salt | 1 tbsp | 51 | 2 | 2 | 1 | 0 | 5 | 0 | 0 |
| almonds, honey-roasted | 1 tbsp | 53 | 2 | 3 | 1 | n/a | 4 | 0 | 12 |
| almonds, natural, sliced | 1 tbsp | 35 | 1 | 1 | 1 | 0 | 3 | 0 | 0 |
| almonds, oil-roasted, with salt | 1 tbsp | 60 | 2 | 2 | 1 | 0 | 5 | 0 | 33 |
| almonds, oil-roasted, without salt | 1 tbsp | 60 | 2 | 2 | 1 | 0 | 5 | 0 | 0 |
| brazil nut, dried | 1 large | 31 | 1 | 1 | 0 | 0 | 3 | 1 | 0 |
| brazil nut butter, natural | 1 tbsp | 95 | 2 | 2 | 1 | n/a | 10 | 2 | 0 |
| brazil nuts, dried | 1 tbsp | 57 | 1 | 1 | 1 | 0 | 6 | 1 | 0 |
| cashew butter, orange | 1 tbsp | 83 | 3 | 6 | 1 | n/a | 6 | 1 | 0 |
| cashew butter, organic | 1 tbsp | 83 | 3 | 6 | 1 | n/a | 6 | 1 | 0 |
| cashew butter, plain, with salt | 1 tbsp | 94 | 3 | 4 | 0 | 1 | 8 | 2 | 98 |
| cashew butter, plain, without salt | 1 tbsp | 94 | 3 | 4 | 0 | n/a | 8 | 2 | 2 |
| cashew nuts, dry-roasted, with salt | 1 tbsp | 49 | 1 | 3 | 0 | 0 | 4 | 1 | 55 |
| cashew nuts, dry-roasted, without salt | 1 tbsp | 49 | 1 | 3 | 0 | 0 | 4 | 1 | 1 |
| cashew nuts, raw | 4 | 39 | 1 | 2 | 0 | 0 | 3 | 1 | 1 |
| chestnuts, Chinese, cooked | 0.25 oz | 11 | 0 | 2 | 0 | n/a | 0 | 0 | 0 |
| chestnuts, Chinese, dried | 0.25 oz | 26 | 0 | 6 | 0 | n/a | 0 | 0 | 0 |
| chestnuts, Chinese, raw | 0.25 oz | 16 | 0 | 3 | 0 | n/a | 0 | 0 | 0 |
| chestnuts, Chinese, roasted | 0.25 oz | 17 | 0 | 4 | 0 | n/a | 0 | 0 | 0 |
| chestnuts, European, cooked | 0.25 oz | 9 | 0 | n/a | n/a | 0 | 0 | 2 | n/a |
| chestnuts, European, dried, peeled | 0.25 oz | 26 | 0 | 6 | n/a | n/a | 0 | 0 | 3 |
| chestnuts, European, dried, unpeeled | 0.25 oz | 27 | 0 | 5 | 1 | n/a | 0 | 0 | 3 |

| FOOD ITEM | SERVING SIZE | CALORIES | PRO (g) | CARB (g) | FIBER (g) | SUGAR (g) | FAT (g) | SAT FAT (g) | SOD (mg) |
|---|---|---|---|---|---|---|---|---|---|
| chestnuts, European, raw, peeled | 0.25 oz | 14 | 0 | 3 | n/a | n/a | 0 | 0 | 0 |
| chestnuts, European, roasted | 1 tbsp | 22 | 0 | 5 | 0 | 1 | 0 | 0 | 0 |
| chestnuts, Japanese, roasted | 1 tbsp | 14 | 0 | 3 | 0 | n/a | 0 | 0 | 1 |
| coconut, dried, shredded, unsweetened | 1 tbsp | 18 | 0 | 1 | 0 | 0 | 3 | 1 | 1 |
| coconut, fresh, shredded | 1 tbsp | 18 | 0 | 1 | 0 | 0 | 3 | 1 | 1 |
| flaxseeds | 1 tbsp | 45 | 1 | 1 | 1 | 0 | 4 | 0 | 0 |
| hazelnut butter | 1 tbsp | 90 | 3 | 3 | 2 | n/a | 8 | 1 | 0 |
| hazelnuts (filberts), blanched | 0.5 oz | 89 | 2 | 2 | 2 | 0 | 9 | 1 | 0 |
| hazelnuts (filberts), blanched, dried | 10 | 88 | 2 | 2 | 1 | 1 | 9 | 1 | 0 |
| hazelnuts (filberts), dried, chopped | 1 tbsp | 45 | 1 | 1 | 1 | 0 | 4 | 0 | 0 |
| hazelnuts (filberts), dried, ground | 1 tbsp | 29 | 1 | 1 | 0 | 3 | 0 | 0 | 0 |
| hazelnuts (filberts), dry-roasted, without salt | 6 | 46 | 1 | 1 | 1 | 0 | 4 | 0 | 0 |
| macadamia nuts, dry-roasted, with salt | 1 tbsp | 60 | 1 | 1 | 0 | 6 | 1 | 1 | 22 |
| macadamia nuts, dry-roasted, without salt | 1 tbsp | 60 | 1 | 1 | 0 | 6 | 1 | 1 | 0 |
| mixed nuts, dry-roasted, with salt | 1 tbsp | 51 | 1 | 2 | 1 | 0 | 4 | 1 | 57 |
| mixed nuts, dry-roasted, without salt | 1 tbsp | 51 | 1 | 2 | 1 | n/a | 4 | 1 | 1 |
| mixed nuts, oil-roasted, with peanuts, with salt | 1 tbsp | 55 | 1 | 2 | 1 | 0 | 5 | 1 | 37 |
| mixed nuts, oil-roasted, with peanuts, without salt | 1 tbsp | 55 | 1 | 2 | 1 | 0 | 5 | 1 | 1 |
| mixed nuts, oil-roasted, without peanuts, with salt | 1 tbsp | 55 | 1 | 2 | 1 | 0 | 5 | 1 | 28 |
| mixed nuts, oil-roasted, without peanuts, without salt | 1 tbsp | 55 | 1 | 2 | 1 | n/a | 5 | 1 | 1 |
| peanut butter, chocolate silk | 1 tbsp | 95 | 3 | 7 | 1 | 6 | 8 | 2 | 58 |
| peanut butter, creamy | 1 tbsp | 94 | 4 | 3 | 1 | 1 | 8 | 2 | 73 |
| peanut butter, crunchy, reduced-fat | 1 tbsp | 95 | 4 | 8 | 1 | 2 | 6 | 1 | 110 |
| peanut butter, extra-crunchy | 1 tbsp | 95 | 4 | 4 | 1 | 2 | 8 | 2 | 65 |

| FOOD ITEM | SERVING SIZE | CALORIES | PRO (g) | CARB (g) | FIBER (g) | SUGAR (g) | FAT (g) | SAT FAT (g) | SOD (mg) |
|---|---|---|---|---|---|---|---|---|---|
| peanut butter, natural | 1 tbsp | 100 | 4 | 4 | 1 | 1 | 8 | 1 | 60 |
| peanut butter, reduced-fat | 1 tbsp | 81 | 4 | 5 | 1 | 2 | 5 | 1 | 89 |
| peanut butter, reduced-sodium | 1 tbsp | 101 | 4 | 4 | 1 | 1 | 8 | 2 | 32 |
| peanut butter, super chunk, roasted honey nut | 1 tbsp | 95 | 4 | 4 | 1 | 2 | 9 | 2 | 63 |
| peanuts, dry-roasted, with salt | 1 tbsp | 53 | 2 | 2 | 1 | 0 | 4 | 1 | 73 |
| peanuts, dry-roasted, without salt | 1 tbsp | 53 | 2 | 2 | 1 | 0 | 5 | 1 | 1 |
| peanuts, shelled, cooked, with salt | 1 tbsp | 36 | 2 | 2 | 1 | 0 | 2 | 0 | 84 |
| pecans, dried, chopped | 1 tbsp | 51 | 1 | 1 | 1 | 0 | 5 | 0 | 0 |
| pecans, dried, halved | 1 tbsp | 47 | 1 | 1 | 1 | 0 | 5 | 0 | 0 |
| pecans, dry-roasted, with salt | 1 tbsp | 48 | 1 | 1 | 1 | 0 | 5 | 0 | 26 |
| pecans, dry-roasted, without salt | 1 tbsp | 48 | 1 | 1 | 1 | 0 | 5 | 0 | 0 |
| pecans, honey-roasted | 1 tbsp | 46 | 1 | 2 | 1 | 1 | 5 | 0 | 23 |
| pecans, oil-roasted, with salt | 1 tbsp | 49 | 1 | 1 | 1 | 0 | 5 | 0 | 27 |
| pecans, oil-roasted, without salt, halved | 1 tbsp | 49 | 1 | 1 | n/a | n/a | 5 | 1 | 0 |
| pecans, raw, halved | 1 tbsp | 48 | 1 | 1 | 0 | 0 | 5 | 0 | 0 |
| pecans, unsalted fancy pieces | 1 tbsp | 53 | 1 | 1 | 1 | 0 | 5 | 1 | 0 |
| pine nuts (pignolia), dried | 1 tbsp | 57 | 1 | 1 | 0 | 0 | 6 | 0 | 0 |
| pine pinyon nuts | 1 tbsp | 54 | 1 | 2 | 1 | n/a | 5 | 0 | 6 |
| pistachio butter, natural | 1 tbsp | 90 | 3 | 5 | 2 | n/a | 7 | 1 | 0 |
| pistachio butter, organic | 1 tbsp | 90 | 3 | 5 | 2 | n/a | 7 | 1 | 0 |
| pistachio nuts, dry-roasted, with salt | 1 tbsp | 45 | 2 | 2 | 1 | 1 | 4 | 0 | 32 |
| pistachio nuts, dry-roasted, without salt | 1 tbsp | 46 | 2 | 2 | 1 | 1 | 4 | 0 | 1 |
| pistachio nuts, raw | 1 tbsp | 45 | 2 | 2 | 1 | 1 | 4 | 0 | 0 |
| pumpkin and squash seed kernels, dried (pepitas) | 1 oz | 153 | 7 | 5 | 1 | 0 | 13 | 2 | 5 |
| pumpkin and squash seed kernels, roasted, with salt | 1 tbsp | 74 | 5 | 2 | 1 | 0 | 6 | 1 | 82 |
| pumpkin and squash seed kernels, roasted, without salt | 1 oz | 147 | 9 | 4 | 1 | 0 | 12 | 2 | 5 |

| FOOD ITEM | SERVING SIZE | CALORIES | PRO (g) | CARB (g) | FIBER (g) | SUGAR (g) | FAT (g) | SAT FAT (g) | SOD (mg) |
|---|---|---|---|---|---|---|---|---|---|
| pumpkin seeds, dry-roasted | 1 tbsp | 47 | 2 | 2 | 0 | 0 | 4 | 1 | 2 |
| pumpkin seeds, raw | 1 tbsp | 63 | 3 | 1 | 0 | 0 | 5 | 1 | 2 |
| sesame seed paste (tahini) | 1 tbsp | 95 | 3 | 4 | 1 | n/a | 8 | 1 | 2 |
| sesame seed paste (tahini), raw | 1 tbsp | 86 | 3 | 4 | 1 | n/a | 7 | 1 | 11 |
| sesame seed paste (tahini), roasted | 1 tbsp | 95 | 4 | 2 | 1 | 1 | 9 | 1 | 5 |
| sesame seeds, dried, kernels | 1 tbsp | 59 | 2 | 1 | 1 | 0 | 6 | 1 | 4 |
| sesame seeds, dried, whole | 1 tbsp | 52 | 2 | 2 | 1 | 0 | 4 | 1 | 1 |
| sesame seeds, ground | 1 tbsp | 51 | 2 | 1 | 1 | 0 | 4 | n/a | 17 |
| sunflower seed butter, with salt | 1 tbsp | 93 | 3 | 4 | 4 | 2 | 8 | 1 | 83 |
| sunflower seed butter, without salt | 1 tbsp | 93 | 3 | 4 | 1 | n/a | 8 | 1 | 0 |
| sunflower seeds, dry-roasted, with salt | 1 tbsp | 47 | 2 | 3 | 1 | 0 | 4 | 0 | 33 |
| sunflower seeds, dry-roasted, without salt | 1 tbsp | 47 | 2 | 3 | 1 | 0 | 4 | 0 | 0 |
| sunflower seeds, hulled | 1 tbsp | 43 | 2 | 2 | 1 | 0 | 4 | 0 | 0 |
| sunflower seeds, oil-roasted, with salt | 1 tbsp | 50 | 2 | 3 | 1 | 0 | 4 | 1 | 35 |
| sunflower seeds, oil-roasted, without salt | 1 tbsp | 50 | 2 | 3 | 1 | 0 | 4 | 1 | 0 |
| walnuts, black, dried, chopped | 1 tbsp | 48 | 2 | 1 | 1 | 0 | 5 | 0 | 0 |
| walnuts, English, dried, chopped | 1 tbsp | 49 | 1 | 1 | 1 | 0 | 5 | 0 | 0 |
| walnuts, English, dried, ground | 1 tbsp | 33 | 1 | 1 | 0 | 0 | 3 | 0 | 0 |
| walnuts, English, dried, halved | 1 tbsp | 41 | 1 | 1 | 0 | 0 | 4 | 0 | 0 |
| watermelon seeds, dried | 1 tbsp | 38 | 2 | 1 | 0 | n/a | 3 | 1 | 7 |

## PASTA

| FOOD ITEM | SERVING SIZE | CALORIES | PRO (g) | CARB (g) | FIBER (g) | SUGAR (g) | FAT (g) | SAT FAT (g) | SOD (mg) |
|---|---|---|---|---|---|---|---|---|---|
| acini di peppe pasta, semolina, dry | 1 oz | 103 | 4 | 21 | 1 | 1 | 0 | 0 | 1 |
| alphabet pasta, egg, dry | 1 oz | 106 | 4 | 20 | 1 | 1 | 1 | 0 | 6 |

*Note: For most pasta shapes, 1 ounce of dry pasta makes approximately ½ cup cooked.

| FOOD ITEM | SERVING SIZE | CALORIES | PRO (g) | CARB (g) | FIBER (g) | SUGAR (g) | FAT (g) | SAT FAT (g) | SOD (mg) |
|---|---|---|---|---|---|---|---|---|---|
| alphabet pasta, semolina, dry | 1 oz | 102 | 4 | 21 | 1 | 1 | 1 | 0 | 1 |
| angel hair pasta, corn, dry | 1 oz | 105 | 2 | 23 | 0 | 0 | 1 | 0 | 8 |
| angel hair pasta, semolina, dry | 1 oz | 102 | 4 | 21 | 1 | 1 | 1 | 0 | 1 |
| angel hair pasta, semolina, garlic-parsley, dry, organic | 1 oz | 104 | 3 | 20 | 1 | 1 | 1 | 0 | 2 |
| angel hair pasta, semolina, tomato-basil, dry, organic | 1 oz | 105 | 3 | 20 | 1 | 1 | 1 | 0 | 0 |
| angel hair pasta, whole wheat, dry, organic | 1 oz | 106 | 4 | 21 | 3 | 1 | 1 | 0 | 5 |
| bow-tie pasta, egg, dry | 1 oz | 106 | 4 | 20 | 1 | 1 | 1 | 0 | 6 |
| bow-tie pasta, semolina, dry | 1 oz | 103 | 4 | 21 | 1 | 1 | 0 | 0 | 1 |
| cannelloni pasta, white rice, dry | 1 oz | 107 | 2 | 22 | 0 | 0 | 0 | 0 | 0 |
| capellini pasta, semolina, dry | 1 oz | 103 | 4 | 21 | 1 | 1 | 0 | 0 | 1 |
| cavatelli pasta, semolina, dry | 1 oz | 103 | 4 | 21 | 1 | 1 | 0 | 0 | 1 |
| coiled fideo pasta, semolina, dry | 1 oz | 103 | 4 | 21 | 1 | 1 | 0 | 0 | 1 |
| conchigliette pasta, lentil bean, Papadini, wheat-free, gluten-free, dry | 1 oz | 95 | 7 | 16 | 3 | 0 | 0 | 0 | 47 |
| ditalini pasta, semolina, dry | 1 oz | 103 | 4 | 21 | 1 | 1 | 0 | 0 | 12 |
| egg pasta, homemade | ½ cup | 92 | 4 | 17 | 3 | n/a | 1 | 0 | 59 |
| eggless pasta, fresh, cooked | ½ cup | 70 | 2 | 14 | 1 | n/a | 1 | 0 | 42 |
| elbow pasta, corn, dry | 1 oz | 99 | 2 | 21 | 2 | 0 | 1 | 0 | 7 |
| elbow pasta, semolina, dry | 1 oz | 102 | 4 | 21 | 1 | 1 | 1 | 0 | 1 |
| elbow twist pasta, semolina, dry | 1 oz | 102 | 4 | 21 | 1 | 1 | 1 | 0 | 1 |
| fettuccine pasta (tagliatelle), brown rice, dry | 1 oz | 106 | 2 | 21 | 1 | 0 | 0 | 0 | 0 |
| fettuccine pasta (tagliatelle), rice, dry | 1 oz | 104 | 2 | 23 | 1 | 0 | 0 | 0 | 7 |
| fettuccine pasta (tagliatelle), semolina, dry | 1 oz | 103 | 4 | 21 | 1 | 1 | 0 | 0 | 1 |
| fettuccine pasta (tagliatelle), spinach, dry | 1 oz | 98 | 4 | 20 | 1 | 1 | 1 | 0 | 9 |
| fettuccine pasta (tagliatelle), white rice, dry | 1 oz | 102 | 2 | 22 | 0 | 0 | 0 | 0 | 0 |

| FOOD ITEM | SERVING SIZE | CALORIES | PRO (g) | CARB (g) | FIBER (g) | SUGAR (g) | FAT (g) | SAT FAT (g) | SOD (mg) |
|---|---|---|---|---|---|---|---|---|---|
| fideo pasta, semolina, dry | 1 oz | 103 | 4 | 21 | 1 | 1 | 0 | 0 | 1 |
| gemelli pasta, semolina, dry | 1 oz | 102 | 4 | 21 | 1 | 1 | 1 | 0 | 1 |
| lasagna pasta, rice, dry | 1 oz | 104 | 2 | 22 | 0 | 0 | 0 | 0 | 6 |
| lasagna pasta, semolina, dry | 1 oz | 102 | 4 | 21 | 1 | 1 | 1 | 0 | 1 |
| linguine pasta, lentil bean, Papadini, wheat-free, gluten-free, dry | 1 oz | 95 | 7 | 16 | 3 | 0 | 0 | 0 | 47 |
| linguine pasta, semolina, dry | 1 oz | 103 | 4 | 21 | 1 | 1 | 0 | 0 | 1 |
| macaroni pasta, low-protein, wheat-free, dry | 1 oz | 97 | 0 | 24 | 0 | 0 | 0 | 0 | 0 |
| manicotti pasta, semolina, dry | 1 oz | 103 | 4 | 21 | 1 | 1 | 0 | 0 | 1 |
| mostaccioli pasta, semolina, dry | 1 oz | 102 | 4 | 21 | 1 | 1 | 1 | 0 | 1 |
| orzo pasta, lentil bean, Papadini, wheat-free, gluten-free, dry | 1 oz | 95 | 7 | 16 | 3 | 0 | 0 | 0 | 47 |
| orzo pasta, semolina, dry | 1 oz | 103 | 4 | 21 | 1 | 1 | 0 | 0 | 1 |
| pastina pasta, semolina, dry | 1 oz | 103 | 4 | 21 | 1 | 1 | 0 | 0 | 1 |
| penne pasta, lentil bean, Papadini, wheat-free, gluten-free, dry | 1 oz | 95 | 7 | 16 | 3 | 0 | 0 | 0 | 47 |
| penne pasta, rice, dry | 1 oz | 104 | 2 | 23 | 1 | 0 | 0 | 0 | 7 |
| penne pasta, semolina, dry | 1 oz | 103 | 4 | 21 | 1 | 1 | 0 | 0 | 1 |
| penne pasta, whole wheat, dry, organic | 1 oz | 106 | 4 | 21 | 3 | 1 | 1 | 0 | 5 |
| pot pie squares pasta, egg, dry | 1 oz | 106 | 4 | 20 | 1 | 1 | 1 | 0 | 6 |
| radiatore pasta, semolina, dry | 1 oz | 102 | 4 | 21 | 1 | 1 | 1 | 0 | 1 |
| ribbon pasta, eggless, dry, organic | 1 oz | 106 | 4 | 21 | 1 | 1 | 1 | 0 | 3 |
| ribbon pasta, semolina, dry | 1 oz | 103 | 4 | 21 | 1 | 1 | 0 | 0 | 1 |
| rigatoni pasta, semolina, dry | 1 oz | 102 | 4 | 21 | 1 | 1 | 1 | 0 | 1 |
| rotelle pasta, semolina, dry | 1 oz | 102 | 4 | 21 | 1 | 1 | 1 | 0 | 1 |
| rotelle pasta, spinach, dry | 1 oz | 98 | 4 | 20 | 1 | 1 | 1 | 0 | 9 |

## PASTA (cont.)

| FOOD ITEM | SERVING SIZE | CALORIES | PRO (g) | CARB (g) | FIBER (g) | SUGAR (g) | FAT (g) | SAT FAT (g) | SOD (mg) |
|---|---|---|---|---|---|---|---|---|---|
| rotini pasta, lentil bean, Papadini, wheat-free, gluten-free, dry | 1 oz | 95 | 7 | 16 | 3 | 0 | 0 | 0 | 47 |
| shell pasta, large, low-protein, wheat-free, dry | 1 oz | 97 | 0 | 24 | 0 | 0 | 0 | 0 | 0 |
| shell pasta, large, white rice, dry | 1 oz | 107 | 2 | 22 | 0 | 0 | 0 | 0 | 0 |
| shell pasta, semolina, cooked | ½ cup | 91 | 3 | 18 | 1 | 0 | 1 | 0 | 1 |
| shell pasta, semolina, dry | 1 oz | 103 | 4 | 21 | 1 | 1 | 0 | 0 | 1 |
| shell pasta, small, low-protein, wheat-free, dry | 1 oz | 97 | 0 | 24 | 0 | 0 | 0 | 0 | 0 |
| shell pasta, small, white rice, dry | 1 oz | 107 | 2 | 22 | 0 | 0 | 0 | 0 | 0 |
| spaghetti pasta, brown rice, dry | 1 oz | 106 | 2 | 21 | 1 | 0 | 0 | 0 | 0 |
| spaghetti pasta, corn, dry | 1 oz | 99 | 2 | 21 | 2 | 0 | 1 | 0 | 7 |
| spaghetti pasta, lentil bean, Papadini, wheat-free, gluten-free, dry | 1 oz | 95 | 7 | 16 | 3 | 0 | 0 | 0 | 47 |
| spaghetti pasta, semolina, dry, organic | 1 oz | 106 | 4 | 22 | 1 | 1 | 1 | 0 | 3 |
| spaghetti pasta, spinach, dry, organic | 1 oz | 106 | 4 | 22 | 2 | 1 | 1 | 0 | 10 |
| spaghetti pasta, whole wheat, dry, organic | 1 oz | 100 | 5 | 20 | 5 | 1 | 1 | 0 | 5 |
| spirals pasta, rice, dry | 1 oz | 104 | 2 | 23 | 1 | 0 | 0 | 0 | 7 |
| tortiglioni pasta, semolina, dry | 1 oz | 103 | 4 | 21 | 1 | 1 | 0 | 0 | 1 |
| tubettini pasta, semolina, dry | 1 oz | 103 | 4 | 21 | 1 | 1 | 0 | 0 | 1 |
| vermicelli pasta, semolina, dry | 1 oz | 102 | 4 | 21 | 1 | 1 | 1 | 0 | 1 |
| vermicelli pasta, soy, dry | 1 oz | 94 | 0 | 23 | 1 | 5 | 0 | 0 | 1 |
| vermicelli pasta, white rice, dry | 1 oz | 102 | 2 | 22 | 0 | 0 | 0 | 0 | 0 |
| wagon wheels pasta, semolina, dry | 1 oz | 103 | 4 | 21 | 1 | 1 | 0 | 0 | 1 |
| ziti pasta, semolina, dry | 1 oz | 103 | 4 | 21 | 1 | 1 | 0 | 0 | 1 |
| zitoni pasta, semolina, dry | 1 oz | 102 | 4 | 21 | 1 | 1 | 1 | 0 | 1 |

| FOOD ITEM | SERVING SIZE | CALORIES | PRO (g) | CARB (g) | FIBER (g) | SUGAR (g) | FAT (g) | SAT FAT (g) | SOD (mg) |
|---|---|---|---|---|---|---|---|---|---|
| **Chicken** | | | | | | | | | |
| chicken, breast, boneless, without skin, stewed | 3 oz | 128 | 25 | 0 | 0 | 0 | 3 | 1 | 54 |
| chicken, breast, boneless, without skin, raw | 4 oz | 132 | 25 | 0 | 0 | 0 | 3 | 1 | 55 |
| chicken, breast, oven-roasted, fat-free, sliced | 3 oz | 67 | 14 | 2 | 0 | 0 | 0 | 0 | 924 |
| chicken, breast, with bone, with skin, raw | 4 oz | 195 | 24 | 0 | 0 | 0 | 10 | 3 | 71 |
| chicken, breast, with bone, with skin, roasted | 3 oz | 168 | 25 | 0 | 0 | 0 | 7 | 2 | 60 |
| chicken, drumstick, with skin, cooked | 3 oz | 174 | 22 | 0 | 0 | 0 | 9 | 2 | 65 |
| chicken, drumstick, with skin, raw | 4 oz | 183 | 22 | 0 | 0 | 0 | 10 | 3 | 94 |
| chicken, drumstick, without skin, cooked | 3 oz | 146 | 24 | 0 | 0 | 0 | 5 | 1 | 91 |
| chicken, drumstick, without skin, raw | 4 oz | 135 | 23 | 0 | 0 | 0 | 4 | 1 | 100 |
| chicken, ground, raw | 4 oz | 150 | 18 | 0 | 0 | 0 | 9 | 3 | 65 |
| chicken, thigh, boneless, without skin, cooked | 3 oz | 166 | 21 | 0 | 0 | 0 | 8 | 2 | 64 |
| chicken, thigh, boneless, without skin, raw | 4 oz | 164 | 21 | 0 | 0 | 0 | 8 | 2 | 63 |
| chicken, thigh, with bone, with skin, raw | 4 oz | 189 | 15 | 0 | 0 | 0 | 14 | 4 | 68 |
| chicken, thigh, with bone, with skin, roasted | 3 oz | 149 | 15 | 0 | 0 | 0 | 9 | 3 | 51 |
| chicken frankfurter | 1 | 116 | 6 | 3 | 0 | 0 | 9 | 2 | 617 |
| chicken liver paté | 1 oz | 57 | 4 | 2 | 0 | 0 | 4 | 1 | 109 |
| chicken lunch meat, deli | 1 oz | 30 | 6 | 1 | 0 | 1 | 1 | 0 | 180 |
| chicken lunch meat, deli, breast, browned | 1 oz | 30 | 6 | 1 | 0 | 1 | 1 | 0 | 180 |
| chicken meatball | 1 | 48 | 6 | 2 | 0 | n/a | 2 | 1 | 36 |
| chicken spread, canned | 1 oz | 41 | 1 | 3 | n/a | n/a | 3 | 1 | 133 |
| **Game** | | | | | | | | | |
| duck, breast, wild, without skin, raw | 4 oz | 139 | 23 | 0 | 0 | 0 | 5 | 2 | 65 |
| duck, breast, young, without bones, without skin, broiled | 3 oz | 119 | 23 | 0 | 0 | 0 | 2 | 0 | 89 |
| duck, Chinese pressed | 3 oz | 163 | 6 | 16 | 1 | n/a | 8 | 3 | 77 |

| FOOD ITEM | SERVING SIZE | CALORIES | PRO (g) | CARB (g) | FIBER (g) | SUGAR (g) | FAT (g) | SAT FAT (g) | SOD (mg) |
|---|---|---|---|---|---|---|---|---|---|
| duck, domesticated, whole, without skin, roasted | 3 oz | 171 | 20 | 0 | 0 | 0 | 10 | 4 | 55 |
| duck, mallard, raw | 4 oz | 172 | 26 | 0 | 0 | 0 | 2 | 0 | n/a |
| duck, whole, roasted, chopped | 3 oz | 287 | 16 | 0 | 0 | 0 | 24 | 8 | 50 |
| duck, whole, without skin, raw | 4 oz | 150 | 21 | 0 | 0 | 0 | 7 | 3 | 84 |
| duck, widgeon, raw | 4 oz | 174 | 26 | 0 | 0 | 0 | 2 | n/a | n/a |
| duck, wild, whole, with skin, raw | 4 oz | 239 | 20 | 0 | 0 | 0 | 17 | 6 | 64 |
| duckling, Peking, breast, with skin, roasted | 3 oz | 172 | 21 | 0 | 0 | 0 | 9 | 2 | 71 |
| duckling, Peking, breast, without skin, broiled | 3 oz | 119 | 23 | 0 | 0 | 0 | 2 | 0 | 89 |
| emu, fan filet, broiled | 3 oz | 131 | 27 | 0 | 0 | 0 | 2 | 1 | 45 |
| emu, ground, broiled | 3 oz | 139 | 24 | 0 | 0 | 0 | 4 | 1 | 55 |
| emu, ground, raw | 4 oz | 152 | 26 | 0 | 0 | 0 | 5 | 1 | 64 |
| emu, thigh, raw | 4 oz | 124 | 26 | 0 | 0 | 0 | 2 | 1 | 81 |
| emu, top loin, broiled | 3 oz | 129 | 25 | 0 | 0 | 0 | 3 | 1 | 49 |
| goose, liver, raw | 4 oz | 151 | 19 | 7 | 0 | n/a | 5 | 2 | 159 |
| goose, liver, smoked | 1 oz | 131 | 3 | 1 | 0 | n/a | 12 | 4 | 198 |
| goose, snow, raw | 4 oz | 137 | 26 | 0 | 0 | 0 | 4 | n/a | n/a |
| goose, whole, boneless, roasted, with skin | 3 oz | 259 | 21 | 0 | 0 | 0 | 18 | 6 | 60 |
| goose, whole, roasted | 3 oz | 259 | 21 | 0 | 0 | 0 | 19 | 6 | 60 |
| goose, whole, without skin, raw | 4 oz | 183 | 26 | 0 | 0 | 0 | 8 | 3 | 99 |
| ostrich, fan, raw | 4 oz | 133 | 25 | 0 | 0 | 0 | 3 | 1 | 85 |
| ostrich, ground, 3% fat, cooked | 3 oz | 121 | 23 | 0 | 0 | 0 | 3 | n/a | 64 |
| ostrich, ground, broiled | 3 oz | 149 | 22 | 0 | 0 | 0 | 6 | 2 | 68 |
| ostrich, ground, raw | 4 oz | 187 | 23 | 0 | 0 | 0 | 10 | 2 | 82 |
| ostrich, round, raw | 4 oz | 132 | 25 | 0 | 0 | 0 | 3 | 1 | 82 |
| ostrich, tenderloin, raw | 4 oz | 139 | 25 | 0 | 0 | 0 | 4 | 2 | 98 |
| ostrich, top loin, cooked | 3 oz | 132 | 24 | 0 | 0 | 0 | 3 | 1 | 65 |
| pheasant, breast, without skin, raw | 4 oz | 151 | 28 | 0 | 0 | 0 | 4 | 1 | 37 |

| FOOD ITEM | SERVING SIZE | CALORIES | PRO (g) | CARB (g) | FIBER (g) | SUGAR (g) | FAT (g) | SAT FAT (g) | SOD (mg) |
|---|---|---|---|---|---|---|---|---|---|
| **Game (cont.)** | | | | | | | | | |
| pheasant, leg, without skin, raw | 4 oz | 152 | 25 | 0 | 0 | 0 | 5 | 2 | 51 |
| pheasant, whole, cooked | 3 oz | 210 | 28 | 0 | 0 | 0 | 10 | 3 | 37 |
| pheasant, whole, raw | 4 oz | 205 | 26 | 0 | 0 | 0 | 11 | 3 | 45 |
| pheasant, whole, without skin, raw | 4 oz | 151 | 27 | 0 | 0 | 0 | 4 | 1 | 42 |
| quail, breast, without skin, raw | 4 oz | 139 | 26 | 0 | 0 | 0 | 3 | 1 | 62 |
| quail, whole, cooked | 3 oz | 199 | 21 | 0 | 0 | 0 | 12 | 3 | 44 |
| quail, whole, with skin, raw | 4 oz | 218 | 22 | 0 | 0 | 0 | 14 | 4 | 60 |
| quail, whole, without skin, raw | 4 oz | 152 | 25 | 0 | 0 | 0 | 5 | 2 | 58 |
| squab, whole, with skin, raw | 4 oz | 333 | 21 | 0 | 0 | 0 | 27 | 10 | 61 |
| squab, whole, without skin, raw | 4 oz | 161 | 20 | 0 | 0 | 0 | 9 | 2 | 58 |
| squab meat, light, without skin, raw | 4 oz | 152 | 25 | 0 | 0 | 0 | 5 | 1 | 62 |
| **Turkey** | | | | | | | | | |
| Jennie-O Turkey Store Breakfast Sausage Links | 56 g | 140 | 9 | 0 | 0 | 0 | 11 | 3 | 360 |
| Jennie-O Turkey Store Breakfast Sausage Patties | 64 g | 160 | 10 | 0 | 0 | 0 | 13 | 3.5 | 420 |
| Jennie-O Turkey Store Deli Thin Turkey Breast Lunchmeat—Sun Dried Tomato | 56 g | 50 | 9 | 2 | 0 | 0 | 1.5 | 0 | 410 |
| Jennie-O Turkey Store Extra Lean Ground | 112 g | 120 | 26 | 0 | 0 | 0 | 1.5 | 0.5 | 80 |
| Jennie-O Turkey Store Extra Lean Turkey Bacon | 15 g | 20 | 3 | 0 | 0 | 0 | 0.5 | 0 | 140 |
| Jennie-O Turkey Store Fresh Italian Dinner Sausage | 109 g | 160 | 17 | 0 | 0 | 0 | 10 | 2.5 | 650 |
| Jennie-O Turkey Store Fresh Tenderloins | 112 g | 120 | 26 | 0 | 0 | 0 | 1.5 | 0 | 75 |
| Jennie-O Turkey Store Frozen Premium 1/3 lb White Turkey Burger | 149 g | 250 | 27 | 0 | 0 | 0 | 17 | 4 | 750 |
| Jennie-O Turkey Store Frozen Seasoned Turkey Burger | 112 g | 160 | 20 | 0 | 0 | 0 | 9 | 2.5 | 280 |
| Jennie-O Turkey Store Lean Ground | 112 g | 160 | 23 | 0 | 0 | 0 | 8 | 2.5 | 80 |
| Jennie-O Turkey Store Lean Turkey Burger Patties | 112 g | 160 | 23 | 0 | 0 | 0 | 8 | 2.5 | 80 |

| FOOD ITEM | SERVING SIZE | CALORIES | PRO (g) | CARB (g) | FIBER (g) | SUGAR (g) | FAT (g) | SAT FAT (g) | SOD (mg) |
|---|---|---|---|---|---|---|---|---|---|
| Jennie-O Turkey Store Marinated Tenderloin— Roast | 112 g | 110 | 21 | 4 | 0 | 1 | 1 | 0 | 840 |
| Jennie-O Turkey Store Oven Ready Bone-in Turkey Breast—Homestyle | 112 g | 130 | 22 | 0 | 0 | 0 | 4 | 1 | 420 |
| Jennie-O Turkey Store Oven Ready Whole Turkey— Homestyle | 112 g | 160 | 20 | 0 | 0 | 0 | 9 | 3 | 370 |
| Jennie-O Turkey Store Turkey Breast Cutlets | 112 g | 120 | 26 | 0 | 0 | 0 | 1.5 | 0 | 75 |
| turkey, breast, fat-free, honey-roasted, without skin | 1 oz | 29 | 5 | 1 | 0 | 1 | 0 | 0 | 335 |
| turkey, breast, 97% fat-free, smoked | 1 oz | 27 | 6 | 0 | 0 | 0 | 0 | 0 | 329 |
| turkey, breast, strip, raw | 4 oz | 120 | 28 | 0 | 0 | 0 | 1 | 0 | 100 |
| turkey, breast, tenderloin, raw | 4 oz | 120 | 28 | 0 | 0 | 0 | 2 | 0 | 65 |
| turkey, breast, with skin, raw | 4 oz | 178 | 25 | 0 | 0 | 0 | 8 | 2 | 67 |
| turkey, breast, with skin, roasted | 3 oz | 161 | 24 | 0 | 0 | 0 | 6 | 2 | 54 |
| turkey, dark meat, with skin, raw | 4 oz | 181 | 21 | 0 | 0 | 0 | 10 | 3 | 81 |
| turkey, dark meat, with skin, roasted | 3 oz | 188 | 23 | 0 | 0 | 0 | 10 | 3 | 65 |
| turkey, dark meat, without skin, raw | 4 oz | 142 | 23 | 0 | 0 | 0 | 5 | 2 | 87 |
| turkey, dark meat, without skin, roasted | 3 oz | 159 | 24 | 0 | 0 | 0 | 6 | 2 | 67 |
| turkey, drumstick, with skin, smoked | 3 oz | 177 | 24 | 0 | 0 | 0 | 8 | 3 | 847 |
| turkey, drumstick, without skin, cooked | 3 oz | 159 | 24 | 0 | 0 | 0 | 6 | 2 | 67 |
| turkey, giblets, raw | 1 | 315 | 47 | 5 | 0 | 0 | 10 | 3 | 212 |
| turkey, gizzard, raw | 1 | 139 | 22 | 0 | 0 | 0 | 5 | 1 | 81 |
| turkey, ground, 11% fat, sausage | 3 oz | 146 | 14 | 0 | 0 | 0 | 10 | 3 | 517 |
| turkey, heart, raw | 1 | 34 | 5 | 0 | 0 | 0 | 1 | 0 | 27 |
| turkey, leg, with skin, raw | 4 oz | 163 | 22 | 0 | 0 | 0 | 8 | 2 | 84 |
| turkey, leg, with skin, roasted | 3 oz | 177 | 24 | 0 | 0 | 0 | 8 | 3 | 65 |
| turkey, light meat, with skin, raw | 4 oz | 180 | 25 | 0 | 0 | 0 | 8 | 2 | 67 |
| turkey, light meat, with skin, roasted | 3 oz | 168 | 24 | 0 | 0 | 0 | 7 | 2 | 54 |

| FOOD ITEM | SERVING SIZE | CALORIES | PRO (g) | CARB (g) | FIBER (g) | SUGAR (g) | FAT (g) | SAT FAT (g) | SOD (mg) |
|---|---|---|---|---|---|---|---|---|---|
| **Turkey (cont.)** | | | | | | | | | |
| turkey, light meat, with skin, smoked | 3 oz | 177 | 24 | 0 | 0 | 0 | 8 | 2 | 847 |
| turkey, light meat, without skin, raw | 3 oz | 98 | 20 | 0 | 0 | 0 | 1 | 0 | 54 |
| turkey, light meat, without skin, roasted | 3 oz | 134 | 25 | 0 | 0 | 3 | 1 | 0 | 54 |
| turkey, light meat, without skin, smoked | 3 oz | 145 | 25 | 0 | 0 | 4 | 1 | 0 | 847 |
| turkey, liver, raw | 4 oz | 263 | 20 | 3 | 0 | 0 | 19 | 6 | 81 |
| turkey, neck, without skin, raw | 1 | 243 | 36 | 0 | 0 | 0 | 10 | 3 | 167 |
| turkey, wing, with skin, smoked | 3 oz | 195 | 23 | 0 | 0 | 0 | 11 | 3 | 847 |
| turkey croquette | 3 oz | 219 | 14 | 11 | 0 | 0 | 13 | 3 | 176 |
| turkey egg roll | 1 | 103 | 4 | 9 | 1 | n/a | 6 | 1 | 164 |
| turkey frankfurter | 1 | 102 | 6 | 1 | 0 | 0 | 8 | 3 | 642 |
| turkey jerky, hot and spicy | 1 oz | 71 | 14 | 3 | 0 | 3 | 1 | 0 | 486 |
| turkey jerky, original | 1 oz | 81 | 14 | 3 | 0 | 3 | 1 | 0 | 557 |
| turkey jerky, teriyaki | 1 oz | 81 | 14 | 4 | 0 | 4 | 1 | 0 | 586 |
| turkey meat loaf | 4-oz slice | 184 | 22 | 8 | 1 | n/a | 7 | 2 | 139 |
| turkey meatball | 1 oz | 48 | 6 | 2 | 0 | 0 | 2 | 1 | 36 |
| turkey nugget | 0.6-oz piece | 47 | 4 | 3 | 0 | 0 | 2 | 1 | 155 |
| turkey pastrami lunch meat | 1 oz | 35 | 5 | 1 | 0 | 1 | 1 | 0 | 278 |
| turkey pepperoni, sliced | 1 oz | 69 | 9 | 1 | 0 | 0 | 3 | 1 | 527 |
| turkey sausage, raw | 1 oz | 44 | 5 | 0 | 0 | 0 | 2 | 1 | 168 |
| turkey sausage, smoked, hot | 1 oz | 45 | 4 | 1 | 0 | 1 | 2 | 1 | 263 |

## SEAFOOD

| FOOD ITEM | SERVING SIZE | CALORIES | PRO (g) | CARB (g) | FIBER (g) | SUGAR (g) | FAT (g) | SAT FAT (g) | SOD (mg) |
|---|---|---|---|---|---|---|---|---|---|
| crab, Alaskan, king crab leg, raw | 4 oz | 95 | 21 | 0 | 0 | 0 | 1 | 0 | 948 |
| crab, Alaskan, king crab leg, steamed | 3 oz | 83 | 16 | 0 | 0 | 0 | 1 | 0 | 912 |
| crab, baked | 3 oz | 117 | 16 | 0 | 0 | n/a | 5 | 1 | 270 |
| crab, blue, canned, drained | ½ cup | 67 | 14 | 0 | 0 | 0 | 1 | 0 | 225 |

| FOOD ITEM | SERVING SIZE | CALORIES | PRO (g) | CARB (g) | FIBER (g) | SUGAR (g) | FAT (g) | SAT FAT (g) | SOD (mg) |
|---|---|---|---|---|---|---|---|---|---|
| crab, blue, cooked | 3 oz | 101 | 20 | 0 | 0 | 0 | 1 | 0 | 334 |
| crab, blue, flaked, steamed | 3 oz | 87 | 17 | 0 | 0 | 0 | 2 | 0 | 237 |
| crab, blue, raw | 4 oz | 99 | 20 | 0 | 0 | 1 | 0 | 0 | 332 |
| crab, Dungeness, raw | 4 oz | 98 | 20 | 1 | 0 | n/a | 1 | 0 | 335 |
| crab, Dungeness, steamed | 3 oz | 94 | 19 | 1 | 0 | n/a | 1 | n/a | 321 |
| crab, king, leg, baked | 3 oz | 117 | 16 | 0 | 0 | n/a | 5 | 1 | 270 |
| crab, imitation (surimi) | 3 oz | 87 | 10 | 9 | 0 | 0 | 1 | 0 | 715 |
| crab, queen, raw | 3 oz | 102 | 21 | 0 | 0 | 0 | 1 | 0 | 611 |
| crab, queen, steamed | 3 oz | 98 | 20 | 0 | 0 | 0 | 1 | 0 | 588 |
| crab, sautéed | 3 oz | 117 | 16 | 0 | 0 | 0 | 5 | 1 | 270 |
| crab, snow, leg, baked | 3 oz | 117 | 16 | 0 | 0 | 0 | 5 | 1 | 270 |
| crayfish, farmed, raw | 4 oz | 82 | 17 | 0 | 0 | 0 | 1 | 0 | 70 |
| crayfish, farmed, steamed | 3 oz | 74 | 15 | 0 | 0 | 0 | 1 | 0 | 83 |
| crayfish, wild, raw | 4 oz | 87 | 18 | 0 | 0 | 0 | 1 | 0 | 66 |
| crayfish, wild, steamed | 3 oz | 70 | 14 | 0 | 0 | 0 | 1 | 0 | 80 |
| lobster, baked, diced | 3 oz | 99 | 17 | 1 | 0 | 0 | 3 | 1 | 335 |
| lobster, cooked | 3 oz | 81 | 17 | 1 | 0 | 0 | 1 | 0 | 324 |
| lobster, Northern, raw | 4 oz | 102 | 21 | 1 | 0 | 0 | 1 | 0 | 336 |
| lobster, Northern, steamed | 3 oz | 83 | 17 | 1 | 0 | 0 | 1 | 0 | 323 |
| lobster, spiny, raw | 4 oz | 127 | 23 | 3 | 0 | n/a | 2 | 0 | 201 |
| lobster, spiny, steamed, no shell | 3 oz | 122 | 22 | 3 | 0 | n/a | 2 | 0 | 193 |
| lobster, whole or diced, baked | 3 oz | 99 | 17 | 1 | 0 | n/a | 3 | 1 | 335 |
| shrimp, canned, drained | 3 oz | 102 | 20 | 1 | 0 | 0 | 2 | 0 | 144 |
| shrimp, cooked | 3 oz | 101 | 21 | 0 | 0 | 0 | 2 | 0 | 253 |
| shrimp, deveined | 1 oz | 23 | 5 | 0 | 0 | 0 | 0 | 0 | 335 |
| shrimp, dried | 1 oz | 86 | 17 | 1 | 0 | n/a | 1 | 0 | 122 |
| shrimp, imitation (surimi) | 3 oz | 86 | 11 | 8 | 0 | n/a | 1 | 0 | 600 |
| shrimp, popcorn, baked, with margarine, with salt | 3 oz | 132 | 21 | 1 | 0 | n/a | 4 | 1 | 183 |
| shrimp, raw | 1 small | 5 | 1 | 0 | 0 | 0 | 0 | 0 | 7 |
| shrimp, raw | 1 medium | 6 | 1 | 0 | 0 | 0 | 0 | 0 | 9 |

| FOOD ITEM | SERVING SIZE | CALORIES | PRO (g) | CARB (g) | FIBER (g) | SUGAR (g) | FAT (g) | SAT FAT (g) | SOD (mg) |
|---|---|---|---|---|---|---|---|---|---|
| shrimp, raw | 1 large | 7 | 1 | 0 | 0 | 0 | 0 | 0 | 10 |
| shrimp, sautéed | 3 oz | 132 | 21 | 1 | 0 | n/a | 4 | 1 | 183 |
| shrimp, steamed | 1 large | 5 | 1 | 0 | 0 | 0 | 0 | 0 | 12 |
| shrimp with butter sauce | 3 oz | 194 | 16 | 1 | 0 | n/a | 14 | 8 | 245 |

## SNACKS

| FOOD ITEM | SERVING SIZE | CALORIES | PRO (g) | CARB (g) | FIBER (g) | SUGAR (g) | FAT (g) | SAT FAT (g) | SOD (mg) |
|---|---|---|---|---|---|---|---|---|---|
| Baked Cheetos Crunchy Cheese Flavored Snacks | 1 oz | 130 | 2 | 19 | 0 | 1 | 5 | 1 | 240 |
| Baked Cheetos Crunchy 100 Calories Mini Bites Cheese Flavored Snacks | 1 package | 100 | 2 | 14 | 0 | 0 | 4 | 1 | 180 |
| Baked Cheetos Flamin' Hot Cheese Flavored Snacks | 1 package | 200 | 4 | 29 | 0 | 0 | 8 | 1 | 360 |
| Baked Doritos Nacho Cheese | 1 oz | 120 | 2 | 21 | 2 | 1 | 4 | 1 | 220 |
| Baked Lay's Cheddar & Sour Cream Flavored Potato Crisps | 1 oz | 120 | 2 | 21 | 2 | 3 | 3 | 1 | 210 |
| Baked Lay's KC Masterpiece BBQ Flavor Potato Crisps | 1 oz | 120 | 2 | 22 | 2 | 2 | 3 | 0 | 210 |
| Baked Lay's Original Potato Crisps | 1 oz | 110 | 2 | 23 | 2 | 2 | 2 | 0 | 150 |
| Baked Lay's Sour Cream & Onion Flavored Potato Crisps | 1 oz | 120 | 2 | 21 | 2 | 3 | 3 | 0 | 210 |
| Baked Ruffles Original Potato Crisps | 1 oz | 120 | 2 | 21 | 2 | 2 | 3 | 0 | 200 |
| Baked Tostitos Bite Sized Tortilla Chips | 1 oz | 110 | 3 | 24 | 2 | 0 | 1 | 0 | 200 |
| breakfast bar, chocolate chip | 1 | 150 | 2 | 24 | 1 | 11 | 6 | 2 | 80 |
| breakfast bar, peanut butter–chocolate chip | 1 | 150 | 3 | 22 | 1 | 10 | 5 | 2 | 85 |
| breakfast bar, raisin coconut | 1 | 199 | 4 | 29 | 1 | 12 | 8 | 5 | 120 |
| cheese puff | 1 oz | 158 | 2 | 15 | 1 | 1 | 10 | 2 | 298 |
| cheese puff, crunchy | 1 oz | 160 | 2 | 15 | 1 | 1 | 10 | 3 | 290 |
| cheese puff, low-carb | 1 oz | 142 | 10 | 7 | 0 | 0 | 1 | 1 | 435 |
| cheese puff, low-fat, with corn | 1 oz | 122 | 2 | 21 | 3 | 2 | 3 | 1 | 364 |
| cheese puff, original bakes | 1 oz | 162 | 2 | 13 | 0 | 1 | 11 | 2 | 192 |
| Chex Party Mix | 1 oz | 123 | 3 | 21 | 1 | 2 | 3 | 1 | 265 |

| FOOD ITEM | SERVING SIZE | CALORIES | PRO (g) | CARB (g) | FIBER (g) | SUGAR (g) | FAT (g) | SAT FAT (g) | SOD (mg) |
|---|---|---|---|---|---|---|---|---|---|
| corn chips | 1 oz | 145 | 2 | 18 | 0 | n/a | 8 | 6 | 290 |
| corn chips, barbecue flavored | 1 oz | 150 | 2 | 16 | 1 | 1 | 9 | 1 | 290 |
| corn chips, French onion flavored | 1 oz | 140 | 2 | 18 | 2 | 3 | 7 | 1 | 160 |
| corn chips, white, bite-size | 1 oz | 140 | 2 | 17 | 1 | 0 | 8 | 1 | 110 |
| corn chips, whole grain | 1 oz | 140 | 2 | 19 | 2 | 0 | 6 | 1 | 70 |
| Corn Nuts, barbecue | 1 oz | 124 | 3 | 20 | 2 | n/a | 4 | 1 | 277 |
| Corn Nuts, nacho cheese | 1 oz | 124 | 3 | 20 | 2 | n/a | 4 | 1 | 180 |
| Corn Nuts, original | 1 oz | 122 | 3 | 20 | 2 | 0 | 5 | 1 | 182 |
| Corn Nuts, plain | 1 oz | 126 | 2 | 20 | 2 | 0 | 4 | 1 | 244 |
| Corn Nuts, ranch | 1 oz | 132 | 3 | 19 | 2 | 0 | 5 | 1 | 243 |
| Fruit Leather, apple, organic | 1 | 45 | 0 | 12 | 1 | 11 | 0 | 0 | 0 |
| Fruit Leather, apricot | 1 | 45 | 0 | 11 | 1 | 7 | 0 | 0 | 0 |
| Fruit Leather, berry | 1 | 80 | 0 | 17 | 0 | 10 | 1 | 0 | 50 |
| Fruit Leather, grape, organic | 1 | 45 | 0 | 12 | 1 | 11 | 0 | 0 | 0 |
| Fruit Leather, mango | 1 | 45 | 0 | 11 | 1 | 9 | 0 | 0 | 0 |
| Fruit Roll-Ups, cherry | 1 | 53 | 0 | 12 | 0 | 5 | 1 | 0 | 40 |
| Fruit Roll-Ups, grape | 1 | 53 | 0 | 12 | 0 | 5 | 1 | 0 | 58 |
| Fruit Roll-Ups, strawberry | 1 | 52 | 0 | 12 | 0 | 5 | 1 | 0 | 49 |
| Goldfish Crackers | approx 25 | 65 | 1 | 10 | 1 | 3 | 3 | 1 | 57 |
| Goldfish Party Mix | ¼ cup | 85 | 3 | 11 | 1 | 2 | 4 | 1 | 180 |
| granola bar, almond, crunchy, low-fat | 1 | 82 | 2 | 16 | 1 | n/a | 2 | 0 | 61 |
| granola bar, almond, hard | 1 | 117 | 2 | 15 | 1 | n/a | 6 | 3 | 60 |
| granola bar, apple-cinnamon, low-fat | 1 | 106 | 1 | 21 | 1 | 9 | 2 | 1 | 68 |
| granola bar, banana nut | 1 | 95 | 2 | 14 | 1 | 6 | 4 | 1 | 80 |
| granola bar, blueberry, fat-free | 1 | 140 | 2 | 35 | 3 | 14 | 0 | 0 | 10 |
| granola bar, blueberry yogurt, chewy | 1 | 140 | 2 | 26 | 1 | 13 | 4 | 2 | 130 |
| granola bar, carob chip | 1 | 80 | 2 | 15 | 1 | 7 | 2 | 0 | 0 |
| granola bar, chocolate | 1 | 158 | 2 | 23 | 1 | n/a | 7 | 3 | 61 |
| granola bar, chocolate chocolate chip, low-fat | 1 | 103 | 2 | 22 | 1 | 7 | 2 | 1 | 66 |

| FOOD ITEM | SERVING SIZE | CALORIES | PRO (g) | CARB (g) | FIBER (g) | SUGAR (g) | FAT (g) | SAT FAT (g) | SOD (mg) |
|---|---|---|---|---|---|---|---|---|---|
| granola bar, chocolate chip, fat-free | 1 | 140 | 2 | 35 | 3 | 14 | 0 | 0 | 10 |
| granola bar, chocolate chip, hard | 1 | 103 | 2 | 17 | 1 | n/a | 4 | 3 | 81 |
| granola bar, chocolate chunk, low-fat, chewy | 1 | 111 | 2 | 22 | 1 | 10 | 2 | 1 | 79 |
| granola bar, date and almond, fat-free | 1 | 140 | 2 | 35 | 3 | 14 | 0 | 0 | 10 |
| granola bar, Dutch apple, low-fat, chewy | 1 | 100 | 2 | 22 | 2 | 12 | 1 | 0 | 15 |
| granola bar, fruit and nut | 1 | 72 | 1 | 16 | 2 | 12 | 0 | 0 | 3 |
| granola bar, fruit-filled, fat-free | 1 | 97 | 2 | 22 | 2 | 16 | 0 | 0 | 5 |
| granola bar, honey nut, low-fat | 1 | 96 | 2 | 22 | 1 | 6 | 2 | 0 | 68 |
| granola bar, multigrain, chewy | 1 | 78 | 1 | 16 | 1 | 5 | 1 | 0 | 90 |
| granola bar, nut raisin, soft | 1 | 129 | 2 | 18 | 2 | n/a | 6 | 3 | 72 |
| granola bar, oatmeal, low-fat, chewy | 1 | 110 | 1 | 22 | 1 | 10 | 2 | 0 | 69 |
| granola bar, oatmeal raisin, low-fat | 1 | 110 | 1 | 22 | 1 | 10 | 2 | 0 | 69 |
| granola bar, peanut, diet | 1 | 220 | 8 | 35 | 1 | 15 | 6 | 4 | 320 |
| granola bar, peanut crunch, low-fat, chewy | 1 | 110 | 3 | 19 | 2 | 10 | 3 | 0 | 80 |
| granola bar, raisin, fat-free | 1 | 140 | 2 | 35 | 3 | 14 | 0 | 0 | 10 |
| granola bar, raspberry, fat-free | 1 | 140 | 2 | 35 | 3 | 14 | 0 | 0 | 10 |
| granola bar, s'mores, low-fat, chewy | 1 | 111 | 1 | 22 | 1 | 10 | 2 | 1 | 82 |
| granola bar, strawberry, fat-free | 1 | 140 | 2 | 35 | 3 | 14 | 0 | 0 | 10 |
| granola bar, vanilla yogurt, chewy | 1 | 140 | 2 | 26 | 1 | 13 | 4 | 2 | 130 |
| granola bar, wild berry, low-fat, chewy | 1 | 100 | 2 | 22 | 2 | 10 | 1 | 0 | 5 |
| jerky, beef | 1 oz | 126 | 9 | 3 | 3 | 0 | 8 | 3 | 662 |
| jerky, teriyaki | 1 oz | 81 | 13 | 5 | 0 | 1 | 1 | 0 | 648 |
| jerky, turkey | 1 oz | 81 | 14 | 3 | 0 | 3 | 1 | 0 | 557 |
| jerky, venison | 0.5 oz | 48 | 5 | 2 | 0 | 0 | 2 | 1 | 410 |
| popcorn, air-popped | 1 cup | 31 | 1 | 6 | 1 | 0 | 0 | 0 | 1 |
| popcorn, caramel | 1 oz | 122 | 1 | 22 | 1 | 15 | 4 | 1 | 58 |

| FOOD ITEM | SERVING SIZE | CALORIES | PRO (g) | CARB (g) | FIBER (g) | SUGAR (g) | FAT (g) | SAT FAT (g) | SOD (mg) |
|---|---|---|---|---|---|---|---|---|---|
| popcorn, caramel, fat-free | 1 oz | 108 | 1 | 26 | 1 | 18 | 0 | 0 | 81 |
| popcorn, caramel, with peanuts | ½ cup | 85 | 1 | 17 | 1 | 10 | 2 | 0 | 63 |
| popcorn, cheese | ½ cup | 29 | 1 | 3 | 1 | n/a | 2 | 0 | 49 |
| popcorn, honey-butter, unpopped | 0.5 oz | 79 | 1 | 6 | 1 | 0 | 5 | 1 | 67 |
| popcorn, light, unpopped | 0.5 oz | 61 | 2 | 9 | 2 | 0 | 2 | 1 | 162 |
| popcorn, microwaveable, 94% fat-free | 0.5 oz | 44 | 1 | 9 | 1 | 0 | 1 | 0 | 138 |
| popcorn, microwaveable, light butter | 0.5 oz | 52 | 1 | 9 | 1 | 0 | 2 | 1 | 145 |
| popcorn, microwaveable, low-fat, low-sodium | 0.5 oz | 61 | 2 | 10 | 2 | 0 | 1 | 0 | 69 |
| popcorn, oil-popped, low-fat | 0.5 oz | 60 | 2 | 10 | 2 | 0 | 1 | 0 | 125 |
| popcorn, oil-popped, with salt | 1 cup | 55 | 1 | 6 | 1 | 0 | 3 | 1 | 97 |
| popcorn, oil-popped, without salt | 0.5 oz | 74 | 1 | 8 | 1 | 0 | 4 | 1 | 0 |
| popcorn, original, kettle | 1 cup | 80 | 1 | 16 | 2 | 10 | 1 | 0 | 160 |
| popcorn, Smartfood Reduced Fat White Cheddar Cheese Flavored Popcorn | 1 cup | 47 | 1 | 6 | 1 | 0 | 2 | 1 | 93 |
| popcorn, Smartfood White Cheddar Cheese Flavored Popcorn | 1 cup | 95 | 2 | 9 | 1 | 3 | 6 | 1 | 155 |
| popcorn, white, air-popped | 1 cup | 31 | 1 | 6 | 1 | n/a | 0 | 0 | 0 |
| pork skin cracklins | 0.5 oz | 41 | 7 | 1 | 1 | 0 | 6 | 2 | 557 |
| pork skins, barbecue flavored | 0.5 oz | 76 | 8 | 0 | n/a | 0 | 5 | 2 | 378 |
| pork skins, plain | 0.5 oz | 77 | 9 | 0 | 0 | 0 | 4 | 2 | 261 |
| potato chips, baked | 1 cup | 56 | 1 | 9 | 1 | 1 | 2 | 0 | 110 |
| potato chips, barbecue flavor | 0.5 oz | 70 | 1 | 7 | 1 | n/a | 5 | 1 | 106 |
| potato chips, barbecue flavor, baked | 0.5 oz | 60 | 1 | 11 | 1 | 1 | 2 | 0 | 105 |
| potato chips, Cheddar cheese flavored, reduced-fat | 0.5 oz | 70 | 1 | 9 | 1 | 0 | 4 | 0 | 120 |
| potato chips, cheese and jalapeño flavored, reduced-fat | 0.5 oz | 75 | 1 | 9 | 1 | 1 | 4 | 1 | 175 |
| potato chips, fat-free | 0.5 oz | 54 | 1 | 12 | 1 | 1 | 0 | 0 | 91 |

| FOOD ITEM | SERVING SIZE | CALORIES | PRO (g) | CARB (g) | FIBER (g) | SUGAR (g) | FAT (g) | SAT FAT (g) | SOD (mg) |
|---|---|---|---|---|---|---|---|---|---|
| potato chips, honey barbecue flavored, reduced-fat | 0.5 oz | 70 | 1 | 10 | 1 | 1 | 3 | 0 | 125 |
| potato chips, light | 0.5 oz | 71 | 1 | 9 | 1 | 1 | 4 | 1 | 61 |
| potato chips, reduced-fat | 0.5 oz | 67 | 1 | 9 | 1 | 0 | 3 | 1 | 70 |
| potato chips, reduced-fat, unsalted | 0.5 oz | 69 | 1 | 10 | 1 | 0 | 3 | 1 | 1 |
| potato chips, rippled, reduced-fat | 0.5 oz | 70 | 1 | 9 | 1 | 0 | 3 | 0 | 55 |
| potato chips, sour cream and onion flavored | 0.5 oz | 75 | 1 | 7 | 1 | n/a | 5 | 1 | 89 |
| potato chips, unsalted | 0.5 oz | 76 | 1 | 8 | 1 | 0 | 5 | 2 | 1 |
| pretzel, hard | 1 | 23 | 1 | 5 | 0 | 0 | 0 | 0 | 81 |
| pretzel, hard, chocolate-coated | 1 | 50 | 1 | 8 | 0 | n/a | 2 | 1 | 63 |
| pretzel, hard, rods | 1 | 36 | 1 | 7 | 0 | 0 | 0 | 0 | 122 |
| pretzel, hard, tiny twist, fat-free | 0.5 oz | 50 | 2 | 12 | 1 | 1 | 0 | 0 | 210 |
| pretzel, hard, twist, unsalted | 1 | 23 | 1 | 5 | 0 | 0 | 0 | 0 | 17 |
| pretzel, hard, wheat-free | 0.5 oz | 65 | 0 | 10 | 0 | 0 | 3 | 0 | n/a |
| pretzel, hard, whole wheat | 0.5 oz | 51 | 2 | 12 | 1 | n/a | 0 | 0 | 29 |
| pretzel, hard, yogurt-covered | 1 | 19 | 0 | 3 | 0 | 0 | 1 | 1 | 36 |
| pretzel, soft | 1 small | 210 | 5 | 43 | 1 | 0 | 2 | 0 | 870 |
| pretzel, soft | 1 medium | 389 | 9 | 80 | 2 | 0 | 4 | 1 | 1615 |
| pretzel, soft | 1 large | 483 | 12 | 99 | 2 | 0 | 4 | 1 | 2008 |
| pretzel, soft, almond | 1 | 350 | 9 | 72 | 2 | 15 | 2 | 1 | 390 |
| pretzel, soft, almond, with butter | 1 | 400 | 9 | 72 | 2 | 15 | 8 | 5 | 400 |
| pretzel, soft, bagel-shaped, fat-free | 1 | 28 | 1 | 6 | 0 | 0 | 0 | 0 | 65 |
| pretzel, soft, cinnamon sugar | 1 | 350 | 9 | 74 | 2 | 16 | 2 | 0 | 410 |
| pretzel, soft, garlic | 1 | 320 | 9 | 66 | 2 | 9 | 1 | 0 | 830 |
| pretzel, soft, jalapeño | 1 | 270 | 8 | 58 | 2 | 8 | 1 | 0 | 780 |
| pretzel, soft, original | 1 | 391 | 12 | 83 | 3 | 12 | 1 | 0 | 1035 |
| pretzel, soft, Parmesan herb | 1 | 390 | 11 | 74 | 4 | 10 | 5 | 3 | 780 |
| pretzel, soft, sesame | 1 | 350 | 11 | 63 | 3 | 9 | 6 | 1 | 840 |

| FOOD ITEM | SERVING SIZE | CALORIES | PRO (g) | CARB (g) | FIBER (g) | SUGAR (g) | FAT (g) | SAT FAT (g) | SOD (mg) |
|---|---|---|---|---|---|---|---|---|---|
| pretzel, soft, sour cream and onion | 1 | 310 | 9 | 66 | 2 | 9 | 1 | 0 | 920 |
| pretzel, soft, whole wheat | 1 | 408 | 13 | 84 | 8 | 12 | 2 | 0 | 1283 |
| pretzel and cheese snacks | 1 oz | 103 | 3 | 12 | 0 | 1 | 4 | 2 | 391 |
| pretzel crackers | 1 oz | 104 | 3 | 21 | 1 | 1 | 1 | 0 | 406 |
| pretzel sticks, fat-free | 0.5 oz | 55 | 2 | 12 | 1 | 1 | 0 | 0 | 265 |
| pretzel thins, fat-free | 0.5 oz | 55 | 1 | 12 | 1 | 1 | 0 | 0 | 260 |
| rice cake, apple cinnamon | 1 mini | 8 | 0 | 2 | 0 | 1 | 0 | 0 | 7 |
| rice cake, banana nut | 1 | 50 | 1 | 11 | 0 | 5 | 0 | 0 | 44 |
| rice cake, banana nut | 1 mini | 11 | 0 | 2 | 0 | 1 | 0 | 0 | 8 |
| rice cake, brown rice, buckwheat, with salt | 1 | 34 | 1 | 7 | 0 | 0 | 0 | 0 | 10 |
| rice cake, brown rice, buckwheat, without salt | 1 | 34 | 1 | 7 | 0 | 0 | 0 | 0 | 0 |
| rice cake, brown rice, multigrain | 1 | 35 | 1 | 7 | 0 | 0 | 0 | 0 | 23 |
| rice cake, brown rice, multigrain, without salt | 1 | 35 | 1 | 7 | 0 | 0 | 0 | 0 | 0 |
| rice cake, brown rice, plain, with salt | 1 | 35 | 1 | 7 | 0 | 0 | 0 | 0 | 39 |
| rice cake, brown rice, plain, without salt | 1 | 35 | 1 | 7 | 0 | 0 | 0 | 0 | 2 |
| rice cake, brown rice, rye | 1 | 35 | 1 | 7 | 0 | 0 | 0 | 0 | 10 |
| rice cake, brown rice, sesame seed, with salt | 1 | 35 | 1 | 7 | 0 | 0 | 0 | 0 | 20 |
| rice cake, brown rice, sesame seed, without salt | 1 | 35 | 1 | 7 | 0 | 0 | 0 | 0 | 0 |
| rice cake, brown rice and corn | 1 | 35 | 1 | 7 | 0 | 0 | 0 | 0 | 26 |
| rice cake, caramel corn | 1 mini | 13 | 0 | 3 | 0 | 1 | 0 | 0 | 14 |
| rice cake, Cheddar | 1 mini | 8 | 0 | 1 | 0 | 0 | 0 | 0 | 23 |
| rice cake, cheese and coconut | 0.5 oz | 32 | 0 | 7 | n/a | n/a | 0 | n/a | n/a |
| rice cake, chocolate crunch | 1 | 61 | 1 | 12 | 0 | 4 | 1 | 0 | 34 |
| rice cake, chocolate crunch | 1 mini | 13 | 0 | 3 | 0 | 1 | 0 | 0 | 7 |
| rice cake, cinnamon streusel | 1 | 57 | 1 | 12 | 0 | 4 | 1 | 0 | 22 |
| rice cake, double sesame | 1 | 25 | 1 | 5 | 0 | 1 | 0 | 0 | 43 |
| rice cake, garlic sesame | 1 | 25 | 1 | 5 | 0 | 0 | 0 | 0 | 43 |

| FOOD ITEM | SERVING SIZE | CALORIES | PRO (g) | CARB (g) | FIBER (g) | SUGAR (g) | FAT (g) | SAT FAT (g) | SOD (mg) |
|---|---|---|---|---|---|---|---|---|---|
| rice cake, honey nut | 1 | 80 | 2 | 18 | 1 | 2 | 1 | 0 | 2 |
| rice cake, honey nut | 1 mini | 8 | 0 | 2 | 0 | 1 | 0 | 0 | 11 |
| rice cake, lemon sesame | 1 | 81 | 2 | 17 | 1 | 0 | 1 | 0 | 23 |
| rice cake, lemon sesame, organic | 1 | 83 | 2 | 18 | 1 | 0 | 1 | 0 | 24 |
| rice cake, multigrain | 1 | 65 | 2 | 15 | 1 | 0 | 0 | 0 | 22 |
| rice cake, peanut butter | 1 | 61 | 1 | 12 | 0 | 5 | 1 | 0 | 61 |
| rice cake, popcorn, organic | 1 | 70 | 1 | 16 | n/a | n/a | 0 | 0 | 55 |
| rice cake, seaweed, organic | 1 | 80 | 2 | 17 | 1 | 1 | 0 | 0 | 95 |
| rice cake, sesame tamari, organic | 1 | 78 | 2 | 16 | 2 | 0 | 1 | 0 | 125 |
| rice cake, teriyaki sesame | 1 | 25 | 1 | 5 | 0 | 1 | 0 | 0 | 23 |
| rice cake, toasted sesame | 1 | 78 | 2 | 17 | 2 | 0 | 1 | 0 | 70 |
| rice cake, unsalted | 1 mini | 8 | 0 | 2 | 0 | n/a | 0 | 0 | 1 |
| rice cake, white Cheddar | 1 mini | 10 | 0 | 2 | 0 | 0 | 0 | 0 | 34 |
| sesame stick, baked | 1 ea | 9 | 0 | 1 | 0 | 0 | 0 | 0 | 25 |
| sesame stick, honey roasted | 0.5 oz | 80 | 1 | 7 | 1 | 1 | 5 | 1 | 165 |
| sesame stick, wheat, with salt | 0.5 oz | 77 | 2 | 7 | 0 | 0 | 5 | 1 | 211 |
| sesame stick, wheat, without salt | 0.5 oz | 77 | 2 | 7 | n/a | n/a | 5 | 1 | 4 |
| taro chips | 0.5 oz | 71 | 0 | 10 | 1 | 1 | 4 | 1 | 48 |
| taro chips, spiced | 0.5 oz | 65 | 1 | 10 | 1 | 1 | 3 | 0 | 85 |
| taro chips, sweet potato | 0.5 oz | 70 | 1 | 9 | 2 | 1 | 4 | 1 | 35 |
| tortilla chips, baked, light | 0.5 oz | 66 | 1 | 10 | 1 | 0 | 2 | 0 | 142 |
| tortilla chips, baked, low-fat | 0.5 oz | 59 | 2 | 11 | 1 | 0 | 1 | 0 | 59 |
| tortilla chips, baked, without salt | 0.5 oz | 55 | 2 | 12 | 1 | 0 | 1 | 0 | 0 |
| tortilla chips, low-fat, without salt | 0.5 oz | 59 | 2 | 11 | 1 | 0 | 1 | 0 | 2 |
| tortilla chips, nacho, reduced-fat | 0.5 oz | 63 | 1 | 10 | 1 | n/a | 2 | 0 | 142 |
| trail mix | 0.5 oz | 65 | 2 | 6 | 1 | n/a | 4 | 1 | 32 |
| wasabi peas, Trader Joe's | ⅓ cup | 80 | 1 | 12 | 1 | 4 | 3 | 1 | 190 |

# SOUPS, SAUCES, AND GRAVIES

| FOOD ITEM | SERVING SIZE | CALORIES | PRO (g) | CARB (g) | FIBER (g) | SUGAR (g) | FAT (g) | SAT FAT (g) | SOD (mg) |
|---|---|---|---|---|---|---|---|---|---|
| gravy, au jus | 2 tbsp | 5 | 0 | 1 | 0 | n/a | n/a | 0 | 0 |
| gravy, beef | 1 tbsp | 13 | 0 | 1 | 0 | n/a | 1 | 0 | 97 |
| gravy, biscuit | 1 tbsp | 77 | 0 | 9 | 0 | 0 | 5 | 0 | 247 |
| gravy, chicken | 1 tbsp | 12 | 1 | 1 | n/a | n/a | 1 | 0 | 85 |
| gravy, mushroom | 1 tbsp | 7 | 0 | 1 | 0 | n/a | 0 | 0 | 85 |
| gravy, pork | 1 tbsp | 10 | 0 | 1 | 0 | 0 | 1 | 0 | 80 |
| gravy, sausage | 1 tbsp | 24 | 1 | 1 | 0 | n/a | 2 | 1 | 51 |
| gravy, Southern | 1 tbsp | 68 | n/a | 9 | 0 | 1 | 4 | 1 | 411 |
| gravy, turkey | 1 tbsp | 8 | 1 | 1 | 0 | 0 | 0 | 0 | 86 |
| sauce, aioli | 2 tbsp | 114 | 0 | 8 | 0 | 2 | 10 | 2 | 210 |
| sauce, Alfredo | 2 tbsp | 55 | 1 | 1 | 0 | 0 | 5 | 2 | 200 |
| sauce, barbecue | 2 tbsp | 24 | 0 | 4 | 0 | 2 | 0 | 0 | 254 |
| sauce, basil pesto, Melissa's | 2 tbsp | 170 | 3 | 2 | 0 | 1 | 17 | 3 | 115 |
| sauce, béarnaise | 2 tbsp | 78 | 0 | 0 | 0 | 0 | 8 | 4 | 112 |
| sauce, béchamel | 2 tbsp | 35 | 0 | 2 | 0 | 0 | 3 | 2 | 287 |
| sauce, cheese | 2 tbsp | 60 | 3 | 2 | 0 | n/a | 5 | 2 | 150 |
| sauce, chili | 1 tbsp | 20 | 0 | 5 | 0 | 4 | 0 | 0 | 480 |
| sauce, Creole | 1 tbsp | 6 | 0 | 1 | n/a | n/a | n/a | n/a | 85 |
| sauce, curry | 1 tbsp | 9 | 0 | 0 | 0 | 0 | 1 | 0 | 49 |
| sauce, enchilada | 1 tbsp | 5 | 0 | 1 | 0 | 0 | 0 | n/a | 99 |
| sauce, green chile | 1 tbsp | 30 | 1 | 7 | 0 | 5 | 0 | 0 | 190 |
| sauce, hoisin | 1 tbsp | 35 | 1 | 7 | 0 | 4 | 1 | 0 | 258 |
| sauce, hollandaise | 1 tbsp | 43 | 1 | 0 | n/a | n/a | 5 | 3 | 39 |
| sauce, marinara | 1 tbsp | 9 | 0 | 1 | 0 | 0 | 0 | 0 | 64 |
| sauce, mole poblano | 1 tbsp | 25 | 1 | 2 | 1 | n/a | 2 | 0 | 20 |
| sauce, mole verde | 1 tbsp | 15 | 1 | 1 | 0 | n/a | 1 | 0 | 48 |
| sauce, mushroom | 1 tbsp | 14 | 0 | 2 | 0 | 2 | 1 | 0 | 65 |
| sauce, nacho | 1 tbsp | 28 | 1 | 1 | 0 | 0 | 2 | 1 | 155 |
| sauce, oyster | 1 tbsp | 5 | 0 | 0 | 1 | 0 | 0 | 0 | 109 |

| FOOD ITEM | SERVING SIZE | CALORIES | PRO (g) | CARB (g) | FIBER (g) | SUGAR (g) | FAT (g) | SAT FAT (g) | SOD (mg) |
|---|---|---|---|---|---|---|---|---|---|
| sauce, pasta, Amy's Organic Family Marinara Pasta Sauce | ½ cup | 80 | 1 | 10 | 3 | 5 | 3 | 0.5 | 590 |
| sauce, pasta, Amy's Organic Garlic Mushroom Pasta Sauce | ½ cup | 120 | 3 | 10 | 3 | 5 | 7 | 2.5 | 680 |
| sauce, pasta, Amy's Organic Low Sodium Marinara Sauce | ½ cup | 40 | 1 | 7 | 1 | 5 | 1 | 0 | 100 |
| sauce, pasta, Amy's Organic Roasted Garlic Pasta Sauce | ½ cup | 130 | 2 | 13 | 3 | 5 | 8 | 1 | 470 |
| sauce, pasta, Amy's Organic Tomato Basil Pasta Sauce | ½ cup | 110 | 2 | 11 | 3 | 6 | 6 | 1 | 580 |
| sauce, pasta, with meat | 1 tbsp | 18 | 1 | 3 | 0 | 2 | 1 | 0 | 66 |
| sauce, pepper | 1 tbsp | 2 | 0 | 0 | 0 | 0 | 0 | 0 | 373 |
| sauce, plum | 1 tbsp | 35 | 0 | 8 | 0 | 0 | 0 | 0 | 103 |
| sauce, puttanesca, Amy's Puttanesca Sauce | ½ cup | 45 | 2 | 6 | 1 | 3 | 2 | 0 | 680 |
| sauce, sofrito | 1 tbsp | 35 | 2 | 1 | 0 | 0 | 3 | 0 | 171 |
| sauce, sour cream | 1 tbsp | 73 | 2 | 7 | n/a | n/a | 4 | 2 | 179 |
| sauce, spaghetti | 1 tbsp | 6 | 0 | 1 | 0 | 1 | 0 | 0 | 49 |
| sauce, spaghetti, sugar-free | 1 tbsp | 8 | 0 | 1 | 0 | 0 | 0 | 0 | 48 |
| sauce, stir-fry, Melissa's | 1 tbsp | 25 | 0 | 6 | 0 | 0 | 0 | 0 | 720 |
| sauce, stroganoff | 1 tbsp | 50 | 2 | 8 | 0 | 0 | 1 | 1 | 574 |
| sauce, sweet and sour | 1 tbsp | 15 | 0 | 4 | 0 | 3 | 0 | 0 | 50 |
| sauce, taco, green | 1 tbsp | 5 | 0 | 1 | 0 | 0 | 0 | 0 | 96 |
| sauce, taco, red | 1 tbsp | 7 | 0 | 1 | 0 | 1 | 0 | 0 | 103 |
| sauce, tamari | 1 tbsp | 10 | 2 | 0 | 0 | 0 | 0 | 0 | 920 |
| sauce, teriyaki | 1 tbsp | 15 | 1 | 3 | 0 | 2 | 0 | 0 | 689 |
| sauce, tomato, with salt | ½ cup | 39 | 2 | 9 | 2 | 5 | 0 | 0 | 642 |
| sauce, tomato, without salt | ½ cup | 37 | 2 | 9 | 2 | n/a | 0 | 0 | 13 |
| sauce, tomato-chili | 1 tbsp | 18 | 0 | 3 | 1 | 2 | 0 | 0 | 228 |
| sauce, white | 1 tbsp | 27 | 1 | 1 | 0 | 0 | 2 | 1 | 78 |
| soup, bean and bacon | 1 cup | 158 | 9 | 24 | 6 | n/a | 3 | 1 | 994 |
| soup, bean and ham, low-sodium | 1 cup | 99 | 5 | 18 | 4 | 5 | 1 | 0 | 310 |

| FOOD ITEM | SERVING SIZE | CALORIES | PRO (g) | CARB (g) | FIBER (g) | SUGAR (g) | FAT (g) | SAT FAT (g) | SOD (mg) |
|---|---|---|---|---|---|---|---|---|---|
| soup, bean and pork | 1 cup | 183 | 8 | 24 | 8 | 4 | 6 | 2 | 1005 |
| soup, beef and country vegetable | 1 cup | 143 | 12 | 15 | n/a | n/a | 4 | 1 | 810 |
| soup, beef and mushroom | 1 cup | 100 | 6 | 12 | n/a | 4 | 2 | n/a | n/a |
| soup, beef and mushroom, low-sodium | 1 cup | 173 | 11 | 19 | 1 | n/a | 6 | 4 | 63 |
| soup, beef and onion | 1 cup | 89 | 2 | 17 | 1 | 2 | 2 | 1 | 2150 |
| soup, beef and vegetable | 1 cup | 120 | 9 | 17 | n/a | n/a | 2 | 1 | 1259 |
| soup, beef barley | 1 cup | 90 | 7 | 15 | 0 | 0 | 1 | 0 | 970 |
| soup, beef broth | 1 cup | 17 | 3 | 0 | 0 | 0 | 1 | 0 | 782 |
| soup, beef broth, 99% fat-free | 1 cup | 15 | 3 | 0 | 0 | 0 | 0 | 0 | 450 |
| soup, beef broth, fat-free | 1 cup | 10 | 2 | 0 | 0 | 0 | 0 | 0 | 120 |
| soup, beef broth, low-sodium | 1 cup | 38 | 5 | 1 | 0 | 1 | 1 | 0 | 72 |
| soup, beef noodle | 1 cup | 34 | 2 | 6 | 1 | n/a | 1 | 0 | 1035 |
| soup, beef stroganoff | 1 cup | 173 | 9 | 16 | 2 | 2 | 9 | 3 | 659 |
| soup, black bean | ½ cup | 90 | 5 | 13 | 8 | 2 | 2 | 1 | 580 |
| soup, black bean, low-fat, organic | ½ cup | 70 | 4 | 13 | 3 | 4 | 1 | 0 | 290 |
| soup, borscht | 1 cup | 78 | 3 | 8 | 2 | n/a | 4 | 2 | 496 |
| soup, broccoli-cheese | 1 cup | 180 | 6 | 12 | n/a | n/a | 12 | 4 | 910 |
| soup, cauliflower | 1 cup | 68 | 3 | 11 | n/a | n/a | 2 | 0 | 841 |
| soup, cheese | 1 cup | 231 | 9 | 16 | 1 | n/a | 15 | 9 | 1020 |
| soup, chicken and wild rice | 1 cup | 190 | 6 | 17 | 2 | 3 | 11 | 5 | 990 |
| soup, chicken broth | 1 cup | 15 | 1 | 0 | 0 | 0 | 1 | 0 | 930 |
| soup, chicken broth, fat-free | 1 cup | 25 | 6 | 0 | 0 | 0 | 0 | 0 | 390 |
| soup, chicken broth, low-fat, organic | 1 cup | 25 | 2 | 2 | 0 | 1 | 1 | 1 | 440 |
| soup, chicken broth, low-sodium | 1 cup | 38 | 5 | 3 | 0 | 0 | 1 | 0 | 72 |
| soup, chicken corn chowder | 1 cup | 225 | 7 | 17 | 2 | n/a | 14 | 4 | 678 |
| soup, chicken ham noodle | 1 cup | 112 | 14 | 6 | 0 | n/a | 3 | 1 | 747 |
| soup, chicken mushroom chowder | 1 cup | 192 | 7 | 17 | 3 | n/a | 11 | 3 | 814 |

| FOOD ITEM | SERVING SIZE | CALORIES | PRO (g) | CARB (g) | FIBER (g) | SUGAR (g) | FAT (g) | SAT FAT (g) | SOD (mg) |
|---|---|---|---|---|---|---|---|---|---|
| soup, chicken mushroom, chunky | 1 cup | 122 | 4 | 9 | 0 | n/a | 9 | 2 | 875 |
| soup, chicken noodle | 1 cup | 80 | 6 | 12 | 0 | 0 | 2 | 0 | 890 |
| soup, chicken noodle, chunky | 1 cup | 114 | 8 | 14 | n/a | n/a | 3 | 1 | 875 |
| soup, chicken noodle, low-sodium | 1 cup | 76 | 4 | 11 | 1 | 0 | 2 | 1 | 426 |
| soup, chicken rice | 1 cup | 100 | 6 | 17 | 2 | 2 | 1 | 1 | 990 |
| soup, chicken rice, low-fat | 1 cup | 130 | 8 | 21 | 2 | 4 | 2 | 0 | 390 |
| soup, chicken vegetable | 1 cup | 70 | 3 | 8 | 1 | 1 | 3 | 1 | 889 |
| soup, chicken vegetable, low-sodium | 1 cup | 166 | 12 | 19 | 1 | 2 | 5 | 1 | 84 |
| soup, chicken vegetable, reduced-fat | 1 cup | 96 | 6 | 15 | n/a | n/a | 1 | 0 | 461 |
| soup, chicken with dumplings | 1 cup | 91 | 5 | 6 | 0 | 1 | 5 | 1 | 810 |
| soup, chicken with stars, fat-free | 1 cup | 45 | 3 | 8 | 1 | 0 | 0 | 0 | 713 |
| soup, chicken wild rice | 1 cup | 190 | 6 | 17 | 2 | 3 | 11 | 5 | 990 |
| soup, chili, beef | 1 cup | 183 | 7 | 23 | 10 | 2 | 7 | 4 | 1117 |
| soup, clam chowder, Manhattan-style | 1 cup | 78 | 2 | 12 | 1 | 1 | 2 | 0 | 578 |
| soup, clam chowder, New England–style | 1 cup | 190 | 6 | 20 | 1 | 3 | 10 | 3 | 920 |
| soup, clam chowder, New England–style, reduced-fat | 1 cup | 110 | 6 | 19 | 2 | 2 | 2 | 1 | 860 |
| soup, consommé, beef | 1 cup | 29 | 5 | 2 | 0 | n/a | 0 | 0 | 636 |
| soup, corn chowder, Amy's, organic | 1 cup | 190 | 3 | 25 | 3 | 4 | 10 | 5 | 580 |
| soup, crab | 1 cup | 76 | 5 | 10 | 1 | n/a | 2 | 0 | 1235 |
| soup, crab bisque | ½ cup | 130 | 11 | 6 | 0 | n/a | 6 | 2 | 321 |
| soup, cream of asparagus | 1 cup | 98 | 3 | 12 | 1 | 1 | 5 | 1 | 1108 |
| soup, cream of broccoli, reduced-fat | 1 cup | 70 | 2 | 14 | 2 | 3 | 1 | 1 | 813 |
| soup, cream of celery | 1 cup | 82 | 2 | 8 | 1 | 2 | 5 | 1 | 858 |
| soup, cream of celery, 98% fat-free | ½ cup | 60 | 1 | 8 | 1 | 1 | 3 | 1 | 780 |
| soup, cream of chicken | 1 cup | 101 | 3 | 8 | 0 | 1 | 7 | 2 | 743 |
| soup, cream of chicken, reduced-sodium | 1 cup | 66 | 2 | 11 | 0 | 0 | 2 | 1 | 405 |

| FOOD ITEM | SERVING SIZE | CALORIES | PRO (g) | CARB (g) | FIBER (g) | SUGAR (g) | FAT (g) | SAT FAT (g) | SOD (mg) |
|---|---|---|---|---|---|---|---|---|---|
| soup, cream of chicken with rice | 1 cup | 90 | 3 | 14 | 0 | 3 | 3 | 2 | 860 |
| soup, cream of Mexican pepper pot | 1 cup | 101 | 2 | 9 | 2 | 1 | 6 | 2 | 786 |
| soup, cream of mushroom | 1 cup | 96 | 2 | 8 | 0 | 2 | 7 | 2 | 731 |
| soup, cream of mushroom, Amy's, organic | ¾ cup | 140 | 3 | 13 | 2 | 3 | 9 | 2 | 590 |
| soup, cream of mushroom, low-sodium | 1 cup | 120 | 2 | 9 | 0 | 1 | 8 | 2 | 45 |
| soup, cream of onion | 1 cup | 100 | 2 | 12 | 0 | 4 | 5 | 1 | 862 |
| soup, cream of potato | 1 cup | 68 | 2 | 11 | 0 | n/a | 2 | 1 | 930 |
| soup, cream of shrimp | 1 cup | 96 | 2 | 8 | 0 | 2 | 7 | 2 | 731 |
| soup, cream of tomato | 1 cup | 130 | 3 | 26 | 2 | 18 | 2 | 1 | 760 |
| soup, cream of tomato, Amy's, organic | 1 cup | 100 | 2 | 17 | 3 | 11 | 2 | 2 | 690 |
| soup, cream of tomato, low-sodium | 1 cup | 85 | 2 | 18 | 0 | 7 | 2 | 0 | 49 |
| soup, cream of vegetable | 1 cup | 107 | 2 | 12 | 1 | 0 | 6 | 1 | 1170 |
| soup, escarole | 1 cup | 25 | 1 | 3 | 1 | 1 | 1 | 0 | 930 |
| soup, fiesta herb | 1 cup | 91 | 3 | 18 | 1 | 2 | 1 | 0 | 1761 |
| soup, French onion | 1 cup | 43 | 2 | 6 | 1 | 4 | 1 | 0 | 856 |
| soup, gazpacho | 1 cup | 43 | 7 | 4 | 0 | 2 | 0 | 0 | 687 |
| soup, green pea | 1 cup | 165 | 9 | 27 | 5 | 8 | 3 | 1 | 918 |
| soup, leek | 1 cup | 70 | 2 | 10 | 0 | 2 | 3 | 1 | 850 |
| soup, lentil, Amy's, organic | 1 cup | 150 | 8 | 19 | 9 | 3 | 5 | 1 | 590 |
| soup, lentil, fat-free | ½ cup | 55 | 5 | 13 | 5 | 3 | 0 | 0 | 225 |
| soup, lentil, low-fat, organic | ½ cup | 55 | 4 | 11 | 4 | 2 | 1 | 0 | 280 |
| soup, lentil, vegetarian, Amy's, organic | ½ cup | 75 | 4 | 19 | 5 | 2 | 2 | 0 | 295 |
| soup, lentil vegetable, Amy's, organic | 1 cup | 150 | 7 | 23 | 6 | 5 | 4 | 1 | 680 |
| soup, lobster bisque | ½ cup | 126 | 10 | 6 | 0 | n/a | 7 | 2 | 225 |
| soup, lobster gumbo | ½ cup | 89 | 5 | 10 | 1 | n/a | 4 | 1 | 221 |
| soup, minestrone | 1 cup | 120 | 5 | 22 | 4 | 4 | 2 | 0 | 1050 |
| soup, minestrone, Amy's, organic | 1 cup | 90 | 3 | 17 | 3 | 5 | 2 | 0 | 580 |

| FOOD ITEM | SERVING SIZE | CALORIES | PRO (g) | CARB (g) | FIBER (g) | SUGAR (g) | FAT (g) | SAT FAT (g) | SOD (mg) |
|---|---|---|---|---|---|---|---|---|---|
| soup, minestrone, Amy's, organic, reduced-sodium | 1 cup | 90 | 3 | 17 | 3 | 5 | 2 | 0 | 290 |
| soup, miso with tofu | 1 cup | 220 | 10 | 42 | 0 | 2 | 2 | 0 | 1380 |
| soup, mushroom | 1 cup | 96 | 2 | 11 | 1 | 0 | 5 | 1 | 1020 |
| soup, mushroom barley | 1 cup | 73 | 2 | 12 | 1 | n/a | 2 | 0 | 891 |
| soup, mushroom with beef stock | 1 cup | 73 | 6 | 6 | 0 | n/a | 3 | 1 | 942 |
| soup, onion mushroom | 1 cup | 25 | 0 | 6 | 1 | 1 | 0 | 0 | 480 |
| soup, pasta and three bean, Amy's, organic | 1 cup | 130 | 5 | 19 | 4 | 6 | 5 | 1 | 680 |
| soup, oxtail | 1 cup | 71 | 3 | 9 | 1 | 3 | 3 | 1 | 1210 |
| soup, oyster stew | 1 cup | 135 | 6 | 10 | 0 | n/a | 8 | 5 | 1041 |
| soup, pepper pot | 1 cup | 98 | 6 | 9 | 0 | 1 | 4 | 2 | 914 |
| soup, potato-ham chowder | 1 cup | 192 | 6 | 13 | 1 | n/a | 12 | 4 | 874 |
| soup, potato leek, Amy's, organic | 1 cup | 180 | 2 | 21 | 2 | 2 | 10 | 6 | 580 |
| soup, ramen, Cup of Noodles | 1 package | 140 | 8 | 26 | 4 | 4 | 1 | 0 | 540 |
| soup, savory herb with garlic | 1 cup | 98 | 3 | 19 | 1 | 2 | 1 | 0 | 1502 |
| soup, scotch broth | 1 cup | 75 | 5 | 9 | 1 | 1 | 2 | 1 | 953 |
| soup, shark fin | 1 cup | 99 | 7 | 8 | 0 | n/a | 4 | 1 | 1082 |
| soup, shrimp gumbo | 4 oz | 79 | 5 | 9 | 1 | n/a | 3 | 1 | 160 |
| soup, split pea, Amy's, organic | 1 cup | 100 | 7 | 19 | 4 | 4 | 0 | 0 | 570 |
| soup, split pea, fat-free, organic | ½ cup | 50 | 4 | 10 | 2 | 2 | 0 | 0 | 285 |
| soup, sweet and sour | 1 cup | 72 | 3 | 14 | 2 | n/a | 1 | 0 | 1292 |
| soup, tomato | 1 cup | 161 | 6 | 22 | 3 | 15 | 6 | 3 | 744 |
| soup, tomato beef | 1 cup | 127 | 4 | 19 | 1 | n/a | 4 | 1 | 829 |
| soup, tomato bisque | 1 cup | 179 | 6 | 27 | 0 | n/a | 6 | 3 | 1002 |
| soup, tomato bisque, chunky, Amy's, organic | 1 cup | 120 | 2 | 21 | 2 | 14 | 3 | 2 | 680 |
| soup, tomato garden | 1 cup | 51 | 2 | 9 | 2 | 3 | 1 | 0 | 222 |
| soup, tomato rice | 1 cup | 100 | 1 | 21 | 1 | 9 | 2 | 0 | 700 |
| soup, turkey, chunky | 1 cup | 65 | 5 | 7 | n/a | n/a | 2 | 1 | 443 |

| FOOD ITEM | SERVING SIZE | CALORIES | PRO (g) | CARB (g) | FIBER (g) | SUGAR (g) | FAT (g) | SAT FAT (g) | SOD (mg) |
|---|---|---|---|---|---|---|---|---|---|
| soup, turkey noodle | 1 cup | 64 | 4 | 8 | 1 | n/a | 2 | 1 | 758 |
| soup, turkey vegetable | 1 cup | 68 | 3 | 8 | 0 | n/a | 3 | 1 | 853 |
| soup, vegetable | 1 cup | 70 | 3 | 8 | 1 | 1 | 3 | 1 | 889 |
| soup, vegetable, chunky, Amy's, organic | 1 cup | 60 | 3 | 13 | 3 | 5 | 0 | 0 | 680 |
| soup, vegetable, vegetarian | 1 cup | 62 | 2 | 12 | 3 | 4 | 1 | 0 | 886 |
| soup, vegetable barley, Amy's, organic | 1 cup | 70 | 2 | 13 | 3 | 5 | 1 | 0 | 580 |
| soup, vegetable beef | 1 cup | 78 | 6 | 10 | 0 | 1 | 2 | 1 | 791 |
| soup, vegetable chicken | 1 cup | 50 | 3 | 8 | n/a | n/a | 1 | 0 | 807 |

## SOY FOODS

| FOOD ITEM | SERVING SIZE | CALORIES | PRO (g) | CARB (g) | FIBER (g) | SUGAR (g) | FAT (g) | SAT FAT (g) | SOD (mg) |
|---|---|---|---|---|---|---|---|---|---|
| cheese, Chedarella | 1 oz | 110 | 7 | 0 | 0 | 0 | 9 | 6 | 190 |
| cheese, soy | 1 oz | 8 | 1 | 1 | n/a | n/a | 0 | n/a | n/a |
| cheese, soy, American | 1 oz | 50 | 6 | 0 | 0 | 0 | 3 | 0 | 411 |
| cheese, soy, Cheddar | 1 oz | 50 | 6 | 1 | 1 | 0 | 3 | 0 | 397 |
| cheese, soy, Cheddar, Good Shreds | 1 oz | 61 | 7 | 0 | 0 | 0 | 3 | 0 | 334 |
| cheese, soy, Cheddar, Melissa's, shredded | 1 oz | 63 | 7 | 2 | 1 | 0 | 0 | 0 | 190 |
| cheese, soy, chunk, Melissa's | 1 oz | 63 | 7 | 2 | 1 | 0 | 3 | 0 | 190 |
| cheese, soy, cottage | 4 oz | 171 | 14 | 8 | 0 | 2 | 9 | 1 | 23 |
| cheese, soy, jalapeño jack | 1 oz | 50 | 6 | 0 | 0 | 0 | 3 | 0 | 354 |
| cheese, soy, mozzarella | 1 oz | 42 | 6 | 0 | 0 | 0 | 3 | 0 | 383 |
| cheese, soy, mozzarella, Good Shreds | 1 oz | 61 | 7 | 1 | 0 | 0 | 3 | 0 | n/a |
| cheese, soy, mozzarella, Melissa's, shredded | 1 oz | 63 | 7 | 2 | 1 | 0 | 3 | 0 | 190 |
| cheese, soy, slices, Melissa's | 1 slice (⅔ oz) | 45 | 3 | 3 | 0 | 0 | 2 | 0 | 180 |
| cheese, soy, Swiss | 1 oz | 50 | 6 | 1 | 0 | 0 | 3 | 0 | n/a |
| creamer, soy, French vanilla | 1 tbsp | 20 | 0 | 3 | 0 | 3 | 1 | 0 | 5 |
| creamer, soy, hazelnut | 1 tbsp | 16 | 0 | 1 | 0 | 0 | 1 | 0 | 5 |

| FOOD ITEM | SERVING SIZE | CALORIES | PRO (g) | CARB (g) | FIBER (g) | SUGAR (g) | FAT (g) | SAT FAT (g) | SOD (mg) |
|---|---|---|---|---|---|---|---|---|---|
| creamer, soy, plain | 1 tbsp | 15 | 0 | 1 | 0 | 0 | 1 | 0 | 5 |
| creamer, soy blend | 1 tbsp | 79 | 1 | 9 | 0 | 1 | 5 | 1 | 26 |
| miso | 1 tbsp | 34 | 2 | 5 | 1 | 1 | 1 | 0 | 640 |
| miso, brown | 1 tbsp | 30 | 3 | 3 | 0 | 0 | 0 | 0 | 750 |
| miso, dark red | 1 tbsp | 27 | 2 | 3 | 0 | 2 | 1 | 0 | 740 |
| miso paste, barley | 1 tbsp | 30 | 3 | 3 | 0 | 0 | 0 | 0 | 300 |
| miso paste, brown | 1 tbsp | 30 | 3 | 6 | 3 | 3 | 0 | 0 | 660 |
| miso paste, light yellow | 1 tbsp | 27 | 2 | 3 | 0 | 2 | 1 | 0 | 740 |
| miso paste, mellow yellow | 1 tbsp | 24 | 1 | 4 | 1 | 2 | 0 | 0 | 353 |
| miso paste, white | 1 tbsp | 33 | 1 | 6 | 0 | 3 | 0 | 0 | 467 |
| miso sauce | 1 tbsp | 24 | 1 | 5 | 0 | n/a | 0 | 0 | 254 |
| pasta, soy, elbow | 1 oz | 107 | 13 | 9 | 4 | 2 | 2 | 1 | 102 |
| pasta, soy, penne | 1 oz | 102 | 14 | 9 | 4 | 2 | 2 | 1 | 102 |
| pasta, soy, rotini | 1 oz | 104 | 13 | 9 | 4 | 2 | 2 | 1 | 103 |
| seitan, barbecue | 4 oz | 160 | 24 | 12 | 0 | 3 | 2 | 1 | 360 |
| seitan, teriyaki | 4 oz | 160 | 26 | 10 | 0 | 0 | 2 | 1 | 320 |
| sour cream, soy | 1 tbsp | 20 | 1 | 2 | n/a | n/a | 2 | 0 | 25 |
| tempeh | 4 oz | 219 | 21 | 11 | n/a | n/a | 12 | 3 | 10 |
| tempeh, bacon | 3 oz | 120 | 12 | 9 | 1 | 0 | 4 | 1 | 343 |
| tempeh, barbecue burger | 3 oz | 131 | 11 | 12 | 0 | 3 | 4 | 2 | 196 |
| tempeh, cooked | 4 oz | 222 | 21 | 11 | n/a | n/a | 13 | 4 | 16 |
| tempeh, garden vegetable | 4 oz | 142 | 18 | 9 | 7 | 0 | 4 | 1 | 125 |
| tempeh, tamari grilled vegetable burger | 3 oz | 131 | 12 | 10 | 0 | 2 | 5 | 2 | 284 |
| tempeh, 3-grain | 4 oz | 190 | 12 | 25 | 6 | 2 | 4 | 2 | 17 |
| tempeh, wild rice | 4 oz | 190 | 12 | 25 | 7 | 1 | 4 | 1 | 20 |
| tofu, extra-firm, nigari | 4 oz | 73 | 11 | 2 | 0 | 1 | 7 | 1 | 9 |
| tofu, salted and fermented | 4 oz | 131 | 9 | 6 | 0 | n/a | 9 | 1 | 3258 |
| tofu, silken, extra-firm | 4 oz | 43 | 8 | 1 | 0 | 1 | 1 | 0 | 111 |
| tofu, silken, firm | 4 oz | 70 | 8 | 3 | 0 | 3 | 3 | 0 | 41 |
| tofu, silken, firm, enriched | 4 oz | 95 | 8 | 8 | 4 | 0 | 3 | 0 | 54 |

| FOOD ITEM | SERVING SIZE | CALORIES | PRO (g) | CARB (g) | FIBER (g) | SUGAR (g) | FAT (g) | SAT FAT (g) | SOD (mg) |
|---|---|---|---|---|---|---|---|---|---|
| tofu, silken, firm, light | 4 oz | 42 | 7 | 1 | 0 | 1 | 1 | 0 | 96 |
| tofu, silken, firm, organic | 4 oz | 81 | 8 | 3 | 0 | 0 | 3 | 0 | 54 |
| tofu, silken, soft | 4 oz | 63 | 5 | 3 | 0 | 1 | 3 | 0 | 6 |
| yogurt, soy, apricot-mango | 6 oz | 160 | 4 | 30 | 1 | 20 | 2 | 0 | 20 |
| yogurt, soy, banana-strawberry | 6 oz | 160 | 4 | 30 | 1 | 20 | 2 | 0 | 20 |
| yogurt, soy, black cherry | 6 oz | 160 | 4 | 30 | 1 | 20 | 2 | 0 | 20 |
| yogurt, soy, blueberry | 6 oz | 160 | 4 | 30 | 1 | 20 | 2 | 0 | 20 |
| yogurt, soy, key lime | 6 oz | 170 | 4 | 30 | 1 | 21 | 2 | 0 | 20 |
| yogurt, soy, lemon | 6 oz | 160 | 4 | 31 | 1 | 22 | 2 | 0 | 20 |
| yogurt, soy, lemon-kiwi | 6 oz | 150 | 4 | 29 | 1 | 21 | 2 | 0 | 20 |
| yogurt, soy, mixed berry | 6 oz | 160 | 4 | 31 | 1 | 21 | 2 | 0 | 20 |
| yogurt, soy, peach | 6 oz | 170 | 4 | 32 | 1 | 25 | 2 | 0 | 20 |
| yogurt, soy, plain | 6 oz | 90 | 4 | 17 | 1 | 9 | 2 | 0 | 23 |
| yogurt, soy, raspberry | 6 oz | 160 | 4 | 30 | 1 | 22 | 2 | 0 | 20 |
| yogurt, soy, strawberry | 6 oz | 160 | 4 | 31 | 1 | 22 | 2 | 0 | 20 |
| yogurt, soy, vanilla | 6 oz | 120 | 4 | 23 | 1 | 16 | 2 | 0 | 20 |
| yogurt, tofu | 4 oz | 123 | 5 | 21 | 0 | 2 | 2 | 0 | 46 |

## SPORTS BARS

| FOOD ITEM | SERVING SIZE | CALORIES | PRO (g) | CARB (g) | FIBER (g) | SUGAR (g) | FAT (g) | SAT FAT (g) | SOD (mg) |
|---|---|---|---|---|---|---|---|---|---|
| ABB Steel Bar | 1 bar (65 g) | 250 | 16 | 36 | 1 | 25 | 4 | 3 | 250 |
| Avid Source Protein Bar | 1 bar (60 g) | 240 | 24 | 22 | 1 | 8 | 6 | 1.5 | 230 |
| Balance Bar, almond brownie | 1 bar (50 g) | 200 | 14 | 23 | 2 | 18 | 6 | 1.5 | 115 |
| Balance Bar, chocolate | 1 bar (50 g) | 200 | 14 | 22 | <1 | 18 | 6 | 3.5 | 180 |
| Balance Bar, chocolate peanut butter | 1 bar (50 g) | 200 | 14 | 22 | 1 | 1 | 8 | 4 | 190 |
| Balance Bar, chocolate raspberry fudge | 1 bar (50 g) | 200 | 14 | 22 | 1 | 19 | 6 | 3 | 90 |
| Balance Bar, cookie dough | 1 bar (50 g) | 200 | 15 | 22 | <1 | 18 | 6 | 3.5 | 180 |

| FOOD ITEM | SERVING SIZE | CALORIES | PRO (g) | CARB (g) | FIBER (g) | SUGAR (g) | FAT (g) | SAT FAT (g) | SOD (mg) |
|---|---|---|---|---|---|---|---|---|---|
| Balance Bar, honey peanut | 1 bar (50 g) | 200 | 14 | 24 | <1 | 20 | 6 | 3 | 180 |
| Balance Bar, mocha chip | 1 bar (50 g) | 200 | 14 | 23 | <1 | 19 | 6 | 3.5 | 125 |
| Balance Bar, peanut butter | 1 bar (50 g) | 200 | 14 | 22 | 1 | 17 | 6 | 2.5 | 230 |
| Balance Bar, trail mix, chocolate chip | 1 bar (50 g) | 210 | 14 | 22 | 3 | 14 | 7 | 3 | 310 |
| Balance Bar, trail mix, cinnamon, oats, and honey | 1 bar (50 g) | 210 | 15 | 23 | 3 | 12 | 7 | 2.5 | 230 |
| Balance Bar, trail mix, fruit and nut | 1 bar (50 g) | 210 | 15 | 23 | 2 | 16 | 7 | 2.5 | 240 |
| Balance Bar, yogurt honey peanut | 1 bar (50 g) | 200 | 15 | 22 | <1 | 18 | 6 | 3 | 190 |
| Balance CarbWell Bar, caramel and chocolate | 1 bar (50 g) | 190 | 14 | 23 | 1 | 1 | 7 | 4 | 200 |
| Balance CarbWell Bar, chocolate fudge | 1 bar (50 g) | 190 | 14 | 23 | 2 | 1 | 6 | 4 | 190 |
| Balance Gold Bar, caramel nut blast | 1 bar (50 g) | 210 | 15 | 23 | <1 | 13 | 7 | 4 | 85 |
| Balance Gold Bar, chewy chocolate chip | 1 bar (50 g) | 210 | 15 | 22 | <1 | 15 | 7 | 4 | 140 |
| Balance Gold Bar, chocolate peanut butter | 1 bar (50 g) | 210 | 15 | 22 | <1 | 11 | 7 | 4 | 125 |
| Balance Gold Bar, rocky road | 1 bar (50 g) | 210 | 15 | 22 | 1 | 12 | 7 | 4 | 80 |
| Balance Gold Bar, triple chocolate chaos | 1 bar (50 g) | 200 | 15 | 22 | <1 | 12 | 6 | 4 | 85 |
| Big 100 Bar, chocolate chip cookie dough | 1 bar (100 g) | 360 | 27 | 51 | 2 | 26 | 5 | 3 | 100 |
| Big 100 Bar, chocolate graham cracker chip | 1 bar (100 g) | 360 | 24 | 55 | 2 | 26 | 4 | 1 | 105 |
| Big 100 Bar, peanut butter cookie dough | 1 bar (100 g) | 360 | 27 | 51 | 2 | 25 | 5 | 2 | 260 |
| Big 100 Colossal Bar | 1 bar (100 g) | 400 | 31 | 45 | 2 | 26 | 11 | 6 | 640 |
| Bonanza Bar | 1 bar | 500 | 30 | 60 | 7 | 18 | 16 | 4 | 270 |
| Chef Jay's Trioplex Bar, caramel apple | 1 bar | 335 | 30 | 38 | 6 | 11 | 7 | 3 | 212 |
| Chef Jay's Trioplex Bar, chocolate coconut | 1 bar | 430 | 30 | 45 | 4 | 16 | 15 | 4 | 102 |
| Chef Jay's Trioplex Bar, peanut butter banana | 1 bar | 410 | 30 | 45 | 6 | 16 | 15 | 3.5 | 130 |
| Chef Jay's Trioplex Bar, s'mores | 1 bar | 430 | 30 | 46 | 4 | 16 | 16 | 3 | 130 |

| FOOD ITEM | SERVING SIZE | CALORIES | PRO (g) | CARB (g) | FIBER (g) | SUGAR (g) | FAT (g) | SAT FAT (g) | SOD (mg) |
|---|---|---|---|---|---|---|---|---|---|
| Chef Jay's Trioplex Bar, very berry | 1 bar | 420 | 30 | 45 | 4 | 16 | 16 | 2 | 130 |
| Clif Bar, apricot | 1 bar (68 g) | 230 | 10 | 45 | 5 | 21 | 3 | 0.5 | 125 |
| Clif Bar, banana nut bread | 1 bar (68 g) | 250 | 10 | 43 | 5 | 21 | 6 | 1 | 130 |
| Clif Bar, black cherry almond | 1 bar (68 g) | 250 | 10 | 44 | 5 | 20 | 5 | 1.5 | 110 |
| Clif Bar, black cookies and cream | 1 bar (68 g) | 240 | 10 | 47 | 5 | 21 | 4 | 1.5 | 210 |
| Clif Bar, carrot cake | 1 bar (68 g) | 230 | 10 | 46 | 5 | 21 | 3 | 0.5 | 90 |
| Clif Bar, chocolate brownie bar | 1 bar (68 g) | 240 | 10 | 46 | 5 | 21 | 4 | 1.5 | 150 |
| Clif Bar, chocolate peanut crunch | 1 bar (68 g) | 250 | 11 | 43 | 5 | 20 | 6 | 2 | 210 |
| Clif Bar, crunchy peanut butter | 1 bar (68 g) | 250 | 12 | 40 | 5 | 18 | 6 | 1.5 | 250 |
| Clif Bar, lemon poppy seed | 1 bar (68 g) | 240 | 10 | 46 | 5 | 21 | 3.5 | 1.5 | 110 |
| Clif Bar, oatmeal raisin walnut | 1 bar (68 g) | 240 | 10 | 43 | 5 | 20 | 5 | 1 | 130 |
| Clif Builder's Bar, chocolate | 1 bar (68 g) | 270 | 20 | 30 | 4 | 19 | 5 | 0 | 260 |
| Clif Builder's Bar, cookies and cream | 1 bar (68 g) | 270 | 20 | 30 | 3 | 19 | 8 | 4.5 | 280 |
| Clif Builder's Bar, peanut butter | 1 bar (68 g) | 270 | 20 | 30 | 4 | 19 | 8 | 5 | 260 |
| Colossus Protein Cookies | 1 bar | 250 | 10 | 44 | 5 | 21 | 5 | 2 | 110 |
| Complete Protein Diet Bar | 1 bar | 190 | 20 | 18 | 0 | n/a | 4 | 2 | 180 |
| Detour Bar | 1 bar | 310 | 30 | 25 | 3 | 12 | 10 | 4 | 480 |
| Detour BUZZ! | 1 bar | 330 | 30 | 30 | 4 | 3 | 6 | 0 | 350 |
| Detour Oatmeal Bars | 1 bar | 460 | 30 | 58 | 5 | 9 | 12 | 4 | 180 |
| Doctor's CarbRite Diet Bar | 1 bar | 190 | 21 | 22 | <1 | 0 | 4 | 2 | 140 |
| JoyRide Bar | 1 bar | 340 | 30 | 27 | 2 | 16 | 12 | 9 | 270 |
| Lean Blondie | 1 bar | 170 | 15 | 15 | 1 | 2 | 6 | 2 | 220 |
| Lean Body Cookie Bar | 1 bar | 370 | 30 | 30 | 3 | 12 | 13 | 4 | 310 |
| Lean Body Gold Bar | 1 bar | 300 | 30 | 29 | 1 | 7 | 10 | 6 | 290 |
| Lean Body Protein Bar | 1 bar | 300 | 32 | 28 | <1 | 9 | 7 | 3.5 | 60 |
| Lean Brownie | 1 bar | 170 | 15 | 14 | 2 | 2 | 6 | 3 | 220 |

| FOOD ITEM | SERVING SIZE | CALORIES | PRO (g) | CARB (g) | FIBER (g) | SUGAR (g) | FAT (g) | SAT FAT (g) | SOD (mg) |
|---|---|---|---|---|---|---|---|---|---|
| Lean protein bites, lemon pie | 1 oz | 100 | 13 | 9 | 4 | n/a | 5 | 4 | 160 |
| Lean protein bites, white chocolate netrition.com | 1 oz | 120 | 16 | 2 | 0 | 2 | 4 | 2 | 200 |
| Luna bar, caramel nut brownie | 1 bar (48 g) | 190 | 9 | 27 | 4 | 11 | 6 | 3 | 125 |
| Luna bar, chai tea | 1 bar (48 g) | 180 | 10 | 27 | 2 | 12 | 4 | 3 | 125 |
| Luna bar, iced oatmeal raisin | 1 bar (48 g) | 180 | 10 | 28 | 3 | 10 | 4 | 2.5 | 170 |
| Luna bar, key lime pie | 1 bar (48 g) | 180 | 10 | 26 | 3 | 10 | 4 | 3 | 125 |
| Luna bar, lemon zest | 1 bar (48 g) | 180 | 10 | 26 | 3 | 10 | 4 | 3 | 125 |
| Luna bar, peanut butter cookie | 1 bar (48 g) | 190 | 10 | 25 | 3 | 8 | 6 | 3 | 120 |
| Luna bar, s'mores | 1 bar (48 g) | 180 | 10 | 26 | 3 | 9 | 4 | 3 | 125 |
| Muscle Sandwich | 1 bar | 290 | 13 | 25 | 2 | 15 | 16 | 5 | 140 |
| Myoplex Carb Sense, chocolate chip brownie | 1 bar | 270 | 28 | 24 | 1 | 1 | 8 | 5 | 140 |
| Myoplex Carb Sense, chocolate peanut butter | 1 bar | 250 | 28 | 24 | 1 | 1 | 7 | 5 | 270 |
| Myoplex Carb Sense, cookies and cream | 1 bar | 260 | 28 | 24 | 1 | 2 | 8 | 4.5 | 260 |
| Myoplex Lite Bar, chocolate chip crisp | 1 bar | 190 | 15 | 26 | 4 | 12 | 4.5 | 3 | 260 |
| Myoplex Lite Bar, chocolate peanut butter crisp | 1 bar | 190 | 15 | 25 | 6 | 12 | 5 | 3 | 390 |
| Myoplex Lite Bar, cinnamon roll crisp | 1 bar | 190 | 15 | 28 | 5 | 15 | 4 | 2.5 | 230 |
| Nitro-Tech Bar | 1 bar | 290 | 35 | 33 | 2 | 3 | 6 | 4.5 | 130 |
| Oat-Rageous Bar | 1 bar | 290 | 21 | 42 | 6 | 17 | 5 | 0.5 | 160 |
| Odyssey Protein | 1 bar | 290 | 30 | 29 | 3 | 3 | 9 | 5 | 290 |
| OhYeah! Bar | 1 bar | 380 | 26 | 31 | 4 | 8 | 19 | 7 | 130 |
| One Way Bar | 1 bar | 340 | 30 | 29 | 1 | 12 | 12 | 5 | 450 |
| Opti-Pro Bar | 1 bar | 290 | 20 | 40 | 1 | 27 | 6 | 3.5 | 350 |
| organic food bar, blueberry | 1 bar (68 g) | 310 | 8 | 35 | 6 | 22 | 13 | 2 | 25 |
| organic food bar, chocolate chip | 1 bar (68 g) | 300 | 12 | 36 | 7 | 24 | 12 | 2 | 25 |
| organic food bar, cranberry | 1 bar (68 g) | 310 | 8 | 35 | 6 | 22 | 13 | 2 | 25 |

| FOOD ITEM | SERVING SIZE | CALORIES | PRO (g) | CARB (g) | FIBER (g) | SUGAR (g) | FAT (g) | SAT FAT (g) | SOD (mg) |
|---|---|---|---|---|---|---|---|---|---|
| organic food bar, original | 1 bar (68 g) | 300 | 14 | 34 | 6 | 20 | 12 | 2 | 25 |
| Organic Vegan Whole Food Nutrition Bar | 1 bar (68 g) | 300 | 14 | 34 | 6 | 20 | 12 | 2 | 25 |
| PowerBar Triple Threat | 1 bar (55 g) | 220 | 11 | 32 | 4 | 14 | 5 | 2 | 180 |
| PowerBar Triple Threat, caramel peanut crisp | 1 bar (55 g) | 220 | 11 | 32 | 4 | 14 | 5 | 2 | 210 |
| PowerBar Triple Threat, caramel peanut fusion | 1 bar (55 g) | 230 | 10 | 30 | 4 | 15 | 8 | 4 | 190 |
| PowerBar Triple Threat, chocolate caramel | 1 bar (55 g) | 230 | 10 | 30 | 4 | 15 | 8 | 4.5 | 150 |
| Pria, chocolate peanut crunch powerbar | 1 bar (28 g) | 110 | 5 | 16 | 1 | 10 | 3.5 | 2 | 85 |
| Pria, crème caramel crisp powerbar | 1 bar (28 g) | 110 | 5 | 17 | 1 | 10 | 3 | 2.5 | 90 |
| Pria, double chocolate cookie powerbar | 1 bar (28 g) | 110 | 5 | 16 | 1 | 10 | 3 | 2 | 100 |
| Pria, French vanilla crisp powerbar | 1 bar (28 g) | 110 | 5 | 17 | 1 | 9 | 3 | 2 | 80 |
| Pria, mint chocolate cookie powerbar | 1 bar (28 g) | 110 | 5 | 15 | 1 | 9 | 3.5 | 2.5 | 90 |
| Pria Carb Select, caramel nut brownie | 1 bar (48 g) | 170 | 10 | 21 | 2 | 1 | 8 | 5 | 90 |
| Pria Carb Select, chocolate mocha crisp | 1 bar (35 g) | 130 | 8 | 16 | 4 | 1 | 6 | 3.5 | 115 |
| Pria Carb Select, chocolate peanut butter crisp | 1 bar (35 g) | 130 | 8 | 16 | 4 | 1 | 6 | 3.5 | 140 |
| Pria Carb Select, cookies and caramel | 1 bar (48 g) | 170 | 10 | 22 | 2 | 1 | 7 | 4.5 | 90 |
| Pro 42 Bar | 1 bar | 380 | 42 | 37 | 2 | 1 | 8 | 5 | 100 |
| Promax | 1 bar | 290 | 20 | 36 | 1 | 34 | 6 | 3.5 | 200 |
| Protein 8 | 1 bar | 250 | 30 | 22 | 3 | 1 | 6 | 4.5 | 210 |
| Protein Plus, chocolate crisp powerbar | 1 bar (78 g) | 290 | 23 | 37 | 2 | 18 | 6 | 3.5 | 190 |
| Protein Plus, chocolate peanut butter powerbar | 1 bar (78 g) | 300 | 23 | 39 | 1 | 19 | 6 | 3.5 | 210 |
| Protein Plus, cookies and cream powerbar | 1 bar (78 g) | 300 | 23 | 38 | 1 | 18 | 6 | 3.5 | 170 |
| Protein Plus, vanilla yogurt powerbar | 1 bar (78 g) | 300 | 23 | 38 | 1 | 19 | 6 | 3.5 | 150 |
| Protein Plus Carb Select, chocolate caramel crunch | 1 bar (73 g) | 270 | 20 | 32 | 2 | 1 | 11 | 7 | 170 |
| Protein Plus Carb Select, chocolate peanut butter | 1 bar (73 g) | 270 | 22 | 30 | 2 | 1 | 9 | 4 | 290 |

| FOOD ITEM | SERVING SIZE | CALORIES | PRO (g) | CARB (g) | FIBER (g) | SUGAR (g) | FAT (g) | SAT FAT (g) | SOD (mg) |
|---|---|---|---|---|---|---|---|---|---|
| Protein Plus Carb Select, double chocolate | 1 bar (73 g) | 260 | 22 | 30 | 1 | 1 | 7 | 3.5 | 190 |
| Protein Plus Carb Select, peanut caramel | 1 bar (73 g) | 270 | 22 | 30 | 2 | 1 | 9 | 4 | 290 |
| Pure Protein | 1 bar | 310 | 32 | 24 | 1 | 9 | 10 | 4.5 | 270 |
| Response Bar | 1 bar | 310 | 32 | 24 | 1 | 9 | 10 | 4.5 | 270 |
| Rockin' Roll Bar | 1 bar | 210 | 21 | 20 | 3 | 1 | 8 | 1 | 230 |
| soy protein bar, apple spice yogurt | 1 bar (2 oz) | 220 | 14 | 32 | 1 | 19 | 4 | 3 | 130 |
| soy protein bar, banana nut | 1 bar (2 oz) | 230 | 11 | 41 | 3 | 27 | 3 | 0 | 100 |
| soy protein bar, berry | 1 bar (2 oz) | 230 | 11 | 40 | 3 | 25 | 3 | 0 | 100 |
| soy protein bar, berry yogurt | 1 bar (2 oz) | 220 | 14 | 32 | 1 | 21 | 4 | 3 | 120 |
| soy protein bar, café mocha | 1 bar (2 oz) | 220 | 14 | 34 | 1 | 20 | 4 | 3 | 150 |
| soy protein bar, chocolate | 1 bar (2 oz) | 230 | 11 | 41 | 4 | 23 | 3 | 0 | 110 |
| soy protein bar, chocolate, coated | 1 bar (2 oz) | 220 | 14 | 33 | 1 | 19 | 4 | 3 | 190 |
| soy protein bar, chocolate, uncoated | 1 bar (2 oz) | 210 | 14 | 36 | 2 | 18 | 0 | 0 | 160 |
| soy protein bar, cookies and cream | 1 bar (2 oz) | 220 | 14 | 33 | 2 | 25 | 4 | 3 | 160 |
| soy protein bar, chocolate brownie, high-protein | 1 bar (2 oz) | 234 | 19 | 21 | 0 | 0 | 8 | 3 | 162 |
| soy protein bar, chocolate mint | 1 bar (2 oz) | 234 | 19 | 20 | 0 | 0 | 8 | 3 | 162 |
| soy protein bar, creamy caramel | 1 bar (2 oz) | 230 | 14 | 34 | 1 | 28 | 4 | 3 | 160 |
| soy protein bar, fudge-coated peanut butter | 1 bar (2 oz) | 230 | 14 | 32 | 1 | 20 | 5 | 3 | 150 |
| soy protein bar, honey yogurt peanut | 1 bar (2 oz) | 230 | 14 | 32 | 1 | 20 | 5 | 3 | 150 |
| soy protein bar, oatmeal raisin | 1 bar (2 oz) | 230 | 11 | 41 | 3 | 24 | 3 | 0 | 130 |
| Tiger's milk bar, protein-rich | 1 bar (1 oz) | 145 | 7 | 18 | 1 | 13 | 5 | 1 | 70 |
| Zone Perfect Bar, apple cinnamon | 1 bar | 210 | 15 | 21 | 1 | 14 | 7 | 3 | 280 |
| Zone Perfect Bar, chocolate mint | 1 bar | 210 | 16 | 21 | <1 | 13 | 7 | 5 | 260 |
| Zone Perfect Bar, chocolate peanut butter | 1 bar | 210 | 16 | 21 | <1 | 13 | 7 | 4 | 330 |

| FOOD ITEM | SERVING SIZE | CALORIES | PRO (g) | CARB (g) | FIBER (g) | SUGAR (g) | FAT (g) | SAT FAT (g) | SOD (mg) |
|---|---|---|---|---|---|---|---|---|---|
| Zone Perfect Bar, chocolate raspberry | 1 bar | 210 | 15 | 21 | 1 | 13 | 7 | 4.5 | 260 |
| Zone Perfect Bar, cinnamon roll | 1 bar | 210 | 15 | 22 | <1 | 15 | 7 | 4 | 270 |
| Zone Perfect Bar, double chocolate | 1 bar | 210 | 16 | 21 | 1 | 14 | 7 | 5 | 260 |
| Zone Perfect Bar, fudge graham | 1 bar | 210 | 16 | 21 | 1 | 14 | 7 | 4 | 270 |
| Zone Perfect Bar, strawberry yogurt | 1 bar | 210 | 15 | 21 | 1 | 14 | 7 | 4.5 | 260 |

## SPORTS DRINKS

| FOOD ITEM | SERVING SIZE | CALORIES | PRO (g) | CARB (g) | FIBER (g) | SUGAR (g) | FAT (g) | SAT FAT (g) | SOD (mg) |
|---|---|---|---|---|---|---|---|---|---|
| berry | 8 fl oz | 12 | 0 | 3 | 0 | 3 | 0 | 0 | 31 |
| berry ice | 8 fl oz | 82 | 0 | 21 | 0 | 21 | 0 | 0 | 71 |
| black cherry | 8 fl oz | 12 | 0 | 3 | 0 | 3 | 0 | 0 | 31 |
| cherry rush | 8 fl oz | 62 | 0 | 15 | 0 | 12 | 0 | 0 | 94 |
| citrus cooler | 8 fl oz | 26 | 0 | 6 | 0 | 5 | 0 | 0 | 39 |
| clear cherry chill | 8 fl oz | 71 | 0 | 19 | 0 | 19 | 0 | 0 | 65 |
| cool blue rasp | 8 fl oz | 62 | 0 | 15 | n/a | 13 | 0 | 0 | 94 |
| fruit punch, All Punch | 8 fl oz | 53 | 0 | 15 | 0 | 15 | 0 | 0 | 37 |
| fruit punch, can | 8 fl oz | 72 | 0 | 19 | 0 | 15 | 0 | 0 | 28 |
| grape, All Sport | 8 fl oz | 53 | 0 | 13 | 0 | 13 | 0 | 0 | 37 |
| grape, bottle | 8 fl oz | 12 | 0 | 3 | 0 | 3 | 0 | 0 | 31 |
| kiwi-strawberry, bottle | 8 fl oz | 12 | 0 | 3 | 0 | 3 | 0 | 0 | 31 |
| lemon ice | 8 fl oz | 62 | 0 | 15 | 0 | 13 | 0 | 0 | 94 |
| lemon lime | 8 fl oz | 77 | 0 | 19 | 0 | 14 | 0 | 0 | 53 |
| lemon lime, dry | 1 scoop | 78 | 0 | 20 | n/a | 19 | 0 | 0 | 129 |
| lemon lime, All Sport | 8 fl oz | 47 | 0 | 13 | 0 | 13 | 0 | 0 | 37 |
| low-calorie | 8 fl oz | 26 | 0 | 7 | 0 | 0 | 0 | 0 | 84 |
| melon | 8 fl oz | 12 | 0 | 3 | 0 | 3 | 0 | 0 | 31 |
| midnite thunder | 8 fl oz | 62 | 0 | 15 | 0 | 13 | 0 | 0 | 94 |
| mountain blast | 8 fl oz | 73 | 0 | 19 | n/a | 15 | 0 | 0 | 28 |

| FOOD ITEM | SERVING SIZE | CALORIES | PRO (g) | CARB (g) | FIBER (g) | SUGAR (g) | FAT (g) | SAT FAT (g) | SOD (mg) |
|---|---|---|---|---|---|---|---|---|---|
| orange, All Sport | 8 fl oz | 47 | 0 | 13 | 0 | 13 | 0 | 0 | 37 |
| orange, Gatorade | 8 fl oz | 89 | 0 | 22 | 0 | 19 | 0 | 0 | 14 |
| orange, Gatorade, dry | 1 scoop | 78 | 0 | 20 | n/a | 19 | 0 | 0 | 129 |
| orange edge | 8 fl oz | 71 | 0 | 19 | 0 | 19 | 0 | 0 | 65 |
| peach | 8 fl oz | 12 | 0 | 3 | 0 | 3 | 0 | 0 | 31 |
| Powerade | 8 fl oz | 78 | 0 | 18 | 0 | 15 | 0 | 0 | 54 |
| strawberry kiwi | 8 fl oz | 62 | 0 | 15 | 0 | 13 | 0 | 0 | 94 |
| thunder punch | 8 fl oz | 83 | 0 | 21 | 0 | 21 | 0 | 0 | 71 |
| tropical citrus | 8 fl oz | 12 | 0 | 3 | 0 | 3 | 0 | 0 | 31 |
| tropical punch | 8 fl oz | 62 | 0 | 15 | 0 | 13 | 0 | 0 | 94 |
| watermelon | 8 fl oz | 62 | 0 | 15 | 0 | 13 | 0 | 0 | 94 |
| wild apple | 8 fl oz | 62 | 0 | 15 | 0 | 13 | 0 | 0 | 94 |

## SWEETENERS

| FOOD ITEM | SERVING SIZE | CALORIES | PRO (g) | CARB (g) | FIBER (g) | SUGAR (g) | FAT (g) | SAT FAT (g) | SOD (mg) |
|---|---|---|---|---|---|---|---|---|---|
| agave nectar | 1 tsp | 15 | 0 | 4 | 0 | 4 | 0 | 0 | 4 |
| aspartame | 1 tsp (1 packet) | 13 | n/a | 3 | 0 | 3 | 0 | 0 | 0 |
| barley malt syrup | 1 tsp | 25 | 1 | 6 | 0 | 6 | 0 | 0 | 3 |
| blackstrap molasses | 1 tsp | 16 | 0 | 4 | 0 | 3 | 0 | 0 | 4 |
| brown rice syrup | 1 tsp | 28 | 0 | 7 | 0 | 6 | 0 | 0 | 15 |
| brown sugar, liquid | 1 tsp | 18 | 0 | 5 | 0 | 5 | 0 | 0 | 2 |
| brown sugar, unpacked | 1 tsp | 11 | 0 | 3 | 0 | 3 | 0 | 0 | 1 |
| cane sugar, organic, unrefined | 1 tsp | 16 | 0 | 4 | 0 | 4 | 0 | 0 | 0 |
| corn syrup, dark | 1 tsp | 20 | 0 | 5 | 0 | 2 | 0 | 0 | 11 |
| corn syrup, light | 1 tsp | 19 | 0 | 5 | 0 | 2 | 0 | 0 | 4 |
| Equal | 1 tsp | 13 | n/a | 3 | 0 | 3 | 0 | 0 | 0 |
| fructose, dry | 1 tsp (1 packet) | 15 | 0 | 4 | 0 | 4 | 0 | 0 | 1 |
| honey | 1 tsp | 21 | 0 | 6 | 0 | 0 | 0 | 0 | 0 |
| maple syrup | 1 tsp | 17 | 0 | 4 | 0 | 4 | 0 | 0 | 1 |

| FOOD ITEM | SERVING SIZE | CALORIES | PRO (g) | CARB (g) | FIBER (g) | SUGAR (g) | FAT (g) | SAT FAT (g) | SOD (mg) |
|---|---|---|---|---|---|---|---|---|---|
| molasses, dark | 1 tsp | 17 | 0 | 5 | 0 | 5 | 0 | 0 | 1 |
| molasses, light | 1 tsp | 20 | 0 | 5 | 0 | 5 | 0 | 0 | 3 |
| powdered sugar | 1 tsp | 10 | 0 | 2 | 0 | 2 | 0 | 0 | 3 |
| sorghum syrup | 1 tsp | 17 | 0 | 4 | 0 | 4 | 0 | 0 | 0 |
| Splenda (sucralose) | 1 packet | 3 | 0 | 1 | 0 | 1 | 0 | 0 | 1 |
| stevia | 1 packet | 4 | 0 | 1 | 0 | 0 | 0 | 0 | 0 |
| Sugar Twin (saccharin) | 1 packet | 3 | 0 | 1 | 0 | 1 | 0 | 0 | n/a |
| white sugar | 1 cube | 10 | 0 | 3 | 0 | 3 | 0 | 0 | 3 |
| white sugar | 1 tsp | 16 | 0 | 4 | 0 | 4 | 0 | 0 | 0 |

## VEGETABLES

| FOOD ITEM | SERVING SIZE | CALORIES | PRO (g) | CARB (g) | FIBER (g) | SUGAR (g) | FAT (g) | SAT FAT (g) | SOD (mg) |
|---|---|---|---|---|---|---|---|---|---|
| alfalfa sprouts | ½ cup | 5 | 1 | 1 | 1 | 0 | 0 | 0 | 1 |
| artichoke | 1 medium | 60 | 4 | 13 | 7 | 3 | 0 | 0 | 120 |
| artichoke | 1 large | 76 | 5 | 17 | 9 | 3 | 0 | 0 | 152 |
| artichoke, Jerusalem | ½ cup | 57 | 2 | 13 | 1 | 7 | 0 | 0 | 3 |
| artichoke hearts, cooked, with salt, drained | ½ cup | 42 | 3 | 9 | 5 | 1 | 0 | 0 | 278 |
| artichoke hearts, French, cooked, without salt, drained | ½ cup | 42 | 3 | 9 | 5 | 1 | 1 | 0 | 80 |
| artichoke hearts, Globe, cooked | ½ cup | 42 | 3 | 9 | 5 | 1 | 1 | 0 | 80 |
| artichoke hearts, marinated | ½ cup | 58 | 2 | 7 | 2 | 0 | 3 | 0 | 244 |
| arugula (rocket) | 4 oz | 28 | 3 | 4 | 2 | 2 | 1 | 0 | 31 |
| arugula (rocket), chopped | 1 cup (0.7 oz) | 5 | 1 | 1 | 1 | 0 | 0 | 0 | 5 |
| asparagus, cooked | 4 oz | 25 | 3 | 5 | 2 | 1 | 0 | 0 | 4 |
| asparagus, cooked, from frozen | 4 oz | 20 | 3 | 2 | 2 | 0 | 0 | 0 | 3 |
| asparagus, white, cooked | 4 oz | 27 | 3 | 5 | 3 | 3 | 0 | 0 | 0 |
| asparagus tips | 4 oz | 23 | 2 | 4 | 2 | 2 | 0 | 0 | 2 |
| bamboo shoot, cooked | 1 (5 oz) | 17 | 2 | 3 | 1 | 0 | 0 | 0 | 6 |

| FOOD ITEM | SERVING SIZE | CALORIES | PRO (g) | CARB (g) | FIBER (g) | SUGAR (g) | FAT (g) | SAT FAT (g) | SOD (mg) |
|---|---|---|---|---|---|---|---|---|---|
| bamboo shoot, sliced | 1 cup | 41 | 4 | 8 | 3 | 5 | 0 | 0 | 6 |
| bamboo shoot, sliced, cooked, with salt, drained | 1 cup | 13 | 2 | 2 | 1 | 0 | 0 | 0 | 288 |
| bamboo shoot, sliced, cooked, without salt, drained | 1 cup | 14 | 1 | 2 | 1 | 0 | 0 | 0 | 5 |
| beet, green | 1 cup | 8 | 1 | 2 | 1 | 0 | 0 | 0 | 86 |
| beet, green, cooked, with salt, drained | 1 cup | 39 | 4 | 8 | 4 | 1 | 0 | 0 | 687 |
| beets, cooked, with salt | ½ cup | 37 | 1 | 8 | 2 | 7 | 0 | 0 | 242 |
| beets, cooked, without salt | ½ cup | 37 | 1 | 8 | 2 | 7 | 0 | 0 | 65 |
| beets, julienned, canned | ½ cup | 30 | 1 | 7 | 1 | 6 | 0 | 0 | 230 |
| beets, pickled, whole, canned | ½ cup | 65 | 0 | 17 | 4 | 13 | 0 | 0 | 217 |
| beets, pickled, with onions | ½ cup | 53 | 1 | 13 | 1 | 11 | 0 | 0 | 53 |
| beets, small, whole, canned | ½ cup | 30 | 1 | 7 | 1 | 6 | 0 | 0 | 230 |
| bell pepper, chopped | 1 cup | 39 | 1 | 9 | 3 | 4 | 0 | 0 | 3 |
| bell pepper, chopped, steamed | 1 cup | 37 | 1 | 9 | 2 | 3 | 0 | 0 | 3 |
| bell pepper, chopped, stir-fried | 1 cup | 37 | 1 | 9 | 2 | 3 | 0 | 0 | 3 |
| bell pepper, green | 1 medium | 30 | 1 | 7 | 2 | 4 | 0 | 0 | 0 |
| bell pepper, green, dehydrated | 1 oz | 90 | 5 | 20 | 6 | 10 | 1 | 0 | 53 |
| bell pepper, red | 1 medium | 31 | 1 | 7 | 2 | 5 | 0 | 0 | 2 |
| bell pepper, red, dehydrated | 1 oz | 88 | 4 | 20 | 5 | 7 | 1 | 0 | 9 |
| bell pepper, rings, fresh | 5 | 10 | 0 | 2 | 1 | 1 | 0 | 0 | 2 |
| bell pepper, roasted with brine | 2 oz | 18 | 1 | 3 | 0 | 2 | 0 | 0 | 206 |
| bell pepper, strips, fresh | 10 | 5 | 0 | 1 | 1 | 1 | 0 | 0 | 1 |
| bell pepper, yellow | 1 medium | 31 | 1 | 7 | 2 | 5 | 0 | 0 | 2 |
| bitter gourd (balsam pear), cooked, without salt, drained | 1 cup | 24 | 1 | 5 | 2 | 2 | 0 | 0 | 7 |
| bitter gourd (balsam pear) tip | 1 cup | 14 | 3 | 2 | 0 | 0 | 0 | 0 | 5 |
| borage, cooked, with salt, drained | 3 oz | 21 | 2 | 3 | 1 | 0 | 1 | 0 | 276 |

| FOOD ITEM | SERVING SIZE | CALORIES | PRO (g) | CARB (g) | FIBER (g) | SUGAR (g) | FAT (g) | SAT FAT (g) | SOD (mg) |
|---|---|---|---|---|---|---|---|---|---|
| borage, cooked, without salt, drained | 3 oz | 21 | 2 | 3 | 1 | 0 | 1 | 0 | 75 |
| borage, cut into 1 pieces | 1 cup | 19 | 2 | 3 | 1 | 1 | 1 | 0 | 71 |
| broccoflower | 1 cup | 32 | 3 | 6 | 3 | 0 | 0 | 0 | 23 |
| broccoflower, steamed | 1 cup | 50 | 5 | 10 | 5 | 0 | 0 | 0 | 36 |
| broccoli, Chinese | 1 cup | 23 | 1 | 5 | 1 | 0 | 0 | 0 | 40 |
| broccoli, Chinese, cooked | 1 cup | 19 | 1 | 3 | 2 | 1 | 1 | 0 | 6 |
| broccoli, chopped, cooked | 1 cup | 25 | 2 | 4 | 2 | 1 | 0 | 0 | 20 |
| broccoli, florets | 1 cup | 20 | 2 | 4 | 2 | 0 | 0 | 0 | 19 |
| broccoli, leaves, chopped | 1 cup | 25 | 3 | 5 | 2 | 0 | 0 | 0 | 24 |
| broccoli, spear | 1 5" | 11 | 1 | 2 | 1 | 1 | 0 | 0 | 10 |
| broccoli, stalk | 1 medium | 45 | 5 | 8 | 5 | 3 | 0 | 0 | 55 |
| broccoli, stalk, cooked, with salt, drained | 1 5" | 39 | 4 | 7 | 5 | 2 | 0 | 0 | 367 |
| broccoli, steamed | 1 cup | 44 | 5 | 8 | 5 | 3 | 1 | 0 | 42 |
| broccoli, stir-fried | 1 cup | 44 | 5 | 8 | 5 | 3 | 1 | 0 | 42 |
| broccoli raab | 1 cup | 25 | 3 | 4 | 0 | 1 | 0 | 0 | 25 |
| broccoli raab, cooked | 1 cup | 28 | 3 | 3 | 2 | 0 | 0 | 0 | 48 |
| Brussels sprouts | 1 cup | 38 | 3 | 8 | 3 | 2 | 0 | 0 | 22 |
| Brussels sprouts, baby, with butter sauce, frozen | ½ cup | 45 | 2 | 7 | 3 | 2 | 1 | 1 | 205 |
| Brussels sprouts, cooked, with salt, drained | 1 cup | 56 | 4 | 11 | 4 | 3 | 1 | 0 | 200 |
| Brussels sprouts, cooked, without salt, drained | 1 cup | 65 | 6 | 13 | 6 | 3 | 1 | 0 | 23 |
| Brussels sprouts, frozen | 1 cup | 35 | 3 | 7 | 3 | 0 | 0 | 0 | 9 |
| burdock root | ½ cup | 31 | 1 | 7 | 1 | 1 | 0 | 0 | 2 |
| burdock root, cooked, with salt, drained | ½ cup | 55 | 1 | 13 | 1 | 2 | 0 | 0 | 150 |
| burdock root, cooked, without salt, drained | ½ cup | 55 | 1 | 13 | 1 | 2 | 0 | 0 | 3 |
| butterbur, chopped, canned | 1 cup | 4 | 0 | 0 | 0 | 0 | 0 | 0 | 5 |
| butterbur, cooked, with salt, drained | 1 cup | 9 | 0 | 3 | 2 | 0 | 0 | 0 | 298 |
| butterbur, cooked, without salt, drained | 1 cup | 10 | 0 | 3 | 2 | 0 | 0 | 0 | 5 |

| FOOD ITEM | SERVING SIZE | CALORIES | PRO (g) | CARB (g) | FIBER (g) | SUGAR (g) | FAT (g) | SAT FAT (g) | SOD (mg) |
|---|---|---|---|---|---|---|---|---|---|
| butterhead lettuce | 1 5" head | 25 | 2 | 4 | 2 | 2 | 0 | 0 | 8 |
| butterhead lettuce | 5 small leaves | 3 | 0 | 1 | 0 | 0 | 0 | 0 | 1 |
| butterhead lettuce | 5 medium leaves | 5 | 1 | 1 | 0 | 0 | 0 | 0 | 2 |
| butterhead lettuce | 5 large leaves | 10 | 1 | 2 | 1 | 1 | 0 | 0 | 4 |
| cabbage | 1 small leaf | 4 | 0 | 1 | 0 | 1 | 0 | 0 | 3 |
| cabbage | 1 medium leaf | 6 | 0 | 1 | 1 | 1 | 0 | 0 | 4 |
| cabbage | 1 large leaf | 8 | 0 | 2 | 1 | 1 | 0 | 0 | 6 |
| cabbage | ¼ small head | 43 | 3 | 10 | 4 | 6 | 0 | 0 | 32 |
| cabbage | ¼ medium head | 54 | 3 | 13 | 5 | 7 | 0 | 0 | 41 |
| cabbage, bok choy, cooked, drained | 1 cup | 20 | 3 | 3 | 2 | 1 | 0 | 0 | 58 |
| cabbage, bok choy, shredded, cooked | 1 cup | 20 | 3 | 3 | 2 | 1 | 0 | 0 | 58 |
| cabbage, chopped | 1 cup | 21 | 1 | 5 | 2 | 3 | 0 | 0 | 16 |
| cabbage, coleslaw | ¼ cup | 21 | 0 | 4 | 1 | 0 | 1 | 0 | 7 |
| cabbage, cooked, drained | ¼ large head | 69 | 3 | 14 | 6 | 9 | 1 | 0 | 25 |
| cabbage, Japanese, pickled | ½ cup | 23 | 1 | 4 | 2 | 1 | 0 | 0 | 208 |
| cabbage, Korean, pickled (kimchee) | ½ cup | 16 | 1 | 3 | 1 | 1 | 0 | 0 | 498 |
| cabbage, Napa cooked | 1 cup | 13 | 1 | 2 | 2 | 0 | 0 | 0 | 12 |
| cabbage, pak choi, cooked, drained | 1 cup | 20 | 3 | 3 | 2 | 1 | 0 | 0 | 58 |
| cabbage, red | ⅛ medium head | 33 | 2 | 8 | 2 | 4 | 0 | 0 | 29 |
| cabbage, red | ⅛ large head | 45 | 2 | 11 | 3 | 6 | 0 | 0 | 39 |
| cabbage, red, pickled | ¼ cup | 55 | 0 | 14 | 0 | 14 | 0 | 0 | 7 |
| cabbage, red, raw | ⅛ small head | 22 | 1 | 5 | 2 | 3 | 0 | 0 | 20 |
| cabbage, red, raw | ¼ small head | 44 | 2 | 10 | 3 | 6 | 0 | 0 | 38 |
| cabbage, red, sweet & sour | ¼ cup | 55 | 0 | 14 | 1 | 14 | 0 | 0 | 7 |
| cabbage, savoy, shredded | 1 cup | 19 | 1 | 4 | 2 | 2 | 2 | 0 | 20 |

| FOOD ITEM | SERVING SIZE | CALORIES | PRO (g) | CARB (g) | FIBER (g) | SUGAR (g) | FAT (g) | SAT FAT (g) | SOD (mg) |
|---|---|---|---|---|---|---|---|---|---|
| cabbage, shredded | 1 cup | 17 | 1 | 4 | 2 | 2 | 0 | 0 | 13 |
| cabbage, shredded, cooked, with salt, drained | 1 cup | 20 | 3 | 3 | 2 | 1 | 0 | 0 | 459 |
| cabbage, swamp, chopped | 1 cup | 11 | 1 | 2 | 1 | 0 | 0 | 0 | 63 |
| cabbage, swamp shoot | 1 | 2 | 0 | 0 | 0 | 0 | 0 | 0 | 15 |
| cardoon, cooked, with salt, drained | 1 cup | 32 | 1 | 8 | 2 | 0 | 0 | 0 | 602 |
| cardoon, cooked, without salt, drained | 1 cup | 32 | 1 | 8 | 2 | 0 | 0 | 0 | 257 |
| cardoon, shredded | 1 cup | 36 | 1 | 9 | 3 | 3 | 0 | 0 | 303 |
| carrot | 1 medium | 25 | 1 | 6 | 2 | 3 | 0 | 0 | 42 |
| carrot, baby | 1 medium | 4 | 0 | 1 | 1 | 1 | 0 | 0 | 8 |
| carrot, baby | 1 large | 5 | 0 | 12 | 0 | 1 | 0 | 0 | 12 |
| carrot, baby | ½ cup | 27 | 1 | 6 | 1 | 3 | 0 | 0 | 30 |
| carrot, chopped | ½ cup | 26 | 1 | 6 | 2 | 3 | 0 | 0 | 44 |
| carrots, cooked, with salt, drained | ½ cup | 27 | 1 | 6 | 2 | 3 | 1 | 0 | 236 |
| carrots, cooked, without salt, drained | ½ cup | 27 | 0 | 6 | 2 | 3 | 1 | 0 | 43 |
| carrots, glazed | ¼ cup | 54 | 0 | 7 | 1 | 5 | 3 | 1 | 58 |
| carrots, grated | ½ cup | 23 | 1 | 5 | 2 | 3 | 0 | 0 | 38 |
| cassava | ¼ cup | 82 | 1 | 29 | 1 | 1 | 0 | 0 | 7 |
| cassava, bitter, dried | 1 oz | 94 | 0 | 23 | 0 | 0 | 0 | 0 | n/a |
| cassava, yuca blanca, chopped, cooked | ¼ cup | 55 | 0 | 13 | 1 | 0 | 0 | 0 | 5 |
| cauliflower | ¼ small head | 17 | 1 | 4 | 2 | 2 | 0 | 0 | 20 |
| cauliflower | ¼ medium head | 36 | 3 | 8 | 4 | 4 | 0 | 0 | 43 |
| cauliflower | ¼ large head | 53 | 4 | 11 | 5 | 5 | 0 | 0 | 63 |
| cauliflower, cooked, with salt, drained | 1 cup | 34 | 3 | 7 | 5 | 2 | 0 | 0 | 457 |
| cauliflower, cooked, without salt, drained | 1 cup | 29 | 2 | 5 | 3 | 2 | 0 | 0 | 19 |
| cauliflower, florets | 1 cup | 38 | 3 | 7 | 4 | 2 | 1 | 0 | 25 |
| cauliflower, florets, cooked | 1 cup | 39 | 3 | 7 | 5 | 2 | 1 | 0 | 26 |
| cauliflower, green | 1 cup | 20 | 2 | 4 | 2 | 2 | 0 | 0 | 15 |

| FOOD ITEM | SERVING SIZE | CALORIES | PRO (g) | CARB (g) | FIBER (g) | SUGAR (g) | FAT (g) | SAT FAT (g) | SOD (mg) |
|---|---|---|---|---|---|---|---|---|---|
| cauliflower, green, florets | 1 cup | 26 | 3 | 5 | 3 | 3 | 0 | 0 | 20 |
| celery, chopped | 1 cup | 17 | 1 | 4 | 2 | 1 | 0 | 0 | 95 |
| celery, pickled | ½ cup | 11 | 0 | 3 | 1 | 1 | 0 | 0 | 196 |
| celery root (celeriac) | ½ cup | 33 | 1 | 7 | 1 | 1 | 0 | 0 | 78 |
| celery root (celeriac), cooked, with salt, drained | ½ cup | 21 | 1 | 5 | 1 | 1 | 0 | 0 | 230 |
| celery root (celeriac), cooked, without salt, drained | ½ cup | 21 | 1 | 5 | 1 | 1 | 0 | 0 | 47 |
| celery | 1 small stalk | 8 | 0 | 1 | 1 | 1 | 0 | 0 | 49 |
| celery | 1 medium stalk | 9 | 0 | 2 | 1 | 1 | 0 | 0 | 50 |
| celery | 1 large stalk | 10 | 1 | 3 | 1 | 1 | 0 | 0 | 51 |
| celery, cooked | 1 stalk | 7 | 0 | 2 | 1 | 1 | 0 | 0 | 34 |
| celery, cut into 4 strips | 1 cup | 17 | 1 | 4 | 2 | 2 | 0 | 0 | 99 |
| chayote squash | 1 cup | 22 | 1 | 5 | 2 | 2 | 0 | 0 | 3 |
| chayote squash, cooked, with salt | 1 cup | 38 | 1 | 8 | 4 | n/a | 1 | 0 | 379 |
| chayote squash, cooked, without salt | 1 cup | 38 | 1 | 8 | 4 | n/a | 1 | 0 | 2 |
| cherry tomatoes, red | 1 cup | 27 | 1 | 6 | 2 | 4 | 0 | 0 | 7 |
| cherry tomatoes, yellow | 1 cup | 22 | 1 | 4 | 1 | 3 | 0 | 0 | 34 |
| chicory, green, chopped | 1 cup | 41 | 3 | 8 | 7 | 1 | 1 | 0 | 81 |
| chicory, red, shredded | 1 cup | 9 | 1 | 2 | 0 | 0 | 0 | 0 | 9 |
| chicory root | 1 cup | 66 | 1 | 16 | 2 | n/a | 0 | 0 | 45 |
| chrysanthemum, garland, cooked, drained | 1 cup | 20 | 2 | 4 | 2 | 2 | 0 | 0 | 53 |
| chrysanthemum, garland, steamed | 1 | 3 | 0 | 0 | 0 | 0 | 0 | 0 | 17 |
| chrysanthemum, leaves, chopped | 1 cup | 12 | 2 | 2 | 2 | 0 | 0 | 0 | 60 |
| collard greens, chopped | 1 cup | 11 | 1 | 2 | 1 | 0 | 0 | 0 | 7 |
| collard greens, chopped, cooked, with salt, drained | 1 cup | 49 | 4 | 9 | 5 | 1 | 1 | 0 | 479 |
| collard greens, with ham | ½ cup | 39 | 3 | 3 | 2 | n/a | 2 | 1 | 261 |
| collard greens, with pork | ½ cup | 39 | 3 | 3 | 2 | n/a | 2 | 1 | 261 |
| corn, sweet white | ½ cup | 66 | 2 | 15 | 2 | 2 | 1 | 0 | 12 |

| FOOD ITEM | SERVING SIZE | CALORIES | PRO (g) | CARB (g) | FIBER (g) | SUGAR (g) | FAT (g) | SAT FAT (g) | SOD (mg) |
|---|---|---|---|---|---|---|---|---|---|
| corn, sweet white | 1 small ear | 63 | 2 | 14 | 2 | 2 | 1 | 0 | 11 |
| corn, sweet white | 1 large ear | 123 | 5 | 27 | 4 | 5 | 2 | 0 | 21 |
| corn, sweet yellow | ½ cup | 66 | 2 | 15 | 2 | 2 | 1 | 0 | 12 |
| corn, sweet yellow | 1 small ear | 63 | 2 | 14 | 2 | 2 | 1 | 0 | 11 |
| corn, sweet yellow | 1 large ear | 123 | 5 | 27 | 4 | 5 | 2 | 0 | 21 |
| corn, sweet yellow, cooked, with salt | ½ cup | 66 | 2 | 16 | 2 | 3 | 1 | 0 | 201 |
| cowpeas, canned, with pork | ½ cup | 100 | 3 | 20 | 4 | 1 | 2 | 1 | 420 |
| cowpeas, cooked, with salt, drained | ½ cup | 100 | 7 | 17 | 3 | 1 | 1 | 0 | 218 |
| cowpeas, cooked, without salt, drained | ½ cup | 100 | 7 | 17 | 3 | 1 | 1 | 0 | 16 |
| cowpeas, frozen | ½ cup | 112 | 7 | 20 | 5 | 4 | 1 | 0 | 4 |
| cowpeas, leafy tips | 1 cup | 12 | 2 | 1 | 0 | 0 | 0 | 0 | 3 |
| cucumber | 1 (8") | 45 | 2 | 11 | 2 | 5 | 0 | 0 | 6 |
| cucumbers, bitter, cooked, drained | 1 cup | 24 | 1 | 5 | 2 | 2 | 0 | 0 | 7 |
| cucumbers, peeled, pared, chopped | 1 cup | 16 | 1 | 3 | 1 | 2 | 0 | 0 | 3 |
| cucumbers, peeled, sliced | 1 cup | 14 | 1 | 3 | 1 | 2 | 0 | 0 | 2 |
| cucumber, sliced unpeeled | 1 cup | 16 | 1 | 4 | 1 | 2 | 0 | 0 | 2 |
| dandelion greens | 1 cup | 25 | 1 | 5 | 2 | 2 | 0 | 0 | 42 |
| dandelion greens, chopped, cooked, with salt, drained | 1 cup | 35 | 2 | 7 | 3 | 3 | 1 | 0 | 294 |
| dandelion greens, chopped, cooked, without salt, drained | 1 cup | 35 | 2 | 7 | 3 | 3 | 1 | 0 | 46 |
| dandelion leaf | 1 cup | 27 | 1 | 6 | 1 | 0 | 0 | 0 | 43 |
| eggplant, cubed, cooked, with salt, drained | 1 cup | 35 | 1 | 9 | 2 | 3 | 0 | 0 | 237 |
| eggplant, cubed, cooked, without salt, drained | 1 cup | 35 | 1 | 9 | 2 | 3 | 0 | 0 | 1 |
| eggplant, Japanese, cooked | 1 cup | 30 | 2 | 8 | 3 | 5 | 0 | 0 | 0 |
| eggplant, peeled | 1 | 110 | 5 | 26 | 15 | 11 | 1 | 0 | 9 |
| eggplant, pickled | ½ cup | 33 | 1 | 7 | 2 | 3 | 0 | 0 | 1138 |
| eggplant, unpeeled | 1 | 132 | 6 | 31 | 19 | 13 | 1 | 0 | 11 |

## VEGETABLES (cont.)

| FOOD ITEM | SERVING SIZE | CALORIES | PRO (g) | CARB (g) | FIBER (g) | SUGAR (g) | FAT (g) | SAT FAT (g) | SOD (mg) |
|---|---|---|---|---|---|---|---|---|---|
| endive | ½ head | 44 | 3 | 9 | 8 | 1 | 1 | 0 | 56 |
| endive, Belgian | 1 head (2 oz) | 10 | 1 | 2 | 2 | 0 | 0 | 0 | 1 |
| endive, Belgian, chopped | 1 cup | 15 | 1 | 4 | 3 | 0 | 0 | 0 | 2 |
| endive, chopped | 1 cup | 9 | 1 | 2 | 2 | 0 | 0 | 0 | 11 |
| endive, curly | ½ head | 44 | 3 | 9 | 8 | 1 | 1 | 0 | 56 |
| endive, curly, chopped | 1 cup | 9 | 1 | 2 | 2 | 0 | 0 | 0 | 11 |
| epazote | 5 sprigs | 3 | 0 | 1 | 0 | 0 | 0 | 0 | 4 |
| epazote | 1 cup | 4 | 0 | 1 | 0 | 0 | 0 | 0 | 6 |
| eppaw | ¼ cup | 38 | 1 | 8 | 0 | 0 | 0 | 0 | 3 |
| fennel bulb | 4 oz | 35 | 1 | 8 | 4 | 0 | 0 | 0 | 59 |
| fennel bulb, sliced | 1 cup | 27 | 1 | 7 | 3 | 0 | 0 | 0 | 45 |
| fiddlehead fern | 2 oz | 19 | 3 | 3 | n/a | n/a | n/a | n/a | 1 |
| fiddlehead fern, frozen | 2 oz | 19 | 2 | 3 | n/a | n/a | 0 | n/a | n/a |
| garlic | 1 clove | 4 | 0 | 1 | 0 | 0 | 0 | 0 | 0 |
| garlic, chopped | 1 tsp | 4 | 0 | 0 | 0 | 0 | 0 | 0 | 0 |
| gingerroot, grated | 1 tbsp | 5 | 0 | 1 | 0 | 0 | 0 | 0 | 1 |
| gingerroot, slices | 3 | 5 | 0 | 1 | 0 | 0 | 0 | 0 | 1 |
| gourd, bottle, cooked, with salt | 1 cup | 22 | 1 | 5 | 1 | 0 | 0 | 0 | 347 |
| gourd, calabash, cooked | 1 cup | 22 | 1 | 5 | 1 | 0 | 0 | 0 | 3 |
| gourd, dishcloth, cooked | ½ cup | 100 | 1 | 26 | 1 | 0 | 1 | 0 | 38 |
| gourd, strip, dried (kanpyo) | ¼ cup | 35 | 1 | 9 | 1 | 0 | 0 | 0 | 2 |
| gourd, wax, cooked, without salt | 1 cup | 25 | 1 | 5 | 2 | 2 | 0 | 0 | 187 |
| grape leaves | 1 cup | 13 | 1 | 2 | 2 | 1 | 0 | 0 | 1 |
| grape leaves, canned | 1 | 3 | 0 | 0 | 0 | 0 | 0 | 0 | 114 |
| green beans | 1 cup | 38 | 2 | 8 | 3 | 2 | 0 | 0 | 2 |
| green beans, frozen | 1 cup | 38 | 2 | 9 | 4 | 2 | 0 | 0 | 12 |
| green beans, Italian, frozen | 1 cup | 66 | 4 | 15 | 6 | 5 | 0 | 0 | 6 |
| green beans, with almonds, frozen | 1 cup | 77 | 3 | 9 | 3 | 4 | 4 | 0 | 526 |

| FOOD ITEM | SERVING SIZE | CALORIES | PRO (g) | CARB (g) | FIBER (g) | SUGAR (g) | FAT (g) | SAT FAT (g) | SOD (mg) |
|---|---|---|---|---|---|---|---|---|---|
| green beans, with bacon | 4 oz | 60 | 1 | 6 | 3 | 2 | 4 | 2 | 390 |
| jicama (yambean), chopped | ½ cup | 25 | 0 | 6 | 3 | 1 | 0 | 0 | 3 |
| jicama (yambean), cooked, with salt | ½ cup | 19 | 0 | 4 | 2 | n/a | 0 | 0 | 121 |
| jicama (yambean), sliced | 1 cup | 45 | 1 | 11 | 6 | 2 | 0 | 0 | 5 |
| jicama (yambean), sliced, cooked | ½ cup | 19 | 0 | 4 | 2 | n/a | 0 | 0 | 2 |
| jute, cooked, with salt | ½ cup | 16 | 2 | 3 | 1 | 0 | 0 | 0 | 107 |
| jute, cooked, without salt | ½ cup | 16 | 2 | 3 | 1 | 0 | 0 | 0 | 5 |
| kale, curly, chopped | 1 cup | 34 | 2 | 7 | 1 | n/a | 0 | 0 | 29 |
| kale, curly, cooked, without salt | 1 cup | 36 | 2 | 7 | 3 | 2 | 1 | 0 | 30 |
| kale, frozen | 1 cup | 39 | 4 | 7 | 3 | 2 | 1 | 0 | 326 |
| kale, Scotch, chopped | 1 cup | 28 | 2 | 6 | 1 | 1 | 0 | 0 | 47 |
| kale, Scotch, cooked, with salt | 1 cup | 36 | 2 | 7 | 3 | 2 | 1 | 0 | 365 |
| kohlrabi, chopped | 1 cup | 36 | 2 | 8 | 5 | 4 | 0 | 0 | 27 |
| kohlrabi, sliced | 5 slices | 22 | 1 | 5 | 3 | 2 | 0 | 0 | 16 |
| kohlrabi, sliced, cooked | 1 cup | 48 | 3 | 11 | 2 | 5 | 0 | 0 | 35 |
| lambsquarters, chopped | 1 cup | 24 | 2 | 4 | 2 | n/a | 0 | 0 | 24 |
| lambsquarters, cooked, with salt | 1 cup | 58 | 6 | 9 | 4 | 1 | 1 | 0 | 52 |
| leeks, chopped | 1 cup | 54 | 1 | 13 | 2 | 3 | 0 | 0 | 18 |
| leeks, chopped, cooked, with salt | 1 cup | 32 | 1 | 8 | 1 | 1 | 0 | 0 | 256 |
| leeks, chopped, cooked, without salt | 1 cup | 32 | 1 | 8 | 1 | 1 | 0 | 0 | 10 |
| leeks, sliced | 10 slices | 37 | 1 | 8 | 1 | 2 | 0 | 0 | 12 |
| lentil sprouts | ¼ cup | 20 | 2 | 4 | 1 | n/a | 0 | 0 | 2 |
| lettuce, bibb | 4 small leaves | 3 | 0 | 0 | 0 | 0 | 0 | 0 | 1 |
| lettuce, bibb | 4 medium leaves | 5 | 1 | 1 | 0 | 0 | 0 | 0 | 2 |
| lettuce, bibb | 4 large leaves | 8 | 1 | 1 | 1 | 1 | 0 | 0 | 3 |
| lettuce, bibb | 1 5" head | 21 | 2 | 4 | 2 | 2 | 0 | 0 | 8 |

| FOOD ITEM | SERVING SIZE | CALORIES | PRO (g) | CARB (g) | FIBER (g) | SUGAR (g) | FAT (g) | SAT FAT (g) | SOD (mg) |
|---|---|---|---|---|---|---|---|---|---|
| lettuce, Boston | 4 medium leaves | 4 | 0 | 1 | 0 | 0 | 0 | 0 | 2 |
| lettuce, Boston | 1 5" head | 21 | 2 | 4 | 2 | 2 | 0 | 0 | 8 |
| lettuce, butterhead | 4 medium leaves | 4 | 0 | 1 | 0 | 0 | 0 | 0 | 2 |
| lettuce, butterhead | 1 5" head | 21 | 2 | 4 | 2 | 2 | 0 | 0 | 8 |
| lettuce, celtuce | 4 leaves | 6 | 0 | 1 | 0 | 0 | 0 | 0 | 4 |
| lettuce, crisphead | 4 medium leaves | 4 | 0 | 1 | 0 | 1 | 0 | 0 | 3 |
| lettuce, iceberg | 5 large leaves | 10 | 1 | 2 | 1 | 1 | 0 | 0 | 8 |
| lettuce, iceberg, chopped | 1 cup | 8 | 1 | 2 | 1 | 1 | 0 | 0 | 6 |
| lettuce, iceberg, shredded | 1 cup | 10 | 1 | 2 | 1 | 1 | 0 | 0 | 7 |
| lettuce, looseleaf | 5 leaves | 8 | 1 | 1 | 1 | 0 | 0 | 0 | 14 |
| lettuce, looseleaf, shredded | 1 cup | 8 | 1 | 2 | 1 | 0 | 0 | 0 | 16 |
| lettuce, manoa, chopped | 1 cup | 8 | 1 | 1 | 1 | n/a | 0 | 0 | 4 |
| lettuce, red leaf | 4 inner leaves | 2 | 0 | 0 | 0 | 0 | 0 | 0 | 3 |
| lettuce, red leaf | 1 head | 49 | 4 | 7 | 3 | 1 | 1 | 0 | 77 |
| lettuce, red leaf, shredded | 1 cup | 4 | 0 | 1 | 0 | 0 | 0 | 0 | 7 |
| lettuce, romaine | 4 leaves | 13 | 1 | 2 | 1 | 1 | 0 | 0 | 0 |
| lettuce, romaine | 5 inner leaves | 9 | 1 | 2 | 1 | 1 | 0 | 0 | 4 |
| lettuce, romaine, chopped | 1 cup | 8 | 1 | 2 | 1 | 1 | 0 | 0 | 5 |
| lotus root, seeds | 1 oz | 25 | 1 | 5 | n/a | n/a | 0 | 0 | 0 |
| lotus root, sliced into 2.5" pieces | 5 | 30 | 1 | 7 | 2 | n/a | 0 | 0 | 16 |
| mache (lamb's lettuce) | 1 cup | 20 | 1 | 4 | 1 | 0 | 0 | 0 | 16 |
| malabar spinach, cooked | 1 cup | 10 | 1 | 1 | 1 | n/a | 0 | 0 | 24 |
| mountain yam, cubed | ½ cup | 46 | 1 | 11 | 2 | n/a | 0 | 0 | 9 |
| mountain yam, cubed, steamed, with salt | ½ cup | 59 | 1 | 14 | 1 | n/a | 0 | 0 | 180 |
| mountain yam, cubed, steamed, without salt | ½ cup | 59 | 1 | 15 | 2 | n/a | 0 | 0 | 9 |
| mung bean sprouts | ½ cup | 16 | 2 | 3 | 1 | 2 | 0 | 0 | 3 |
| mung bean sprouts, cooked with salt | ½ cup | 13 | 1 | 3 | 1 | 2 | 0 | 0 | 152 |

| FOOD ITEM | SERVING SIZE | CALORIES | PRO (g) | CARB (g) | FIBER (g) | SUGAR (g) | FAT (g) | SAT FAT (g) | SOD (mg) |
|---|---|---|---|---|---|---|---|---|---|
| mung bean sprouts, cooked, without salt | ½ cup | 13 | 1 | 3 | 1 | 2 | 0 | 0 | 5 |
| mung bean sprouts, stir-fried | ½ cup | 31 | 3 | 7 | 1 | n/a | 0 | 0 | 6 |
| mushrooms, brown Italian | 5 | 15 | 2 | 3 | 0 | 1 | 0 | 0 | 4 |
| mushrooms, chanterelle, dried | 4 pieces | 30 | 2 | 4 | 2 | 0 | 0 | 0 | 0 |
| mushrooms, cremini | 5 | 15 | 2 | 3 | 0 | 1 | 0 | 0 | 4 |
| mushrooms, enoki | 5 medium | 6 | 0 | 1 | 0 | 0 | 0 | 0 | 0 |
| mushrooms, enoki | 5 large | 11 | 1 | 2 | 1 | 0 | 0 | 0 | 1 |
| mushrooms, morel, dried | 4 | 20 | 1 | 3 | 0 | 0 | 0 | 0 | 0 |
| mushrooms, oyster | 1 oz | 10 | 1 | 2 | 1 | 0 | 0 | 0 | 5 |
| mushrooms, oyster, dried | 4 | 20 | 1 | 3 | 0 | 0 | 0 | 0 | 0 |
| mushrooms, pickled | 4 | 5 | 0 | 1 | 0 | 0 | 0 | 0 | 1 |
| mushrooms, porcini, dried | 4 | 12 | 1 | 1 | 2 | 1 | 0 | 0 | 0 |
| mushrooms, portobello | 2 oz | 15 | 1 | 3 | 1 | 1 | 0 | 0 | 3 |
| mushrooms, portobello, dried | 4 | 5 | 1 | 1 | 0 | 0 | 0 | 0 | 0 |
| mushrooms, portobello, grilled | 3 oz | 29 | 3 | 4 | 2 | 0 | 1 | 0 | 9 |
| mushrooms, shiitake, dried | 1 tbsp | 30 | 2 | 5 | 1 | n/a | 0 | 0 | 8 |
| mushrooms, shiitake, cooked | 5 | 50 | 1 | 13 | 2 | 4 | 0 | 0 | 4 |
| mushrooms, shiitake, pieces, cooked | ½ cup | 41 | 1 | 10 | 2 | 3 | 0 | 0 | 3 |
| mushrooms, straw, canned, drained | ½ cup | 29 | 3 | 4 | 2 | n/a | 1 | 0 | 349 |
| mushrooms, straw, Padi, dried | 4 | 10 | 1 | 1 | 0 | 0 | 0 | 0 | 0 |
| mustard greens, chopped | 1 cup | 15 | 2 | 3 | 2 | 1 | 0 | 0 | 14 |
| mustard greens, chopped, cooked | 1 cup | 4 | 5 | 5 | n/a | 0 | 0 | 0 | 42 |
| mustard greens, chopped, cooked, with salt | 1 cup | 21 | 3 | 3 | 3 | 0 | 0 | 0 | 353 |
| mustard greens, frozen | 1 cup | 29 | 4 | 5 | 5 | n/a | 0 | 0 | 42 |
| mustard spinach | 1 cup | 33 | 3 | 6 | 4 | n/a | 0 | 0 | 32 |
| nopales cactus, cooked | 1 cup | 22 | 2 | 5 | 3 | 2 | 0 | 0 | 30 |
| nopales cactus, sliced | 1 cup | 14 | 1 | 3 | 2 | 1 | 0 | 0 | 18 |

| FOOD ITEM | SERVING SIZE | CALORIES | PRO (g) | CARB (g) | FIBER (g) | SUGAR (g) | FAT (g) | SAT FAT (g) | SOD (mg) |
|---|---|---|---|---|---|---|---|---|---|
| okra, cooked | 1 cup | 52 | 4 | 11 | 5 | 5 | 1 | 0 | 6 |
| okra, frozen | 3 oz | 26 | 1 | 6 | 2 | 3 | 0 | 0 | 3 |
| okra pods, cooked | 3 oz | 19 | 2 | 4 | 2 | 2 | 0 | 0 | 5 |
| onion, green (scallions), top, chopped | ½ cup | 12 | 1 | 3 | 2 | 1 | 0 | 0 | 2 |
| onion, green (scallions), top and bulb, chopped | ½ cup | 16 | 1 | 4 | 1 | 1 | 0 | 0 | 8 |
| onion, pearl, chopped | ½ cup | 34 | 1 | 8 | 1 | 3 | 0 | 0 | 2 |
| onion, pearl, cooked | ½ cup | 60 | 1 | 14 | n/a | 4 | 0 | 0 | 18 |
| onion, pearl, diced, cooked | ½ cup | 41 | 1 | 9 | 1 | 4 | 0 | 0 | 3 |
| onion, red | 1 small | 29 | 1 | 7 | 1 | 3 | 0 | 0 | 2 |
| onion, red | 1 medium | 46 | 1 | 11 | 2 | 5 | 0 | 0 | 3 |
| onion, red | 1 large | 63 | 1 | 15 | 2 | 6 | 0 | 0 | 5 |
| onion, red, chopped | ½ cup | 46 | 1 | 11 | 1 | 5 | 0 | 0 | 3 |
| onion, red, sliced | 1 small slice | 4 | 0 | 1 | 0 | 0 | 0 | 0 | 0 |
| onion, red, sliced | 1 medium slice | 6 | 0 | 1 | 0 | 1 | 0 | 0 | 0 |
| onion, red, sliced | 1 large slice | 16 | 0 | 4 | 1 | 2 | 0 | 0 | 1 |
| onion, yellow | 1 small | 29 | 1 | 7 | 1 | 3 | 0 | 0 | 2 |
| onion, yellow | 1 medium | 46 | 1 | 11 | 2 | 5 | 0 | 0 | 3 |
| onion, yellow | 1 large | 63 | 1 | 15 | 2 | 6 | 0 | 0 | 5 |
| onion, yellow, chopped | ½ cup | 34 | 1 | 8 | 1 | 3 | 0 | 0 | 2 |
| onion, yellow, sliced | 1 small slice | 4 | 0 | 1 | 0 | 0 | 0 | 0 | 0 |
| onion, yellow, sliced | 1 medium slice | 6 | 0 | 1 | 0 | 1 | 0 | 0 | 0 |
| onion, yellow, sliced | 1 large slice | 16 | 0 | 4 | 1 | 2 | 0 | 0 | 1 |
| palm, hearts | 1 oz | 33 | 1 | 7 | 1 | 5 | 0 | 0 | 4 |
| palm, hearts, canned | ½ cup | 20 | 2 | 3 | 2 | n/a | 0 | 0 | 311 |
| palm, hearts, sliced, cooked | ½ cup | 75 | 2 | 19 | 1 | n/a | 0 | 0 | 10 |
| parsnips, sliced | ½ cup | 49 | 1 | 12 | 3 | 3 | 0 | 0 | 7 |
| parsnips, sliced, cooked, with salt, drained | ½ cup | 63 | 1 | 15 | 3 | 4 | 0 | 0 | 192 |

| FOOD ITEM | SERVING SIZE | CALORIES | PRO (g) | CARB (g) | FIBER (g) | SUGAR (g) | FAT (g) | SAT FAT (g) | SOD (mg) |
|---|---|---|---|---|---|---|---|---|---|
| parsnips, sliced, cooked, without salt, drained | ½ cup | 55 | 1 | 13 | 3 | 4 | 0 | 0 | 8 |
| peas, green | ½ cup | 59 | 4 | 10 | 4 | 4 | 4 | 0 | 0 |
| peas, green, cooked | ½ cup | 62 | 4 | 11 | 4 | 4 | 0 | 0 | 3 |
| peas, snow | ½ cup | 13 | 1 | 2 | 1 | 1 | 0 | 0 | 1 |
| peas, snow, steamed | ½ cup | 35 | 2 | 6 | 2 | 3 | 0 | 0 | 3 |
| peas, snow, stir-fried | ½ cup | 35 | 2 | 6 | 2 | 3 | 0 | 0 | 3 |
| pepper, ancho, dried | 1 | 47 | 2 | 9 | 4 | n/a | 1 | 0 | 7 |
| pepper, banana | 1 | 12 | 1 | 2 | 2 | 1 | 0 | 0 | 6 |
| pepper, hot chili, green | 1 | 18 | 1 | 4 | 1 | 2 | 0 | 0 | 3 |
| pepper, hot chili, red | 1 | 18 | 1 | 4 | 1 | 2 | 0 | 0 | 4 |
| pepper, hot chili, sun-dried | 2 tbsp | 15 | 0 | 3 | 1 | 1 | 0 | 0 | 4 |
| pepper, hot green, chopped | ¼ cup | 15 | 1 | 4 | 1 | 2 | 0 | 0 | 3 |
| pepper, pasilla, dried | 1 | 24 | 1 | 4 | 2 | n/a | 1 | 0 | 6 |
| pigeon peas, cooked, with salt | ¼ cup | 51 | 3 | 10 | 3 | 0 | 0 | 0 | 101 |
| pigeon peas, cooked, without salt | ¼ cup | 51 | 3 | 10 | 3 | n/a | 0 | 0 | 2 |
| pokeberry, cooked | ½ cup | 17 | 2 | 3 | 1 | 1 | 0 | 0 | 15 |
| pokeberry shoot (poke) | ½ cup | 18 | 2 | 3 | 1 | n/a | 0 | 0 | 18 |
| potato, baked, with skin | 1 small | 115 | 2 | 27 | 5 | 1 | 0 | 0 | 12 |
| potato, baked, with skin | 1 medium | 162 | 4 | 36 | 4 | 3 | 0 | 0 | 12 |
| potatoes, new | 3 oz | 54 | 2 | 11 | 3 | 1 | 0 | 0 | 3 |
| potato, red, baked with skin | 6 oz | 154 | 4 | 33 | 3 | 3 | 0 | 0 | 14 |
| potato, roasted | 1 medium | 132 | 3 | 30 | 3 | 2 | 0 | 0 | 10 |
| potato, russet, baked, with skin | 1 medium | 168 | 5 | 37 | 4 | 2 | 0 | 0 | 14 |
| pumpkin, butter | ¼ cup | 320 | 21 | 8 | 2 | n/a | 26 | 6 | 0 |
| pumpkin, canned, with salt | ½ cup | 42 | 1 | 10 | 4 | 4 | 0 | 0 | 295 |
| pumpkin, canned, without salt | ½ cup | 42 | 1 | 10 | 4 | 4 | 0 | 0 | 6 |
| pumpkin, cooked, mashed, with salt | ½ cup | 25 | 1 | 6 | 1 | 1 | 0 | 0 | 290 |
| pumpkin, cooked, mashed, without salt | ½ cup | 25 | 1 | 6 | 1 | 1 | 0 | 0 | 1 |

| FOOD ITEM | SERVING SIZE | CALORIES | PRO (g) | CARB (g) | FIBER (g) | SUGAR (g) | FAT (g) | SAT FAT (g) | SOD (mg) |
|---|---|---|---|---|---|---|---|---|---|
| pumpkin, cubed | ½ cup | 15 | 1 | 4 | 0 | 1 | 0 | 0 | 1 |
| pumpkin flowers | ½ cup | 2 | 0 | 1 | 0 | 0 | 0 | 0 | 1 |
| pumpkin flowers, cooked, with salt | ½ cup | 10 | 1 | 2 | 1 | 2 | 0 | 0 | 162 |
| pumpkin flowers, cooked, without salt | ½ cup | 10 | 1 | 2 | 1 | 2 | 0 | 0 | 4 |
| pumpkin pie filling mix, canned | ½ cup | 140 | 1 | 36 | 11 | n/a | 0 | 0 | 281 |
| purslane | 1 cup | 7 | 1 | 1 | n/a | n/a | 0 | 0 | 19 |
| purslane, cooked, with salt | ½ cup | 18 | 1 | 2 | 0 | n/a | 0 | 0 | 161 |
| purslane, cooked, without salt | ½ cup | 21 | 2 | 4 | n/a | n/a | 0 | 0 | 51 |
| radicchio | 10 leaves | 18 | 1 | 4 | 1 | 0 | 0 | 0 | 18 |
| radicchio, shredded | 1 cup | 9 | 1 | 2 | 0 | 0 | 0 | 0 | 9 |
| radish, daikon | ½ cup | 15 | 1 | 1 | 0 | 0 | 0 | 0 | 0 |
| radish, red | 1 | 1 | 0 | 0 | 0 | 0 | 0 | 0 | 2 |
| radish, red, sliced | ½ cup | 9 | 0 | 2 | 1 | 1 | 0 | 0 | 23 |
| radish, white icicle, sliced | ½ cup | 7 | 1 | 1 | 1 | n/a | 0 | 0 | 8 |
| radish seed sprout | ½ cup | 8 | 1 | 1 | 1 | n/a | 0 | 0 | 1 |
| rapini | 1 cup | 25 | 3 | 4 | 2 | 1 | 0 | 0 | 25 |
| rutabaga | 1 small | 69 | 2 | 16 | 5 | 11 | 0 | 0 | 38 |
| rutabaga | 1 medium | 139 | 5 | 31 | 10 | 22 | 1 | 0 | 77 |
| rutabaga, cubed | ½ cup | 25 | 1 | 6 | 2 | 4 | 0 | 0 | 14 |
| rutabaga, mashed | ½ cup | 48 | 2 | 10 | 2 | 7 | 0 | 0 | 24 |
| salsify, sliced | ½ cup | 55 | 2 | 12 | 2 | n/a | 0 | 0 | 13 |
| salsify, sliced, cooked, with salt | ½ cup | 46 | 2 | 10 | 2 | 2 | 0 | 0 | 170 |
| salsify, sliced, cooked, without salt | ½ cup | 46 | 2 | 10 | 2 | 2 | 0 | 0 | 11 |
| sauerkraut, Bavarian-style, canned | 1 cup | 30 | 0 | 6 | 2 | 4 | 0 | 0 | 210 |
| sauerkraut, canned, low-sodium | 1 cup | 31 | 1 | 6 | 4 | 3 | 0 | 0 | 437 |
| sauerkraut, refrigerated | ½ cup | 20 | 0 | 4 | 3 | 2 | 0 | 0 | 720 |
| seaweed, agar | ¼ cup | 5 | 0 | 1 | 0 | 0 | 0 | 0 | 2 |
| seaweed, agar, dried | 1 tbsp | 3 | 0 | 1 | 0 | 0 | 0 | 0 | 1 |

| FOOD ITEM | SERVING SIZE | CALORIES | PRO (g) | CARB (g) | FIBER (g) | SUGAR (g) | FAT (g) | SAT FAT (g) | SOD (mg) |
|---|---|---|---|---|---|---|---|---|---|
| seaweed, kelp | ¼ cup | 9 | 0 | 2 | 0 | 0 | 0 | 0 | 47 |
| seaweed, kombu | ¼ cup | 9 | 0 | 2 | 0 | 0 | 0 | 0 | 47 |
| seaweed, nori | ¼ cup | 7 | 1 | 1 | 0 | 0 | 0 | 0 | 10 |
| seaweed, pickled | ¼ cup | 56 | 0 | 15 | 0 | 0 | 0 | 0 | 55 |
| seaweed, spirulina | ¼ cup | 5 | 1 | 0 | 0 | 0 | 0 | 0 | 19 |
| seaweed, wakame | ¼ cup | 5 | 0 | 1 | 0 | 0 | 0 | 0 | 87 |
| sesbania flower | 1 cup | 5 | 0 | 1 | 0 | 0 | 0 | 0 | 3 |
| shallots, chopped | ¼ cup | 29 | 1 | 7 | 0 | 1 | 0 | 0 | 5 |
| shallots, freeze-dried | 1 tbsp | 3 | 0 | 1 | 0 | 0 | 0 | 0 | 1 |
| snap beans, green | 1 cup | 27 | 1 | 7 | 4 | 3 | 0 | 0 | 0 |
| snap beans, green, canned, with salt, drained | 1 cup | 28 | 2 | 6 | 3 | 1 | 0 | 0 | 371 |
| snap beans, green, canned, without salt, drained | 1 cup | 21 | 1 | 5 | 2 | 0 | 0 | 0 | 20 |
| snap beans, yellow, cooked, drained | 1 cup | 38 | 2 | 9 | 4 | 2 | 0 | 0 | 12 |
| snap beans, yellow, frozen | 1 cup | 41 | 2 | 9 | 3 | 2 | 0 | 0 | 4 |
| spaghetti squash, baked | 1 cup | 42 | 1 | 10 | 2 | 4 | 0 | 0 | 28 |
| spaghetti squash, cubed | 1 cup | 31 | 1 | 7 | n/a | n/a | 1 | 0 | 17 |
| spinach | 3 oz | 20 | 2 | 3 | 2 | 0 | 0 | 0 | 67 |
| spinach, baby | 1 cup | 10 | 1 | 3 | 1 | 0 | 0 | 0 | 39 |
| spinach, chopped | 1 cup | 11 | 1 | 2 | 1 | n/a | 0 | 0 | 63 |
| spinach, cooked, with salt | 1 cup | 41 | 5 | 7 | 4 | 1 | 0 | 0 | 551 |
| spinach, cooked, without salt | 1 cup | 41 | 5 | 7 | 4 | 1 | 0 | 0 | 126 |
| squash, acorn, cooked, with salt | ½ cup | 41 | 1 | 11 | 3 | n/a | 0 | 0 | 293 |
| squash, acorn, cooked, without salt, mashed | ½ cup | 42 | 1 | 11 | 3 | n/a | 0 | 0 | 4 |
| squash, butternut, cooked, mashed | ½ cup | 47 | 1 | 12 | 3 | n/a | 0 | 0 | 2 |
| squash, butternut, cubed | ½ cup | 54 | 1 | 14 | 2 | 3 | 0 | 0 | 5 |
| squash, butternut, cubed, baked | ½ cup | 41 | 1 | 11 | 3 | 2 | 0 | 0 | 4 |
| squash, butternut, frozen | ½ cup | 48 | 2 | 12 | 1 | 2 | 0 | 0 | 2 |

| FOOD ITEM | SERVING SIZE | CALORIES | PRO (g) | CARB (g) | FIBER (g) | SUGAR (g) | FAT (g) | SAT FAT (g) | SOD (mg) |
|---|---|---|---|---|---|---|---|---|---|
| squash, crookneck, cooked, with salt | 1 cup | 36 | 2 | 7 | 3 | 4 | 1 | 0 | 289 |
| squash, crookneck, cooked, without salt | 1 cup | 48 | 2 | 11 | 3 | 4 | 0 | 0 | 12 |
| squash, crookneck, sliced | 1 cup | 25 | 1 | 5 | 2 | n/a | 0 | 0 | 3 |
| squash, Hubbard, cooked, mashed | ½ cup | 35 | 2 | 8 | 3 | 3 | 0 | 0 | 6 |
| squash, Hubbard, cubed | ½ cup | 23 | 1 | 5 | n/a | 1 | 0 | 0 | 4 |
| squash, Hubbard, cubed, baked | ½ cup | 60 | 3 | 13 | 3 | n/a | 1 | 0 | 10 |
| squash, scallop, cooked, with salt | ½ cup | 19 | 1 | 4 | 2 | 2 | 0 | 0 | 284 |
| squash, scallop, cooked, without salt | ½ cup | 19 | 1 | 4 | 2 | 2 | 0 | 0 | 1 |
| squash, straightneck, sliced | 1 cup | 25 | 1 | 5 | 2 | n/a | 0 | 0 | 3 |
| squash, summer | 1 medium | 31 | 2 | 7 | 2 | 4 | 0 | 0 | 4 |
| squash, summer | 1 large | 52 | 4 | 11 | 4 | 7 | 1 | 0 | 6 |
| squash, summer, sliced, cooked, with salt | 1 cup | 36 | 2 | 8 | 3 | 5 | 1 | 0 | 427 |
| squash, summer, sliced, cooked, without salt | 1 cup | 36 | 2 | 8 | 3 | 5 | 1 | 0 | 2 |
| squash, winter, cubed | ½ cup | 20 | 1 | 5 | 1 | 1 | 0 | 0 | 2 |
| squash, winter acorn, cubed | ½ cup | 28 | 1 | 7 | 1 | 2 | 0 | 0 | 2 |
| squash, winter acorn, cubed, baked, with salt | ½ cup | 57 | 1 | 15 | 5 | 4 | 0 | 0 | 246 |
| sweet potato, baked, with skin | 1 small | 95 | 2 | 22 | 3 | 16 | 0 | 0 | 10 |
| sweet potato, baked, without skin | 1 medium | 115 | 2 | 27 | 4 | 9 | 0 | 0 | 41 |
| sweet potato, baked, without skin | 1 large | 162 | 4 | 37 | 6 | 15 | 0 | 0 | 65 |
| sweet potato, candied | ½ cup | 122 | 1 | 14 | 2 | n/a | 3 | 1 | 60 |
| sweet potato, canned, with syrup | ½ cup | 106 | 1 | 25 | 3 | 6 | 0 | 0 | 38 |
| sweet potato, cooked, mashed | ½ cup | 125 | 2 | 29 | 4 | 9 | 0 | 0 | 44 |
| sweet potato, mashed, canned | ½ cup | 129 | 3 | 30 | 2 | 7 | 0 | 0 | 96 |
| sweet potato, peeled, cooked with salt | ½ cup | 90 | 2 | 21 | 3 | 8 | 0 | 0 | 246 |
| sweet potato leaves | ½ cup | 6 | 1 | 1 | 0 | 0 | 0 | 0 | 2 |

| FOOD ITEM | SERVING SIZE | CALORIES | PRO (g) | CARB (g) | FIBER (g) | SUGAR (g) | FAT (g) | SAT FAT (g) | SOD (mg) |
|---|---|---|---|---|---|---|---|---|---|
| Swiss chard | 3 leaves | 27 | 3 | 5 | 2 | 2 | 0 | 0 | 307 |
| Swiss chard, chopped | 1 cup | 7 | 1 | 1 | 1 | 0 | 0 | 0 | 77 |
| Swiss chard, chopped, cooked, with salt, drained | 1 cup | 35 | 3 | 7 | 4 | 2 | 0 | 0 | 726 |
| Swiss chard, chopped, cooked, without salt, drained | 1 cup | 35 | 3 | 7 | 4 | 2 | 0 | 0 | 313 |
| taro, cooked | ¼ cup | 50 | 1 | 12 | 2 | n/a | 0 | 0 | 5 |
| taro leaves | 1 cup | 12 | 1 | 2 | n/a | n/a | 0 | 0 | 1 |
| taro shoot, sliced | ½ cup | 10 | 1 | 2 | 0 | 0 | 0 | 0 | 1 |
| taro, Tahitian, cooked, with salt | ½ cup | 30 | 3 | 4 | 1 | n/a | 0 | 0 | 199 |
| tomatillo | 1 medium | 11 | 0 | 2 | 1 | 1 | 0 | 0 | 0 |
| tomatillo, chopped | ½ cup | 21 | 1 | 4 | 1 | 3 | 1 | 0 | 1 |
| tomato, red | 1 medium | 35 | 1 | 7 | 1 | 4 | 1 | 0 | 5 |
| tomato, red, broiled | 1 | 32 | 1 | 7 | 2 | 5 | 1 | 0 | 14 |
| tomato, red, canned | 4 oz | 19 | 1 | 4 | 1 | 3 | 0 | 0 | 145 |
| tomato, red, chopped | ½ cup | 19 | 1 | 4 | 1 | 3 | 0 | 0 | 8 |
| tomato, red, cooked, without salt | ½ cup | 22 | 1 | 5 | 1 | 3 | 0 | 0 | 13 |
| tomato, red, crushed, canned | ½ cup | 39 | 2 | 9 | 2 | n/a | 0 | 0 | 161 |
| tomato, red, diced, canned, with green chili | ½ cup | 18 | 1 | 4 | 1 | n/a | 0 | 0 | 483 |
| tomato, red, diced, canned, without salt | ½ cup | 25 | 1 | 6 | 2 | 4 | 0 | 0 | 50 |
| tomato, red, sliced | 1 slice | 6 | 0 | 1 | 0 | 1 | 0 | 0 | 2 |
| tomato, red, stewed | ½ cup | 35 | 1 | 7 | 2 | 5 | 0 | 0 | 270 |
| tomato, green | 1 | 28 | 1 | 6 | 1 | 5 | 0 | 0 | 16 |
| tomato, green, fried | 1 | 284 | 5 | 19 | 1 | 4 | 22 | 5 | 134 |
| tomato, orange | 1 | 18 | 1 | 4 | 1 | n/a | 0 | 0 | 47 |
| tomato, orange, chopped | ½ cup | 13 | 1 | 3 | 1 | 0 | 0 | 0 | 33 |
| tomato paste, with salt | 1 tbsp | 13 | 1 | 3 | 1 | 2 | 0 | 0 | 129 |
| tomato paste, without salt | 1 tbsp | 13 | 1 | 3 | 1 | 2 | 0 | 0 | 16 |
| tomato puree, without salt | ½ cup | 43 | 2 | 10 | 2 | 5 | 0 | 0 | 32 |

| FOOD ITEM | SERVING SIZE | CALORIES | PRO (g) | CARB (g) | FIBER (g) | SUGAR (g) | FAT (g) | SAT FAT (g) | SOD (mg) |
|---|---|---|---|---|---|---|---|---|---|
| turnip | 1 small | 17 | 1 | 4 | 1 | 2 | 0 | 0 | 41 |
| turnip | 1 medium | 34 | 1 | 8 | 2 | 5 | 0 | 0 | 82 |
| turnip | 1 large | 51 | 2 | 12 | 3 | 7 | 0 | 0 | 123 |
| turnip, cooked, mashed | ½ cup | 25 | 1 | 6 | 2 | 3 | 0 | 0 | 18 |
| turnip, cubed | 1 cup | 36 | 8 | 2 | 5 | 0 | 0 | 0 | 87 |
| turnip, sliced, pickled | 5 slices | 15 | 0 | 4 | 1 | 3 | 0 | 0 | 15 |
| turnip, with greens | 1 cup | 36 | 4 | 5 | 3 | 2 | 0 | 0 | 26 |
| turnip greens, chopped | 1 cup | 18 | 1 | 4 | 2 | 0 | 0 | 0 | 22 |
| turnip greens, cooked | 1 cup | 48 | 5 | 8 | 6 | 1 | 0 | 0 | 25 |
| wasabi, sliced, cooked, with salt | 1 tbsp | 2 | 0 | 0 | 0 | 0 | 0 | 0 | 23 |
| water chestnuts, canned | 1 oz | 14 | 0 | 3 | 3 | 1 | 0 | 0 | 3 |
| water chestnuts, Chinese (matai), canned | ½ cup | 35 | 1 | 9 | 2 | 2 | 0 | 0 | 6 |
| water chestnuts, Chinese (matai), sliced, canned | ½ cup | 35 | 1 | 9 | 2 | 2 | 0 | 0 | 6 |
| watercress | 4 sprigs | 1 | 0 | 0 | 0 | 0 | 0 | 0 | 4 |
| watercress, chopped | 1 cup | 4 | 1 | 0 | 0 | 0 | 0 | 0 | 14 |
| waxgourd (Chinese preserving melon) | 1 cup | 17 | 1 | 4 | 4 | n/a | 0 | 0 | 147 |
| waxgourd (Chinese preserving melon), candied | 1 oz | 81 | 0 | 23 | n/a | n/a | n/a | n/a | n/a |
| waxgourd (Chinese preserving melon), cooked | 1 cup | 25 | 1 | 5 | 2 | 2 | 0 | 0 | 187 |
| winged bean leaves | 1 cup | 75 | 6 | 14 | 3 | n/a | 1 | 0 | 9 |
| winged bean tuber | ¼ cup | 37 | 3 | 7 | n/a | n/a | 0 | 0 | 9 |
| winged beans, cooked | ¼ cup | 63 | 5 | 6 | 1 | n/a | 3 | 0 | 6 |
| yam, cooked, with salt | ¼ cup | 39 | 1 | 9 | 1 | 0 | 0 | 0 | 83 |
| yam, cooked, without salt | ¼ cup | 39 | 1 | 9 | 1 | 0 | 0 | 0 | 3 |
| yams, candied | ¼ cup | 85 | 1 | 23 | 2 | 11 | 0 | 0 | 180 |
| yardlong beans | ¼ cup | 50 | 4 | 9 | 2 | n/a | 0 | 0 | 2 |
| yautia (tannier) | ¼ cup | 33 | 0 | 8 | 1 | n/a | 0 | 0 | 7 |
| zucchini | 1 medium | 35 | 2 | 7 | 2 | 3 | 0 | 0 | 20 |
| zucchini, sliced, steamed | 1 cup | 25 | 2 | 5 | 2 | 0 | 0 | 0 | 5 |

| FOOD ITEM | SERVING SIZE | CALORIES | PRO (g) | CARB (g) | FIBER (g) | SUGAR (g) | FAT (g) | SAT FAT (g) | SOD (mg) |
|---|---|---|---|---|---|---|---|---|---|
| **Arby's** | | | | | | | | | |
| Junior Roast Beef Sandwich | 125 g | 270 | 16 | 34 | 2 | 5 | 10 | 4 | 740 |
| Market Fresh Martha's Vineyard Salad™ | 291 g | 270 | 26 | 22 | 4 | 17 | 8 | 4 | 450 |
| Raspberry Vinaigrette dressing (for Martha's Vineyard Salad) | 64 g | 190 | 0 | 18 | 0 | 16 | 14 | 1.5 | 390 |
| Sliced Almonds (for Martha's Vineyard Salad) | 14 g | 81 | 4 | 2 | 1 | 0 | 7 | 0 | 0 |
| **Au Bon Pain** | | | | | | | | | |
| **Baked Goods** | | | | | | | | | |
| Chocolate Cake Muffin, low-fat | 4.15 oz | 320 | 4 | 74 | 4 | 48 | 2 | 0.5 | 590 |
| Triple Berry Muffin, low-fat | 4.35 oz | 290 | 5 | 61 | 2 | 31 | 2 | 0.5 | 310 |
| **Soups** | | | | | | | | | |
| Black Bean Soup, low-fat | 8 oz | 100 | 10 | | 16 | 2 | 0.5 | 0 | 890 |
| Chicken Noodle soup, low-fat | 8 oz | 100 | 6 | | 1 | 2 | 2 | 0 | 920 |
| Garden Vegetable, low-fat | 8 oz | 50 | 2 | | 2 | 3 | 1 | 0 | 670 |
| Southern Black Eyed Pea | 8 oz | 120 | 8 | | 8 | 3 | 1 | 0 | 630 |
| Southwest Vegetable, low-fat | 8 oz | 70 | 2 | | 2 | 2 | 2 | 0 | 250 |
| Tomato Basil Bisque soup, low-fat | 8 oz | 140 | 4 | | 4 | 12 | 5 | 3.5 | 330 |
| Vegetable Beef Barley, low-fat | 8 oz | 90 | 7 | | 3 | 2 | 1.5 | 1 | 1220 |
| Vegetarian Chili, low-fat | 8 oz | 120 | 9 | | 15 | 5 | 1.5 | 0 | 870 |
| Vegetarian Lentil (low-fat) | 8 oz | 90 | 7 | | 8 | 3 | 1 | 0 | 840 |
| Vegetarian Minestrone, low-fat | 8 oz | 80 | 3 | | 3 | 4 | 1 | 0 | 740 |
| **Miscellaneous** | | | | | | | | | |
| Fruit Cup | 12 oz | 140 | 2 | | 2 | 30 | 1 | 0 | 20 |
| Garden Salad | 7.8 oz | 110 | 5 | | 5 | 3 | 2 | 0 | 300 |
| Muesli | 7 oz | 340 | 9 | | 6 | 26 | 7 | 1.5 | 40 |
| Oatmeal | 1.41 oz | 150 | 5 | | 4 | 1 | 3 | 0.5 | 0 |
| Raspberry Vinaigrette, fat-free | 2.5 oz | 80 | 0 | | 0 | 16 | 0 | 0 | 190 |

| FOOD ITEM | SERVING SIZE | CALORIES | PRO (g) | CARB (g) | FIBER (g) | SUGAR (g) | FAT (g) | SAT FAT (g) | SOD (mg) |
|---|---|---|---|---|---|---|---|---|---|
| **Auntie Anne's®** | | | | | | | | | |
| Auntie Anne's Stix | 6 pieces (120 g) | 290 | 8 | | 1 | 10 | 1 | 0 | 1130 |
| Garlic Pretzel, without butter | 120 g | 320 | 9 | | 2 | 9 | 1 | 0 | 830 |
| Jalapeño Pretzel, without butter | 120 g | 270 | 8 | | 2 | 8 | 1 | 0 | 780 |
| Original Pretzel, without butter | 120 g | 340 | 10 | | 3 | 10 | 1 | 0 | 900 |
| Sour Cream and Onion Pretzel, without butter | 120 g | 310 | 9 | | 2 | 9 | 1 | 0 | 920 |
| Whole Wheat Pretzel, without butter | 120 g | 350 | 11 | | 7 | 10 | 1.5 | 0 | 1100 |
| **Baja Fresh** | | | | | | | | | |
| **Salads and Tacos** | | | | | | | | | |
| Baja Ensalada with Carnitas | 473 g | 370 | 35 | | 7 | 7 | 18 | 6 | 1410 |
| Baja Ensalada with Chicken | 473 g | 310 | 46 | | 7 | 8 | 7 | 2 | 1210 |
| Baja Ensalada with Shrimp | 445 g | 230 | 28 | | 6 | 8 | 6 | 2 | 1110 |
| Baja Ensalada with Steak | 473 g | 450 | 54 | | 6 | 8 | 18 | 7 | 1240 |
| Baja Fish Taco | 140 g | 320 | 8 | | 3 | 2 | 16 | 2.5 | 400 |
| Baja Style Charbroiled Chicken Taco | 117 g | 250 | 13 | | 3 | 2 | 8 | 1 | 240 |
| Baja Style Charbroiled Shrimp Taco | 126 g | 250 | 12 | | 2 | 2 | 8 | 1 | 290 |
| Baja Style Charbroiled Steak Taco | 115 g | 280 | 14 | | 2 | 2 | 10 | 2 | 240 |
| **Sides** | | | | | | | | | |
| Pico de Gallo | 227 g | 50 | 2 | | 3 | 7 | 0.5 | 0 | 890 |
| Salsa | 227 g | 70 | 2 | | 4 | 6 | 2.5 | 0 | 970 |
| Salsa Roja | 227 g | 70 | 3 | | 4 | 6 | 1 | 0 | 1080 |
| Salsa Verde | 227 g | 50 | 2 | | 3 | 7 | 0 | 0 | 1170 |
| Savory Pork Carnitas | 170 g | 300 | 35 | | 2 | 1 | 16 | 6 | 1010 |
| Tortilla Soup, with chicken | 380 g | 320 | 17 | | 4 | 5 | 14 | 4 | 2750 |
| Tortilla Soup, without chicken | 346 g | 270 | 8 | | 4 | 5 | 14 | 4 | 2600 |

| FOOD ITEM | SERVING SIZE | CALORIES | PRO (g) | CARB (g) | FIBER (g) | SUGAR (g) | FAT (g) | SAT FAT (g) | SOD (mg) |
|---|---|---|---|---|---|---|---|---|---|
| **Ben and Jerry's** | | | | | | | | | |
| Berry Berry Extraordinary Sorbet | ½ cup | 100 | 0 | | 1 | 23 | 0 | 0 | 5 |
| Jamaican Me Crazy sorbet | ½ cup | 140 | 0 | | 1 | 32 | 0 | 0 | 10 |
| Lemonade Sorbet | ½ cup | 100 | 0 | | 1 | 21 | 0 | 0 | 5 |
| Mango Lime Sorbet | ½ cup | 100 | 0 | | 1 | 23 | 0 | 0 | 10 |
| Strawberry Kiwi Sorbet | ½ cup | 100 | 0 | | 1 | 23 | 0 | 0 | 10 |
| **Blimpie** | | | | | | | | | |
| **Subs and Salads** | | | | | | | | | |
| Buffalo Chicken Sub* | 6" sub | 320 | 32 | | 2.7 | 7 | 7.4 | 3 | 2108 |
| Chef Salad | Regular size | 212 | 20 | | 3 | 5 | 9 | 4.6 | 961 |
| Grilled Chicken Salad, without dressing | Regular size | 180 | 22 | | 3 | 1 | 7 | 3.5 | 410 |
| Grilled Chicken Sub* | 6" sub | 350 | 26 | | 3 | 7 | 7 | 2 | 750 |
| Roast Beef Sub* | 6" sub | 370 | 28 | | 3 | 7 | 7 | 2.5 | 1090 |
| Seafood Salad | Regular size | 122 | 6 | | 3.2 | 4.5 | 4.4 | 0.7 | 418 |
| Seafood Sub* | 6" sub | 355 | 14 | | 3.8 | 9 | 7.7 | 1.6 | 895 |
| Turkey Sub* | 6" sub | 330 | 17 | | 3 | 7 | 4.5 | 1 | 1270 |
| **Baked Goods** | | | | | | | | | |
| Oatmeal Raisin Cookie | 1 cookie | 190 | 3 | | 1 | 16 | 8 | 2 | 200 |

*As analyzed, subs were prepared on a 6" white roll with lettuce, tomato, and onion. Salads were prepared following their individual specialty recipes.

| FOOD ITEM | SERVING SIZE | CALORIES | PRO (g) | CARB (g) | FIBER (g) | SUGAR (g) | FAT (g) | SAT FAT (g) | SOD (mg) |
|---|---|---|---|---|---|---|---|---|---|
| **Boston Market** | | | | | | | | | |
| **Meals** | | | | | | | | | |
| ¼ Dark Original Rotisserie Chicken | 204 g | 420 | 47 | 1 | 0 | 0 | 26 | 8 | 660 |
| ¼ Dark Original Rotisserie Chicken, no skin | 204 g | 400 | 46 | 1 | 0 | 0 | 21 | 6 | 700 |
| ¼ Dark Simply Seasoned Chicken | 200 g | 420 | 47 | 0 | 0 | 0 | 26 | 8 | 630 |
| ¼ White Original Rotisserie Chicken | 265 g | 510 | 67 | 2 | 0 | 1 | 27 | 9 | 1140 |
| ¼ White Original Rotisserie Chicken, no skin | 264 g | 320 | 60 | 2 | 0 | 2 | 7 | 2 | 950 |
| ¼ White Simply Seasoned Chicken | 261 g | 510 | 67 | 1 | 0 | 1 | 27 | 9 | 1110 |

| FOOD ITEM | SERVING SIZE | CALORIES | PRO (g) | CARB (g) | FIBER (g) | SUGAR (g) | FAT (g) | SAT FAT (g) | SOD (mg) |
|---|---|---|---|---|---|---|---|---|---|
| **Boston Market (cont.)** | | | | | | | | | |
| **Meals (cont.)** | | | | | | | | | |
| Pastry Top Chicken Pot Pie | 425 g | 800 | 31 | 59 | 4 | 4 | 49 | 18 | 910 |
| Roasted Turkey, with gravy | n/a | 250 | 31 | 5 | 0 | 2 | 11 | 2 | 970 |
| USDA Choice Meatloaf | 7.7 oz | 510 | 31 | 4 | 0 | 4 | 35 | 14 | 115 |
| USDA Choice Roasted Sirloin | 5 oz | 270 | 43 | 0 | 0 | 0 | 10 | 3.5 | 290 |
| **Family Meals** | | | | | | | | | |
| Roasted Turkey, with gravy | n/a | 250 | 31 | 5 | 0 | 2 | 11 | 2 | 970 |
| Whole Original Rotisserie Chicken | 3 oz | 160 | 24 | 0 | 0 | 0 | 7 | 2 | 310 |
| Whole Simply Seasoned Rotisserie Chicken | 3 oz | 160 | 24 | 0 | 0 | 0 | 7 | 2 | 300 |
| USDA Choice Meatloaf | 7.7 oz | 510 | 31 | 4 | 0 | 4 | 35 | 14 | 115 |
| USDA Choice Roasted Sirloin | 5 oz | 270 | 43 | 0 | 0 | 0 | 10 | 3.5 | 290 |
| **Soups and Sides** | | | | | | | | | |
| Au Gratin Potatoes | 5.5 oz | 200 | 7 | 18 | 2 | 3 | 12 | 6 | 350 |
| Caesar Salad Dressing | n/a | 360 | 2 | 30 | n/a | n/a | 38 | 6 | 2 |
| Caesar Side Salad | 142 g | 400 | 5 | 7 | 2 | 4 | 40 | 8 | 980 |
| Chicken Noodle Soup | 6 oz | 180 | 15 | 16 | 1 | 1 | 7 | 2 | 200 |
| Chicken Tortilla Soup, with toppings | 6 oz | 350 | 13 | 25 | 1 | 2 | 21 | 7 | 1040 |
| Cinnamon Apples | 5.1 oz | 210 | 0 | 47 | 3 | 42 | 3 | 0 | 15 |
| Coleslaw | 4.4 oz | 220 | 2 | 11 | 2 | 6 | 19 | 3 | 160 |
| Cranberry Walnut Relish, low-fat | 2.7 oz | 120 | 1 | 27 | 2 | 25 | 1.5 | 0 | 0 |
| Creamed Spinach | 6.7 oz | 280 | 9 | 12 | 4 | 1 | 23 | 15 | 580 |
| Fresh Fruit Salad, low-fat | 5 oz | 60 | 1 | 15 | 1 | 13 | 0 | 0 | 20 |
| Fresh Steamed Vegetables, low-fat | 4.8 oz | 35 | 2 | 6 | 2 | 1 | 0.5 | 0 | 140 |
| Fresh Vegetable Stuffing | 4.8 oz | 190 | 3 | 25 | 2 | 4 | 8 | 1 | 580 |
| Garlic Dill New Potatoes, low-fat | 5.5 oz | 140 | 3 | 24 | 3 | 2 | 3 | 1 | 120 |
| Green Beans, low-fat | 3 oz | 50 | 2 | 7 | 3 | 1 | 3 | 1 | 105 |
| Homestyle Mashed Potatoes | 7.8 oz | 210 | 4 | 29 | 3 | 2 | 9 | 6 | 660 |

| FOOD ITEM | SERVING SIZE | CALORIES | PRO (g) | CARB (g) | FIBER (g) | SUGAR (g) | FAT (g) | SAT FAT (g) | SOD (mg) |
|---|---|---|---|---|---|---|---|---|---|
| Macaroni and Cheese | 7.8 oz | 320 | 9 | 38 | 2 | 7 | 12 | 8 | 950 |
| Poultry Gravy | 2 oz | 25 | 0 | 4 | 0 | 1 | 1 | 0 | 350 |
| Spinach Artichoke Dip | 2 oz | 100 | 3 | 3 | 1 | 1 | 8 | 3.5 | 220 |
| Sweet Corn, low-fat | 6.2 oz | 170 | 6 | 37 | 2 | 10 | 4 | 1 | 95 |
| Sweet Potato Casserole | 7 oz | 460 | 4 | 77 | 3 | 39 | 17 | 6 | 210 |
| **Sandwiches** | | | | | | | | | |
| Boston Chicken Carver | 384 g | 750 | 58 | 69 | 3 | 5 | 30 | 8 | 1670 |
| Boston Sirloin Dip Carver | 488 g | 1280 | 81 | 127 | 5 | 8 | 50 | 15 | 1510 |
| Boston Turkey Carver | 389 g | 860 | 58 | 71 | 3 | 6 | 39 | 9 | 1730 |
| Boston Turkey Dip Carver | n/a | 870 | 59 | 73 | 3 | 6 | 39 | 9 | 2380 |
| Meatloaf Carver | 434 g | 960 | 326 | 79 | 4 | 12 | 45 | 18 | 1280 |
| **Salads** | | | | | | | | | |
| Caesar Salad Dressing | n/a | 360 | 2 | 30 | n/a | 1 | 38 | 6 | 2 |
| Caesar Salad Entrée | 206 | 140 | 11 | 8 | 2 | 6 | 8 | 5 | 280 |
| Chopped Salad Dressing | 71 g | 360 | 0 | 2 | 0 | 1 | 39 | 6 | 1710 |
| Market Chopped Salad | 427 g | 270 | 10 | 33 | 8 | 19 | 13 | 3.5 | 310 |
| Roasted Sirloin topping | 3 oz | 160 | 26 | 0 | 0 | 0 | 6 | 2 | 170 |
| Roasted Turkey topping | 3 oz | 140 | 19 | 1 | 0 | 1 | 6 | 1 | 370 |
| Rotisserie Chicken topping | 3 oz | 100 | 20 | 1 | 0 | 1 | 2.5 | 0.5 | 300 |
| **Desserts** | | | | | | | | | |
| Apple Pie | 1 slice | 310 | 3 | 41 | 2 | 17 | 15 | 3 | 480 |
| Chocolate Cake | 1 slice | 650 | 4 | 86 | 2 | 68 | 32 | 8 | 320 |
| Chocolate Chip Fudge Brownie | 1 | 580 | 9 | 88 | 6 | 65 | 23 | 5 | 350 |
| Cornbread | 1 | 130 | 1 | 21 | 0 | 8 | 3.5 | 1 | 220 |
| Nestle Toll House Chocolate Chip Cookie | 1 | 370 | 4 | 49 | 2 | 28 | 19 | 9 | 0 |
| **Burger King*** | | | | | | | | | |
| **Burgers, Chicken, and Sandwiches** | | | | | | | | | |
| Angus Steak Burger | 291 g | 690 | 37 | 55 | 3 | 11 | 36 | 11 | 1350 |
| Angus Steak Burger, low-carb | 201 g | 330 | 29 | 5 | <1 | 3 | 18 | 9 | 830 |

*BURGER KING® trademarks and nutritional information used with permission from Burger King Brands, Inc.

| FOOD ITEM | SERVING SIZE | CALORIES | PRO (g) | CARB (g) | FIBER (g) | SUGAR (g) | FAT (g) | SAT FAT (g) | SOD (mg) |
|---|---|---|---|---|---|---|---|---|---|
| **Burger King (cont.)** | | | | | | | | | |
| **Burgers, Chicken, and Sandwiches (cont.)** | | | | | | | | | |
| Bacon Cheeseburger | 138 g | 360 | 19 | 31 | 1 | 6 | 18 | 8 | 870 |
| Bacon Double Cheeseburger | 194 g | 530 | 32 | 32 | 1 | 6 | 31 | 14 | 1130 |
| BK Big Fish® | 250 g | 630 | 24 | 67 | 4 | 8 | 30 | 6 | 1380 |
| BK Big Fish®, no tartar sauce | 222 g | 470 | 23 | 65 | 3 | 7 | 13 | 3 | 1240 |
| BK™ Chicken Fries | 6 pieces | 260 | 12 | 18 | 2 | 1 | 15 | 3.5 | 650 |
| BK™ Chicken Fries | 9 pieces | 390 | 18 | 26 | 3 | 1 | 23 | 5 | 980 |
| BK Veggie® Burger | 215 g | 420 | 23 | 46 | 7 | 8 | 16 | 2.5 | 1100 |
| BK Veggie® Burger, no mayonnaise | 205 g | 340 | 23 | 46 | 7 | 8 | 8 | 1 | 1030 |
| Cheeseburger | 133 g | 330 | 17 | 31 | 1 | 6 | 16 | 7 | 780 |
| Chicken Tenders® | 4 pieces | 170 | 9 | 11 | 0 | 0 | 10 | 2.5 | 480 |
| Chicken Tenders® | 5 pieces | 210 | 12 | 13 | 0 | 0 | 12 | 3 | 600 |
| Chicken Tenders® | 6 pieces | 250 | 14 | 16 | 0 | 0 | 15 | 3.5 | 720 |
| Chicken Tenders® | 8 pieces | 340 | 19 | 21 | <1 | 1 | 20 | 5 | 960 |
| Double Cheeseburger | 189 g | 500 | 30 | 31 | 1 | 6 | 29 | 14 | 1030 |
| Double Hamburger | 164 g | 410 | 25 | 30 | 1 | 6 | 21 | 9 | 600 |
| Hamburger | 121 g | 290 | 15 | 30 | 1 | 6 | 12 | 4.5 | 560 |
| Original Chicken Sandwich | 219 g | 660 | 24 | 52 | 4 | 5 | 40 | 8 | 1440 |
| Original Chicken Sandwich, no mayonnaise | 190 g | 450 | 23 | 52 | 4 | 5 | 17 | 4 | 1250 |
| Spicy BK Big Fish® | 250 g | 620 | 24 | 67 | 4 | 7 | 29 | 6 | 1540 |
| Tendercrisp® Chicken Sandwich, no sauce or mayonnaise | 258 g | 570 | 25 | 73 | 3.5 | 8 | 21 | 4.5 | 1540 |
| Tendergrill® Chicken Sandwich, with honey mustard | 258 g | 450 | 37 | 53 | 4 | 9 | 10 | 2 | 1210 |
| Whopper®, low-carb | 167 g | 250 | 20 | 3 | 1 | 2 | 18 | 8 | 270 |
| Whopper®, low-carb, with cheese | 192 g | 340 | 25 | 5 | 1 | 2 | 25 | 13 | 700 |
| Whopper®, no mayonnaise | 269 g | 510 | 28 | 51 | 3 | 11 | 22 | 9 | 880 |
| Whopper®, with cheese, no mayonnaise | 294 g | 600 | 32 | 52 | 3 | 11 | 30 | 14 | 1310 |
| Whopper Jr. ® | 158 g | 370 | 15 | 31 | 2 | 6 | 21 | 6 | 570 |

| FOOD ITEM | SERVING SIZE | CALORIES | PRO (g) | CARB (g) | FIBER (g) | SUGAR (g) | FAT (g) | SAT FAT (g) | SOD (mg) |
|---|---|---|---|---|---|---|---|---|---|
| Whopper Jr. ®, no mayonnaise | 147 g | 290 | 15 | 31 | 2 | 6 | 12 | 4.5 | 490 |
| Whopper Jr. ®, with cheese | 170 g | 410 | 18 | 32 | 2 | 6 | 24 | 8 | 780 |
| Whopper Jr. ®, with cheese, no mayonnaise | 149 g | 330 | 17 | 31 | 2 | 6 | 16 | 7 | 710 |
| **Side Orders** | | | | | | | | | |
| French Fries, with salt | small | 230 | 2 | 26 | 2 | 1 | 13 | 3 | 380 |
| French Fries, with salt | medium | 360 | 4 | 41 | 4 | 1 | 20 | 4.5 | 590 |
| Mott's Strawberry Flavored Apple Sauce | 113 g | 90 | 0 | 23 | <1 | 21 | 0 | 0 | 0 |
| Onion Rings | small | 150 | 2 | 19 | 1 | 2 | 7 | 2 | 220 |
| Onion Rings | medium | 320 | 4 | 40 | 3 | 5 | 16 | 4 | 460 |
| **Dipping Sauces** | | | | | | | | | |
| Barbecue Dipping Sauce | 28 g | 40 | 0 | 11 | 0 | 10 | 0 | 0 | 310 |
| Buffalo Dipping Sauce | 28 g | 80 | 0 | 2 | 0 | 1 | 8 | 1.5 | 350 |
| Honey-Flavored Dipping Sauce | 28 g | 90 | 0 | 23 | 0 | 22 | 0 | 0 | 0 |
| Honey Mustard Dipping Sauce | 28 g | 90 | 0 | 8 | 0 | 7 | 6 | 1 | 180 |
| Ranch Dipping Sauce | 28 g | 140 | 1 | 1 | 0 | 1 | 15 | 2.5 | 95 |
| Sweet and Sour Dipping Sauce | 28 g | 45 | 0 | 11 | 0 | 10 | 0 | 0 | 55 |
| Zesty Onion Ring Dipping Sauce | 28 g | 150 | 0 | 3 | <1 | 2 | 15 | 2.5 | 210 |
| **Salads** (without dressing or garlic parmesan croutons) | | | | | | | | | |
| Garden Salad (no chicken) | 184 g | 90 | 5 | 7 | 3 | 3 | 5 | 2.5 | 125 |
| Side Garden Salad | 98 g | 15 | 1 | 3 | 1 | 1 | 0 | 0 | 0 |
| Tendercrisp® Chicken Caesar Salad | 327 g | 400 | 23 | 31 | 3 | 3 | 21 | 6 | 1240 |
| Tendercrisp® Chicken Garden Salad | 306 g | 400 | 22 | 32 | 5 | 5 | 21 | 7 | 1170 |
| Tendergrill™ Chicken Caesar Salad | 299 g | 220 | 31 | 7 | 2 | 1 | 7 | 3 | 710 |
| Tendergrill™ Chicken Garden Salad | 292 g | 240 | 33 | 8 | 4 | 3 | 9 | 3.5 | 720 |
| **Salad Dressings and Toppings** | | | | | | | | | |
| Garlic Parmesan Croutons | 14 g | 60 | 1 | 9 | 0 | 1 | 2 | 0 | 120 |
| Ken's® Border Ranch | 2 oz | 110 | 2 | 7 | 0 | 2 | 8 | 1.5 | 560 |

| FOOD ITEM | SERVING SIZE | CALORIES | PRO (g) | CARB (g) | FIBER (g) | SUGAR (g) | FAT (g) | SAT FAT (g) | SOD (mg) |
|---|---|---|---|---|---|---|---|---|---|
| **Burger King (cont.)** | | | | | | | | | |
| **Salad Dressings and Toppings (cont.)** | | | | | | | | | |
| Ken's® Creamy Caesar Dressing | 2 oz | 210 | 3 | 4 | 0 | 3 | 21 | 4 | 610 |
| Ken's® Honey Mustard Dressing | 2 oz | 270 | 1 | 15 | 0 | 14 | 23 | 3 | 520 |
| Ken's® Light Italian Dressing | 2 oz | 120 | 0 | 5 | 0 | 4 | 11 | 1.5 | 440 |
| Ken's® Ranch Dressing | 2 oz | 190 | 1 | 2 | 0 | 1 | 20 | 3 | 560 |
| **Breakfast** | | | | | | | | | |
| Croissan'wich®, with bacon, egg, and cheese | 122 g | 340 | 15 | 26 | <1 | 5 | 20 | 7 | 890 |
| Croissan'wich®, with egg and cheese | 115 g | 300 | 12 | 26 | <1 | 5 | 17 | 6 | 740 |
| Croissan'wich®, with ham, egg, and cheese | 149 g | 340 | 18 | 26 | 1 | 6 | 18 | 6 | 1230 |
| Croissan'wich®, with sausage and cheese | 106 g | 370 | 14 | 23 | <1 | 4 | 25 | 9 | 810 |
| Croissan'wich®, with sausage, egg, and cheese | 159 g | 470 | 19 | 26 | <1 | 5 | 32 | 11 | 1060 |
| French Toast Sticks | 5 sticks | 390 | 6 | 46 | 2 | 2 | 20 | 4.5 | 440 |
| Hash Browns | small | 230 | 2 | 23 | 2 | 2 | 15 | 4 | 450 |
| Hash Browns | large | 390 | 3 | 38 | 4 | 4 | 25 | 7 | 760 |
| Maple Syrup | 28 g | 80 | 0 | 21 | 0 | 14 | 0 | 0 | 20 |
| **Milk Shakes** | | | | | | | | | |
| Chocolate | small (16 fl oz) | 470 | 8 | 75 | 1 | 72 | 14 | 9 | 350 |
| Chocolate | medium (22 fl oz) | 690 | 11 | 114 | 2 | 110 | 20 | 12 | 560 |
| Strawberry | small (16 fl oz) | 460 | 7 | 73 | 0 | 71 | 14 | 9 | 240 |
| Strawberry | medium (22 fl oz) | 660 | 10 | 111 | 0 | 109 | 19 | 12 | 330 |
| Vanilla | small (16 fl oz) | 400 | 8 | 57 | 0 | 55 | 15 | 9 | 240 |
| Vanilla | medium (22 fl oz) | 560 | 11 | 79 | 0 | 77 | 21 | 13 | 330 |
| **Milk** | | | | | | | | | |
| Hershey's® 1% Low-fat Chocolate Milk | 8 fl oz | 180 | 9 | 31 | 1 | 29 | 2.5 | 1.5 | 140 |
| Hershey's® 1% Low-fat Milk | 8 fl oz | 110 | 8 | 13 | 0 | 12 | 2.5 | 1.5 | 130 |

| FOOD ITEM | SERVING SIZE | CALORIES | PRO (g) | CARB (g) | FIBER (g) | SUGAR (g) | FAT (g) | SAT FAT (g) | SOD (mg) |
|---|---|---|---|---|---|---|---|---|---|
| **Carl's Jr.** | | | | | | | | | |
| **Chicken and Sandwiches** | | | | | | | | | |
| Bacon Swiss Crispy Chicken Sandwich | 268 g | 750 | 31 | 91 | 0 | 0 | 28 | 28 | 1900 |
| Big Hamburger | 309 g | 520 | 25 | 64 | 4 | 18 | 18 | 6 | 1040 |
| Carl's Catch Fish Sandwich™ | 215 g | 560 | 19 | 58 | 2 | 8 | 27 | 7 | 990 |
| Charbroiled BBQ Chicken Sandwich™ | 245 g | 370 | 35 | 47 | 4 | 12 | 4 | 1 | 1070 |
| Charbroiled Chicken Club Sandwich™ | 270 g | 550 | 42 | 43 | 4 | 9 | 23 | 7 | 1330 |
| Charbroiled Santa Fe Chicken Sandwich™ | 266 g | 610 | 38 | 43 | 4 | 9 | 32 | 8 | 1440 |
| Chicken Breast Strips | 3 pieces | 380 | 22 | 27 | 1 | 1 | 21 | 3.5 | 1360 |
| Chicken Breast Strips | 5 pieces | 630 | 37 | 45 | 2 | 1 | 34 | 6 | 2260 |
| Chili Burger | 330 g | 690 | 39 | 57 | 5 | 11 | 35 | 15 | 1400 |
| Double Western Bacon Cheeseburger® | 308 g | 920 | 51 | 65 | 2 | 14 | 50 | 21 | 1730 |
| Famous Star™ with Cheese | 274 g | 650 | 28 | 51 | 3 | 9 | 37 | 12 | 1170 |
| Kid's Hamburger | 119 g | 280 | 14 | 36 | 1 | 5 | 9 | 3.5 | 480 |
| Low Carb Six Dollar Burger, The | 267 g | 490 | 33 | 6 | 2 | 4 | 37 | 16 | 1270 |
| Original Six Dollar Burger™, The | 411 g | 960 | 38 | 61 | 3 | 17 | 62 | 25 | 1690 |
| Six Dollar Bacon Cheese Burger, The | 390 g | 1010 | 44 | 52 | 3 | 12 | 69 | 28 | 1820 |
| Six Dollar Chili Cheese Burger, The | 426 g | 930 | 46 | 57 | 5 | 12 | 57 | 27 | 1960 |
| Six Dollar Guacamole Bacon Burger, The | 437 g | 1120 | 43 | 54 | 6 | 11 | 81 | 29 | 2160 |
| Six Dollar Western Bacon Burger, The | 364 g | 1080 | 45 | 84 | 4 | 20 | 62 | 27 | 2450 |
| Sourdough Bacon Cheeseburger | 207 g | 550 | 31 | 41 | 2 | 6 | 29 | 14 | 500 |
| Spicy Chicken Sandwich | 198 g | 480 | 14 | 48 | 2 | 6 | 26 | 5 | 1220 |
| Super Star™ with Cheese | 376 g | 920 | 48 | 53 | 3 | 10 | 57 | 21 | 1490 |
| Western Bacon Cheeseburger® | 225 g | 660 | 32 | 64 | 2 | 14 | 30 | 12 | 1410 |

| FOOD ITEM | SERVING SIZE | CALORIES | PRO (g) | CARB (g) | FIBER (g) | SUGAR (g) | FAT (g) | SAT FAT (g) | SOD (mg) |
|---|---|---|---|---|---|---|---|---|---|
| **Carl's Jr. (cont.)** | | | | | | | | | |
| **Sides** | | | | | | | | | |
| Chicken Stars | 4 pieces (57 g) | 170 | 9 | 10 | 1 | 0 | 11 | 3 | 320 |
| CrissCut Fries® | 139 g | 410 | 5 | 43 | 4 | 0 | 24 | 5 | 950 |
| French Fries | kids | 250 | 4 | 32 | 3 | 0 | 12 | 2.5 | 150 |
| French Fries | small | 290 | 5 | 37 | 3 | 0 | 14 | 3 | 170 |
| Fried Zucchini | 139 g | 320 | 6 | 31 | 2 | 3 | 19 | 5 | 860 |
| Onion Rings | 128 g | 440 | 7 | 53 | 3 | 5 | 22 | 5 | 700 |
| **Salads** (without salad dressing) | | | | | | | | | |
| Charbroiled Chicken Salad-To-Go™ | 437 g | 330 | 34 | 17 | 5 | 8 | 7 | 4 | 880 |
| Garden Salad-To-Go™ | 151 g | 120 | 3 | 5 | 2 | 3 | 3 | 1.5 | 230 |
| **Salad Dressing** | | | | | | | | | |
| Balsamic Vinaigrette, low-fat | 2 oz | 260 | 13 | 14 | 1 | 1 | 16 | 4 | 470 |
| Blue Cheese Dressing | 2 oz | 320 | 2 | 1 | 0 | 1 | 35 | 6 | 370 |
| House Dressing | 2 oz | 220 | 1 | 3 | 0 | 2 | 22 | 4 | 440 |
| Thousand Island Dressing | 2 oz | 250 | 1 | 7 | 0 | 4 | 24 | 3.5 | 450 |
| **Breakfast** | | | | | | | | | |
| Bacon & Egg Burrito | 203 g | 560 | 29 | 37 | 1 | 1 | 32 | 11 | 980 |
| Breakfast Bowl, low-carb | 315 g | 900 | 58 | 5 | 2 | 2 | 73 | 33 | 2050 |
| Breakfast Burger | 309 g | 830 | 37 | 65 | 3 | 13 | 46 | 15 | 1600 |
| Breakfast Quesadilla | 176 g | 390 | 17 | 38 | 2 | 2 | 18 | 5 | 920 |
| Hash Brown Nuggets | 108 g | 330 | 3 | 32 | 3 | 1 | 21 | 4.5 | 470 |
| Sourdough Breakfast Sandwich, with ham | 188 g | 450 | 28 | 40 | 2 | 4 | 20 | 9 | 950 |
| **Desserts** | | | | | | | | | |
| Chocolate Cake | 85 g | 300 | 3 | 48 | 1 | 37 | 12 | 3 | 350 |
| Chocolate Chip Cookie | 71 g | 350 | 3 | 46 | 1 | 27 | 18 | 7 | 330 |
| Strawberry Swirl Cheesecake | 99 g | 290 | 6 | 30 | 0 | 20 | 17 | 9 | 230 |

| FOOD ITEM | SERVING SIZE | CALORIES | PRO (g) | CARB (g) | FIBER (g) | SUGAR (g) | FAT (g) | SAT FAT (g) | SOD (mg) |
|---|---|---|---|---|---|---|---|---|---|
| **Shakes** | | | | | | | | | |
| Chocolate | small (21 fl oz) | 540 | 15 | 98 | 0 | 86 | 11 | 7 | 360 |
| Strawberry | small (21 fl oz) | 520 | 14 | 93 | 0 | 82 | 11 | 7 | 340 |
| Vanilla | small (21 fl oz) | 470 | 15 | 77 | 0 | 66 | 11 | 7 | 350 |
| **Cinnabon** | | | | | | | | | |
| Apple Minibon | 100 g | 285 | 5 | 53 | 1 | n/a | 5 | 1 | 261 |
| Chocolatebon, with reduced-fat frosting | 1 minibon (98 g) | 345 | 6 | 52 | 2 | n/a | 13 | 3 | 300 |
| Cinnabon Bites | 6 pieces | 520 | 8 | 78 | 2 | 25 | 16 | 4 | 530 |
| Cinnabon CinnaPoppers | 74 g | 368 | 4 | 41 | 2 | 22 | 21 | 11 | 104 |
| Classic Roll | 221 g | 813 | 15 | 117 | 4 | 55 | 32 | 8 | 801 |
| Frosting Cup | 1.4 oz | 180 | 1 | 20 | 0 | 18 | 11 | 3 | 109 |
| Minibon | 92 g | 339 | 6 | 49 | 2 | 22 | 13 | 3 | 337 |
| Strawberry Minibon | 84 g | 240 | 6 | 43 | 2 | 19 | 5 | 1 | 290 |
| **Cold Stone Creamery** | | | | | | | | | |
| Butterscotch Topping, fat-free (at participating locations) | 1 oz | 80 | 0.9 | 19 | 0 | 14 | 0 | 0 | 85 |
| Caramel Topping, fat-free (at participating locations) | 1 oz | 80 | 0.9 | 19 | 0 | 14 | 0 | 0 | 85 |
| Fudge Topping, fat-free (at participating location) | 1 oz | 80 | 0.9 | 20 | 0 | 16 | 0 | 0 | 15 |
| Light Cake Batter (at participating locations) | small (170 g) | 290 | 8 | 51 | 0 | 32 | 7 | 4.5 | 240 |
| Light Cake Batter (at participating locations) | medium (283 g) | 480 | 13 | 85 | 0 | 62 | 12 | 7 | 400 |
| Light Cake Batter (at participating locations) | large (397 g) | 680 | 19 | 120 | 0 | 87 | 17 | 10 | 570 |
| Light Chocolate (at participating locations) | small (170 g) | 260 | 9 | 43 | 1 | 33 | 7 | 4.5 | 130 |
| Light Chocolate (at participating locations) | medium (283 g) | 440 | 15 | 72 | 2 | 55 | 12 | 7 | 220 |
| Light Chocolate (at participating locations) | large (397 g) | 610 | 21 | 101 | 3 | 78 | 17 | 10 | 300 |
| Light Vanilla | small (170 g) | 260 | 8 | 42 | 0 | 34 | 7 | 4.5 | 130 |

| FOOD ITEM | SERVING SIZE | CALORIES | PRO (g) | CARB (g) | FIBER (g) | SUGAR (g) | FAT (g) | SAT FAT (g) | SOD (mg) |
|---|---|---|---|---|---|---|---|---|---|
| **Cold Stone Creamery (cont.)** | | | | | | | | | |
| Light Vanilla | medium (283 g) | 44 | 14 | 70 | 0 | 56 | 11 | 7 | 220 |
| Light Vanilla | large (397 g) | 610 | 19 | 98 | 0 | 79 | 16 | 10 | 300 |
| Sinless Sorbet Lemon | small (170 g) | 180 | 0 | 48 | 0 | 41 | 0 | 0 | 20 |
| Sinless Sorbet Lemon | medium (283 g) | 310 | 0 | 80 | <1 | 68 | 0 | 0 | 30 |
| Sinless Sorbet Lemon | large (397 g) | 430 | 0 | 112 | <1 | 95 | 0 | 0 | 45 |
| Sinless Sorbet Raspberry | small (170 g) | 200 | 0 | 50 | 0 | 43 | 0 | 0 | 20 |
| Sinless Sorbet Raspberry | medium (283 g) | 330 | 0 | 84 | 0 | 72 | 0 | 0 | 35 |
| Sinless Sorbet Raspberry | large (397 g) | 460 | 0 | 118 | <1 | 101 | 0 | 0 | 50 |
| **Dairy Queen** | | | | | | | | | |
| **Ice Cream** | | | | | | | | | |
| Arctic Rush™ Slush | small | 220 | 0 | 56 | 0 | 56.0 | 0 | 0 | 20 |
| Arctic Rush™ Slush | medium | 290 | 0 | 74 | 0 | 74.0 | 0 | 0 | 30 |
| Chocolate Cone | small | 240 | 6 | 37 | 0 | 25 | 8 | 5 | 115 |
| Chocolate Cone | medium | 340 | 8 | 53 | 0 | 34 | 11 | 7 | 160 |
| Dipped Cone | small | 340 | 6 | 42 | 1 | 31 | 17 | 9 | 130 |
| Dilly Bar, Chocolate | 85 g | 210 | 3 | 21 | 0 | 17 | 13 | 7 | 75 |
| Dilly® Bar, Chocolate Mint | 87 g | 240 | 4 | 24 | 0 | 20 | 15 | 9 | 70 |
| Dilly® Bar, Heath | 87 g | 220 | 3 | 25 | 0 | 22 | 13 | 10 | 95 |
| Dilly® Bar, No Sugar Added | 88 g | 190 | 3 | 24 | 5 | 5 | 13 | 10 | 60 |
| DQ® Chocolate Soft Serve | ½ cup | 150 | 4 | 22 | 0 | 17 | 5 | 3.5 | 75 |
| DQ Freez'r®, Lemon | ½ cup | 80 | 0 | 20 | 0 | 20 | 0 | 0 | 10 |
| DQ® Fudge and Vanilla Bar | 66 g | 60 | 4 | 15 | 5 | 5 | 0 | 0 | 70 |
| DQ® Fudge Bar, No Sugar Added | 66 g | 50 | 4 | 13 | 6 | 4 | 0 | 0 | 70 |
| DQ® Vanilla Orange Bar, No Sugar Added | 66 g | 60 | 2 | 18 | 6 | 4 | 0 | 0 | 40 |
| DQ® Vanilla Soft Serve | ½ cup | 140 | 3 | 22 | 0 | 19 | 5 | 3 | 70 |

| FOOD ITEM | SERVING SIZE | CALORIES | PRO (g) | CARB (g) | FIBER (g) | SUGAR (g) | FAT (g) | SAT FAT (g) | SOD (mg) |
|---|---|---|---|---|---|---|---|---|---|
| Hawaiian Blizzard® | small | 440 | 9 | 69 | 1 | 59 | 15 | 10 | 200 |
| Hawaiian Blizzard® | medium | 590 | 11 | 95 | 2 | 80 | 20 | 14 | 270 |
| Hawaiian Blizzard® | large | 820 | 16 | 130 | 2 | 110 | 28 | 19 | 370 |
| Starkiss® | 85 g | 80 | 0 | 21 | 0 | 17 | 0 | 0 | 10 |
| Sundae, Chocolate | small | 280 | 5 | 49 | 0 | 42 | 7 | 4.5 | 140 |
| Sundae, Chocolate | medium | 400 | 8 | 71 | 0 | 61 | 10 | 6 | 210 |
| Sundae, Chocolate | large | 580 | 11 | 100 | 1 | 87 | 15 | 10 | 260 |
| Sundae, Strawberry | small | 240 | 5 | 40 | 0 | 35 | 7 | 4.5 | 110 |
| Sundae, Strawberry | medium | 340 | 7 | 58 | <1 | 51 | 9 | 6 | 160 |
| Sundae, Strawberry | large | 500 | 10 | 83 | <1 | 72 | 15 | 9 | 230 |
| Vanilla Cone | small | 230 | 6 | 38 | 0 | 27 | 7 | 4.5 | 115 |
| Vanilla Cone | medium | 330 | 8 | 53 | 0 | 38 | 9 | 6 | 160 |
| **Sandwiches** | | | | | | | | | |
| BBQ Beef Sandwich | 142 g | 300 | 1 | 37 | 2 | 15 | 9 | 4 | 610 |
| BBQ Pork Sandwich | 142 g | 280 | 17 | 36 | 2 | 8 | 8 | 2 | 790 |
| Chili 'n' Cheese Dog | 142 g | 330 | 14 | 22 | 2 | 4 | 21 | 9 | 1090 |
| DQ Homestyle® Burger | 138 g | 290 | 17 | 29 | 2 | 5 | 12 | 5 | 630 |
| DQ Homestyle® Cheeseburger | 152 g | 340 | 20 | 29 | 2 | 5 | 17 | 8 | 850 |
| DQ Sandwich | 85 g | 200 | 4 | 31 | 1 | 18 | 6 | 3 | 140 |
| Grilled Chicken Sandwich | 181 g | 370 | 23 | 34 | 1 | 5 | 16 | 2 | 1080 |
| Grilled Chicken Sandwich | 206 g | 470 | 24 | 39 | 1 | 6 | 24 | 4 | 1200 |
| Hot Dog | 99 g | 240 | 9 | 19 | 1 | 4 | 14 | 5 | 730 |
| Vegetable Quesadilla | 156 g | 440 | 20 | 34 | 3 | 2 | 25 | 13 | 690 |
| **Sides and Salads** | | | | | | | | | |
| Crispy Chicken Salad, without dressing | 392 g | 350 | 21 | 21 | 6 | 9 | 20 | 6 | 620 |
| French Fries | small | 300 | 3 | 45 | 3 | <1 | 12 | 2.5 | 640 |
| French Fries | medium | 380 | 4 | 56 | 4 | <1 | 15 | 3 | 800 |
| French Fries | large | 480 | 5 | 72 | 5 | <1 | 19 | 4 | 1040 |
| Grilled Chicken Salad, without dressing | 389 g | 240 | 26 | 12 | 4 | 7 | 10 | 5 | 950 |

| FOOD ITEM | SERVING SIZE | CALORIES | PRO (g) | CARB (g) | FIBER (g) | SUGAR (g) | FAT (g) | SAT FAT (g) | SOD (mg) |
|---|---|---|---|---|---|---|---|---|---|
| **Dairy Queen (cont.)** | | | | | | | | | |
| **Sides and Salads (cont.)** | | | | | | | | | |
| Onion Rings | 113 g | 470 | 6 | 45 | 3 | 7 | 30 | 6 | 740 |
| Side Salad | 126 g | 60 | 3 | 6 | 2 | 4 | 2.5 | 1.5 | 60 |

Note: The nutrient values are meant for general information purposes only. Although the information is based on our recommended product preparation procedures, variations may occur due to differences in product procedures between restaurants. Seasonal differences and slight variations among different manufacturers must also be expected. Menu items listed may not be available at all Dairy Queen/Brazier restaurants and only applies to licensed Dairy Queen/Brazier stores within the United States.

| FOOD ITEM | SERVING SIZE | CALORIES | PRO (g) | CARB (g) | FIBER (g) | SUGAR (g) | FAT (g) | SAT FAT (g) | SOD (mg) |
|---|---|---|---|---|---|---|---|---|---|
| **Denny's** | | | | | | | | | |
| **Breakfast** | | | | | | | | | |
| Ham and Jalapeño Scramble | 25 oz | 1110 | 52 | 117 | 7 | n/a | 55 | 19 | 3930 |
| Peach French Toast, without syrup or condiments | 16 oz | 1370 | 53 | 96 | 4 | n/a | 85 | 34 | 2385 |
| Pepper Jack and Smoked Sausage | 27 oz | 1430 | 54 | 118 | 7 | n/a | 92 | 33 | 4270 |
| Zesty Creole Scrambles | 24 oz | 1310 | 45 | 115 | 6 | n/a | 74 | 22 | 3810 |
| **Dinners** | | | | | | | | | |
| Chicken Fried Chicken Dinner | 11 oz | 550 | 41 | 32 | 2 | n/a | 29 | 6 | 2621 |
| Chicken Tangy Lemon Mushroom | 14 oz | 660 | 56 | 10 | 1 | n/a | 43 | 15 | 1780 |
| Mushroom Swiss Chopped Steak | 14 oz | 800 | 46 | 11 | 1 | n/a | 73 | 29 | 1140 |
| Pot Roast Dinner | 7 oz | 266 | 28 | 2 | 0 | n/a | 16 | 6 | 873 |
| Texas Style Steak Tip | 15 oz | 700 | 38 | 48 | 3 | n/a | 40 | 10 | 2290 |
| Tilapia with Creole | 14 oz | 490 | 37 | 40 | 3 | n/a | 23 | 5 | 1710 |

Note: All suppers are without sides or bread.

| FOOD ITEM | SERVING SIZE | CALORIES | PRO (g) | CARB (g) | FIBER (g) | SUGAR (g) | FAT (g) | SAT FAT (g) | SOD (mg) |
|---|---|---|---|---|---|---|---|---|---|
| **Dessert** | | | | | | | | | |
| Hershey's Chocolate Cake | 5 oz | 631 | 5 | 79 | 2 | n/a | 33 | 13 | 420 |
| **Dippin' Dots** | | | | | | | | | |
| Ice | ½ cup (75 g) | 91 | 0 | 23 | 0 | 16 | 0 | 0 | 12 |
| Ice Cream | ½ cup (85 g) | 190 | 4 | 22 | 0 | 22 | 9 | 6 | 70 |
| Ice Cream, Fudge, no sugar added, fat-free | ½ cup (85 g) | 60 | 1 | 14 | 0 | 5 | 0 | 0 | 80 |
| Ice Cream, Vanilla, no sugar added, low-fat | ½ cup (85 g) | 120 | 3 | 17 | 0 | 7 | 4 | 2.5 | 80 |

| FOOD ITEM | SERVING SIZE | CALORIES | PRO (g) | CARB (g) | FIBER (g) | SUGAR (g) | FAT (g) | SAT FAT (g) | SOD (mg) |
|---|---|---|---|---|---|---|---|---|---|
| Sherbet | ½ cup (85 g) | 100 | 1 | 21 | 0 | 21 | 1 | 1 | 15 |
| Yogurt | ½ cup (85 g) | 110 | 4 | 23 | 0 | 19 | 0 | 0 | 90 |
| **El Pollo Loco** | | | | | | | | | |
| **Meals** | | | | | | | | | |
| BRC Burrito | 8 oz | 423 | 18 | 62 | 6 | 4 | 17 | 4 | 1135 |
| Chicken Taco al Carbon | 3 oz | 148 | 9 | 18 | 1 | 0 | 4 | 0 | 223 |
| Chicken Tortilla Soup | small (10 oz) | 222 | 21 | 17 | 1 | 2 | 9 | 2 | 1135 |
| Flame-Grilled Skinless Chicken Breast | 4 oz | 153 | 29 | 0 | 0 | 0 | 4 | 1 | 540 |
| Original Pollo Bowl® | 17 oz | 544 | 32 | 83 | 13 | 3 | 10 | 1 | 2169 |
| Pollo Choice Skinless Breast Meal | 14 oz | 344 | 38 | 16 | 7 | 5 | 16 | 5 | 1063 |
| **Sides** | | | | | | | | | |
| Fresh Vegetables | 4 oz | 68 | 3 | 6 | 4 | 2 | 4 | 1 | 78 |
| Garden Salad | small (5 oz) | 120 | 10 | 8 | 1 | 2 | 12 | 3 | 278 |
| Pinto Beans | 6 oz | 154 | 7 | 24 | 9 | 3 | 4 | 0 | 674 |
| Spanish Rice | 4 oz | 161 | 3 | 33 | 1 | 0 | 1 | 0 | 421 |
| **Johnny Rockets** | | | | | | | | | |
| Chicken Club Salad with Grilled Chicken Breast | 346 g | 440 | 49 | 8 | 3 | 0 | 25 | 65 | 3020 |
| Grilled Breast of Chicken Sandwich | 274 g | 600 | 35 | 54 | 4 | 6 | 29 | 6 | 1040 |
| Streamliner Hamburger | 303 g | 420 | 26 | 50 | 10 | 10 | 16 | 4 | 1290 |
| Turkey Single Hamburger | 307 g | 610 | 25 | 60 | 3 | 12 | 32 | 9 | 810 |
| **KFC** | | | | | | | | | |
| **Salads** | | | | | | | | | |
| Caesar Side Salad, without dressing and croutons | 76 g | 50 | 4 | 2 | 1 | 1 | 3 | 2 | 135 |
| Hidden Valley, The Original Ranch Fat Free Dressing | 43 g | 35 | 1 | 8 | 0 | 2 | 0 | 0 | 410 |
| House Side Salad, without dressing | 83 g | 15 | 1 | 2 | 1 | 1 | 0 | 0 | 5 |
| Roasted BLT Salad, without dressing | 347 g | 210 | 28 | 8 | 4 | 6 | 7 | 2.5 | 900 |

| FOOD ITEM | SERVING SIZE | CALORIES | PRO (g) | CARB (g) | FIBER (g) | SUGAR (g) | FAT (g) | SAT FAT (g) | SOD (mg) |
|---|---|---|---|---|---|---|---|---|---|
| **KFC (cont.)** | | | | | | | | | |
| **Chicken and Sandwiches** | | | | | | | | | |
| Original Recipe Chicken Breast, without skin | 108 g | 140 | 29 | 0 | 0 | 0 | 3 | 1 | 410 |
| Oven Roasted Twister, without sauce | 247 g | 380 | 29 | 45 | 4 | 9 | 8 | 1.5 | 1260 |
| Tender Roast Filet Meal | 321 g | 360 | 33 | 41 | 4 | 4 | 7 | 2 | 2010 |
| Tender Roast Sandwich, without sauce | 177 g | 260 | 31 | 23 | 1 | 0 | 5 | 1.5 | 690 |
| **Side Dishes** | | | | | | | | | |
| Baked Beans | 136 g | 230 | 8 | 46 | 7 | 22 | 1 | 1 | 720 |
| Corn on the Cob (3") | 82 g | 70 | 2 | 13 | 3 | 5 | 1.5 | 0.5 | 5 |
| Corn on the Cob (5.5") | 162 g | 150 | 5 | 26 | 7 | 10 | 3 | 1 | 10 |
| Green Beans | 96 g | 50 | 2 | 7 | 2 | 2 | 1.5 | 0 | 570 |
| Mashed Potatoes, without gravy | 108 g | 110 | 2 | 16 | 1 | 0 | 4 | 1 | 260 |
| Seasoned Rice | 99 g | 150 | 4 | 32 | 2 | 1 | 1 | 0 | 640 |
| **Long John Silver's** | | | | | | | | | |
| Baked Cod | 1 piece (101 g) | 120 | 22 | 1 | 0 | 0 | 4.5 | 1 | 240 |
| Corn Cobette | 1 (95 g) | 90 | 3 | 14 | 3 | 6 | 3 | 0.5 | 0 |
| Rice | 4 oz (113 g) | 180 | 3 | 34 | 3 | 1 | 3.5 | 1 | 540 |
| **Luby's** | | | | | | | | | |
| **Meals** | | | | | | | | | |
| Blackened Chicken Breast | 1 | 350 | n/a | 5 | 2 | n/a | 15 | n/a | n/a |
| Blackened Tilapia | 1 | 270 | n/a | 5 | 2 | n/a | 11 | n/a | n/a |
| Carved Ham | 1 | 300 | n/a | 6 | 0 | n/a | 11 | n/a | n/a |
| Grilled Chicken Breast, with skin | 1 | 400 | n/a | 1 | 0 | n/a | 20 | n/a | n/a |
| Lemon Basil Salmon | 1 | 355 | n/a | 1 | 0 | n/a | 20 | n/a | n/a |
| Pan Grilled Fillet | 1 | 330 | n/a | 19 | 2 | n/a | 12 | n/a | n/a |
| Parmesan Chicken Alfredo | 1 | 435 | n/a | 22 | 1 | n/a | 22 | n/a | n/a |
| Parmesan Crusted Tilapia | 1 | 300 | n/a | 6 | 0 | n/a | 14 | n/a | n/a |
| Roasted Chicken, ½, without skin | 1 | 460 | n/a | 0 | 0 | n/a | 23 | n/a | n/a |
| Roasted Turkey, without skin or gravy | 1 | 280 | n/a | 0 | 0 | n/a | 3 | n/a | n/a |

| FOOD ITEM | SERVING SIZE | CALORIES | PRO (g) | CARB (g) | FIBER (g) | SUGAR (g) | FAT (g) | SAT FAT (g) | SOD (mg) |
|---|---|---|---|---|---|---|---|---|---|
| **Side Dishes** | | | | | | | | | |
| Black-Eyed Peas | 1 | 222 | n/a | 33 | 10 | n/a | 5 | n/a | n/a |
| Blue Lake Green Beans | 1 | 83 | n/a | 9 | 4 | n/a | 5 | n/a | n/a |
| Broccoli | 1 | 80 | n/a | 9 | 5 | n/a | 4 | n/a | n/a |
| Cabbage | 1 | 70 | n/a | 6 | 3 | n/a | 5 | n/a | n/a |
| Carrots | 1 | 94 | n/a | 15 | 3 | n/a | 4 | n/a | n/a |
| Cauliflower, Peas, and Carrots | 1 | 67 | n/a | 7 | 3 | n/a | 4 | n/a | n/a |
| Chicken Noodle Soup Bowl | 1 | 235 | n/a | 21 | 1 | n/a | 9 | n/a | n/a |
| Corn | 1 | 192 | n/a | 38 | 3 | n/a | 5 | n/a | n/a |
| Fresh Green Beans | 1 | 92 | n/a | 10 | 4 | n/a | 5 | n/a | n/a |
| Grapefruit | 1 | 46 | n/a | 12 | 2 | n/a | 0 | n/a | n/a |
| Grilled Chicken Caesar | 1 | 534 | n/a | 17 | 6 | n/a | 30 | n/a | n/a |
| Grilled Chicken Caesar, without dressing | 1 | 370 | n/a | 16 | 6 | n/a | 13 | n/a | n/a |
| Holiday Rice | 1 | 165 | n/a | 30 | 2 | n/a | 3 | n/a | n/a |
| Jell-O | 1 | 100 | n/a | 24 | 0 | n/a | 0 | n/a | n/a |
| Marinated Cucumbers | 1 | 117 | n/a | 13 | 1 | n/a | 8 | n/a | n/a |
| Mediterranean Vegetables | 1 | 140 | n/a | 9 | 1 | n/a | 10 | n/a | n/a |
| Mixed Field Greens, without dressing | 1 | 34 | n/a | 7 | 3 | n/a | 0 | n/a | n/a |
| Mixed Melons | 1 | 67 | n/a | 20 | 2 | n/a | 0 | n/a | n/a |
| Pineapple | 1 | 48 | n/a | 12 | 1 | n/a | 0 | n/a | n/a |
| Pinto Beans | 1 | 190 | n/a | 28 | 11 | n/a | 5 | n/a | n/a |
| Roasted Mixed Vegetables | 1 | 135 | n/a | 16 | 4 | n/a | 8 | n/a | n/a |
| Roll, white | 1 | 130 | n/a | 23 | 1 | n/a | 3 | n/a | n/a |
| Roll, whole wheat | 1 | 170 | n/a | 23 | 2 | n/a | 5 | n/a | n/a |
| Spinach | 1 | 65 | n/a | 5 | 3 | n/a | 4 | n/a | n/a |
| Spinach Salad, without dressing | 1 | 47 | n/a | 5 | 3 | n/a | 2 | n/a | n/a |
| Vegetable Soup Bowl | 1 | 93 | n/a | 15 | 2 | n/a | 9 | n/a | n/a |
| **Dressings** | | | | | | | | | |
| Blue Cheese Dressing | 1 tbsp | 88 | n/a | 0 | 0 | n/a | 9 | n/a | n/a |
| Caesar Dressing | 1 tbsp | 73 | n/a | 0 | 0 | n/a | 8 | n/a | n/a |

| FOOD ITEM | SERVING SIZE | CALORIES | PRO (g) | CARB (g) | FIBER (g) | SUGAR (g) | FAT (g) | SAT FAT (g) | SOD (mg) |
|---|---|---|---|---|---|---|---|---|---|
| **Luby's (cont.)** | | | | | | | | | |
| **Dressings (cont.)** | | | | | | | | | |
| French Dressing | 1 tbsp | 82 | n/a | 5 | 0 | n/a | 7 | n/a | n/a |
| Greek Dressing | 1 tbsp | 31 | n/a | 0 | 0 | n/a | 3 | n/a | n/a |
| Honey Mustard Dressing | 1 tbsp | 75 | n/a | 4 | 0 | n/a | 7 | n/a | n/a |
| Italian Dressing | 1 tbsp | 75 | n/a | 4 | 0 | n/a | 7 | n/a | n/a |
| Ranch Dressing | 1 tbsp | 55 | n/a | 1 | 0 | n/a | 6 | n/a | n/a |
| Thousand Island Dressing | 1 tbsp | 50 | n/a | 2 | 0 | n/a | 5 | n/a | n/a |
| **Nathan's Famous** | | | | | | | | | |
| Fish Sandwich | 217 g | 469 | 14 | 42 | 13 | 14 | 20 | 4 | 750 |
| French Fries | regular (273 g) | 547 | 6 | 47 | 6 | 0 | 38 | 4 | 200 |
| Hot Dog Nuggets | 6 (99 g) | 351 | 5 | 20 | 0 | 5 | 28 | 4 | 400 |
| Nathan's Famous Hot Dog | 100 g | 309 | 11 | 23 | 1 | 0 | 20 | 8 | 684 |
| Onion Rings | small (159 g) | 559 | 3 | 36 | 2 | 5 | 44 | 6 | 576 |
| ¼ Pound Burger | 248 g | 537 | 25 | 42 | 2 | 11 | 30 | 12 | 813 |
| **Olive Garden** | | | | | | | | | |
| Capellini Pomodoro | 1 | 409 | n/a | n/a | 6 | n/a | 9 | n/a | n/a |
| Chicken Giardino | 1 | 408 | n/a | n/a | 4 | n/a | 12 | n/a | n/a |
| Grilled Chicken | 1 kids' entree | 349 | n/a | n/a | 4 | n/a | 11 | n/a | n/a |
| Herb-Grilled Salmon | 1 | n/a | n/a | 18 | 6 | n/a | n/a | n/a | n/a |
| Minestrone Soup | 1 | 164 | n/a | n/a | 5 | n/a | 1 | n/a | n/a |
| Mixed Grill | 1 | n/a | n/a | 19 | 7 | n/a | n/a | n/a | n/a |
| Mussels di Napoli appetizer | 1 | n/a | n/a | 19 | 1 | n/a | n/a | n/a | n/a |
| Pork Filettino | 1 | n/a | n/a | 17 | 7 | n/a | n/a | n/a | n/a |
| Shrimp Primavera | 1 | 483 | n/a | n/a | 6 | n/a | 11 | n/a | n/a |
| Stuffed Mushroom appetizer | 1 | n/a | n/a | 14 | 2 | n/a | n/a | n/a | n/a |
| **Orange Julius®** | | | | | | | | | |
| **Orange Julius® Originals** | | | | | | | | | |
| Bananarilla® | 16 fl oz | 290 | 3 | 56 | 3 | 44 | 7 | 7 | 75 |

| FOOD ITEM | SERVING SIZE | CALORIES | PRO (g) | CARB (g) | FIBER (g) | SUGAR (g) | FAT (g) | SAT FAT (g) | SOD (mg) |
|---|---|---|---|---|---|---|---|---|---|
| Orange Julius® | 16 fl oz | 220 | 1 | 54 | 1 | 50 | 1 | 0 | 10 |
| Orange Julius® | 20 fl oz | 270 | 1 | 68 | 1 | 62 | 1 | 0 | 10 |
| Raspberry Julius® | 16 fl oz | 240 | 1 | 61 | 1 | 52 | 1 | 0 | 25 |
| Raspberry Julius® | 20 fl oz | 300 | 2 | 76 | 1 | 65 | 1.5 | 1 | 35 |
| Strawberry Julius® | 16 fl oz | 220 | 1 | 57 | 1 | 40 | 0 | 0 | 10 |
| Strawberry Julius® | 20 fl oz | 280 | 1 | 72 | 1 | 50 | 1 | 0 | 10 |
| Tropical | 16 fl oz | 290 | 3 | 54 | 3 | 45 | 7 | 7 | 70 |
| **Premium Fruit Smoothies** | | | | | | | | | |
| Blueberrathon | 20 fl oz | 350 | 2 | 89 | 6 | 72 | 1.5 | 0 | 10 |
| Mango Passion | 20 fl oz | 360 | 7 | 80 | 1 | 69 | 0 | 0 | 250 |
| Stawberry Xtreme | 20 fl oz | 410 | 8 | 87 | 1 | 68 | 0.5 | 0 | 250 |
| Tropical Tango | 20 fl oz | 400 | 2 | 90 | 2 | 34 | 3 | 2 | 85 |

Note: This nutritional information presumes and is dependent upon the operator of the franchised restaurant complying with preparation, ingredient, supply, and portioning requirements. Variations may occur due to differences in procedures at stores. Seasonal differences and slight variations among different manufacturers must also be expected. Information provided is only for licensed Orange Julius stores within the United States.

### P.F. Chang's China Bistro

#### Appetizers

| FOOD ITEM | SERVING SIZE | CALORIES | PRO (g) | CARB (g) | FIBER (g) | SUGAR (g) | FAT (g) | SAT FAT (g) | SOD (mg) |
|---|---|---|---|---|---|---|---|---|---|
| Chang's Chicken in Soothing Lettuce Wraps | 1 | 630 | 44 | 92 | n/a | n/a | 8 | 2 | n/a |
| Chang's Spare Ribs | 1 | 1410 | 59 | 47 | n/a | n/a | 109 | 32 | n/a |
| Chang's Vegetarian Lettuce Wraps | 1 | 370 | 14 | 71 | n/a | n/a | 4 | n/a | n/a |
| Crab Wontons | 1 | 520 | 19 | 51 | n/a | n/a | 26 | 8 | n/a |
| Harvest Spring Rolls | 1 | 640 | 15 | 106 | n/a | n/a | 17 | 2 | n/a |
| Northern Style Spare Ribs | 1 | 1090 | 49 | 6 | n/a | n/a | 95 | 27 | n/a |
| Peking Dumplings (Pan-Fried) | 1 | 420 | 20 | 31 | n/a | n/a | 22 | 7 | n/a |
| Peking Dumplings (Steamed) | 1 | 400 | 20 | 31 | n/a | n/a | 20 | 7 | n/a |
| Salt and Pepper Calamari | 1 | 590 | 26 | 35 | n/a | n/a | 37 | 4 | n/a |
| Seared Ahi Tuna | 1 | 220 | 25 | 18 | n/a | n/a | 5 | 0 | n/a |
| Shrimp Dumplings (Pan Fried) | 1 | 360 | 24 | 26 | n/a | n/a | 17 | 2 | n/a |
| Shrimp Dumplings (Steamed) | 1 | 320 | 24 | 26 | n/a | n/a | 12 | 1 | n/a |

| FOOD ITEM | SERVING SIZE | CALORIES | PRO (g) | CARB (g) | FIBER (g) | SUGAR (g) | FAT (g) | SAT FAT (g) | SOD (mg) |
|---|---|---|---|---|---|---|---|---|---|
| **P.F. Chang's China Bistro (cont.)** | | | | | | | | | |
| **Appetizers (cont.)** | | | | | | | | | |
| Vegetable Dumplings (Pan-Fried) | 1 | 340 | 9 | 47 | n/a | n/a | 12 | 1 | n/a |
| Vegetable Dumplings (Steamed) | 1 | 300 | 9 | 47 | n/a | n/a | 8 | 0 | n/a |
| **Soups and Salads** | | | | | | | | | |
| Hot and Sour Soup | 1 cup | 56 | 3 | 2 | n/a | n/a | 4 | 1 | n/a |
| Oriental Chicken Salad | 1 cup | 940 | 60 | 49 | n/a | n/a | 56 | 6 | n/a |
| Peanut Chicken Salad | 1 cup | 1080 | 73 | 47 | n/a | n/a | 69 | 9 | n/a |
| Pin Rice Noodle Soup | 1 cup | 270 | 12 | 55 | n/a | n/a | 2 | 1 | n/a |
| Warm Duck Spinach Salad | 1 cup | 940 | 45 | 44 | n/a | n/a | 66 | 15 | n/a |
| Wild Alaskan Sockeye Salmon Salad | 1 cup | 470 | 33 | 18 | n/a | n/a | 30 | 4 | n/a |
| Wonton Soup | 1 cup | 52 | 3 | 4 | n/a | n/a | 3 | 1 | n/a |
| **Traditions** | | | | | | | | | |
| Almond Cashew Chicken | 1 lunch size | 740 | 62 | 51 | n/a | n/a | 30 | 5 | n/a |
| Beef with Broccoli | 1 lunch size | 760 | 56 | 23 | n/a | n/a | 49 | 12 | n/a |
| Crisp Honey Chicken | 1 lunch size | 860 | 43 | 84 | n/a | n/a | 36 | 3 | n/a |
| Lo Mein Beef | 1 lunch size | 850 | 47 | 90 | n/a | n/a | 34 | 8 | n/a |
| Lo Mein Chicken | 1 lunch size | 720 | 42 | 92 | n/a | n/a | 20 | 3 | n/a |
| Lo Mein Combo | 1 lunch size | 900 | 51 | 94 | n/a | n/a | 35 | 6 | n/a |
| Lo Mein Pork | 1 lunch size | 740 | 39 | 91 | n/a | n/a | 25 | 5 | n/a |
| Lo Mein Shrimp | 1 lunch size | 700 | 39 | 92 | n/a | n/a | 20 | 3 | n/a |
| Lo Mein Vegetable | 1 lunch size | 550 | 21 | 93 | n/a | n/a | 12 | 2 | n/a |
| Moo Goo Gai Pan | 1 lunch size | 610 | 61 | 32 | n/a | n/a | 25 | 4 | n/a |
| Shrimp with Lobster Sauce | 1 lunch size | 490 | 44 | 21 | n/a | n/a | 24 | 5 | n/a |
| **Vegetarian Plates and Sides** | | | | | | | | | |
| Buddha's Feast, Steamed | 1 | 200 | 10 | 44 | n/a | n/a | 2 | 0 | n/a |

| FOOD ITEM | SERVING SIZE | CALORIES | PRO (g) | CARB (g) | FIBER (g) | SUGAR (g) | FAT (g) | SAT FAT (g) | SOD (mg) |
|---|---|---|---|---|---|---|---|---|---|
| Buddha's Feast, Stir-Fried | 1 | 370 | 21 | 64 | n/a | n/a | 7 | 1 | n/a |
| Coconut Curry Vegetables | 1 | 950 | 36 | 79 | n/a | n/a | 63 | 40 | n/a |
| Garlic Snap Peas | 1 | 220 | 6 | 20 | n/a | n/a | 7 | 1 | n/a |
| Shanghai Cucumbers | 1 | 120 | 10 | 8 | n/a | n/a | 6 | 1 | n/a |
| Sichuan Style Asparagus | 1 | 170 | 11 | 29 | n/a | n/a | 4 | 1 | n/a |
| Spinach Stir-Fried with Garlic | 1 | 110 | 12 | 15 | n/a | n/a | 4 | n/a | n/a |
| Stir-Fried Eggplant | 1 | 510 | 8 | 60 | n/a | n/a | 29 | 2 | n/a |
| Vegetarian Ma Po Tofu | 1 | 760 | 45 | 40 | n/a | n/a | 52 | 6 | n/a |
| **Chicken and Duck** | | | | | | | | | |
| Cantonese Roasted Duck | 1 | 1160 | 45 | 109 | n/a | n/a | 59 | 19 | n/a |
| Chang's Spicy Chicken | 1 | 990 | 61 | 70 | n/a | n/a | 51 | 5 | n/a |
| Chicken with Black Bean Sauce | 1 | 640 | 73 | 31 | n/a | n/a | 22 | 3 | n/a |
| Ginger Chicken and Broccoli | 1 | 620 | 63 | 43 | n/a | n/a | 21 | 3 | n/a |
| Ground Chicken and Eggplant | 1 | 890 | 53 | 70 | n/a | n/a | 43 | 6 | n/a |
| Kung Pao Chicken (training table size) | 1 | 930 | 81 | 38 | n/a | n/a | 50 | 7 | n/a |
| Mu Shu Chicken | 1 | 750 | 63 | 55 | n/a | n/a | 31 | 6 | n/a |
| Orange Peel Chicken | 1 | 1090 | 65 | 73 | n/a | n/a | 60 | 5 | n/a |
| Philip's Better Lemon Chicken | 1 | 810 | 62 | 94 | n/a | n/a | 21 | 3 | n/a |
| Sweet and Sour Chicken | 1 | 800 | 43 | 89 | n/a | n/a | 31 | 3 | n/a |
| **Seafood** | | | | | | | | | |
| Cantonese Scallops | 1 | 370 | 42 | 20 | n/a | n/a | 13 | 2 | n/a |
| Cantonese Shrimp | 1 | 380 | 44 | 17 | n/a | n/a | 15 | 2 | n/a |
| Crispy Honey Shrimp | 1 | 860 | 38 | 85 | n/a | n/a | 37 | 3 | n/a |
| Hot Fish (Catfish) | 1 | 960 | 59 | 86 | n/a | n/a | 42 | 7 | n/a |
| Kung Pao Scallops | 1 | 1180 | 70 | 56 | n/a | n/a | 76 | 8 | n/a |
| Kung Pao Shrimp | 1 | 1230 | 80 | 52 | n/a | n/a | 79 | 8 | n/a |
| Lemon Pepper Shrimp | 1 | 520 | 44 | 31 | n/a | n/a | 25 | 3 | n/a |
| Lemon Scallops | 1 | 720 | 44 | 96 | n/a | n/a | 18 | 2 | n/a |

| FOOD ITEM | SERVING SIZE | CALORIES | PRO (g) | CARB (g) | FIBER (g) | SUGAR (g) | FAT (g) | SAT FAT (g) | SOD (mg) |
|---|---|---|---|---|---|---|---|---|---|
| **Traditions (cont.)** | | | | | | | | | |
| **Seafood (cont.)** | | | | | | | | | |
| Oolong Marinated Sea Bass | 1 | 740 | 78 | 39 | n/a | n/a | 30 | 4 | n/a |
| Salt and Pepper Prawns | 1 | 770 | 53 | 28 | n/a | n/a | 50 | 4 | n/a |
| Wild Alaskan Sockeye Salmon Lemon Pepper | 1 | 670 | 53 | 32 | n/a | n/a | 36 | 5 | n/a |
| Wild Alaskan Sockeye Salmon Steamed with Ginger | 1 | 740 | 60 | 49 | n/a | n/a | 36 | 5 | n/a |
| **Meat** | | | | | | | | | |
| Beef a la Sichuan | 1 | 990 | 69 | 55 | n/a | n/a | 55 | 15 | n/a |
| Mongolian Beef | 1 | 1080 | 85 | 18 | n/a | n/a | 72 | 19 | n/a |
| Mu Shu Pork | 1 | 780 | 57 | 53 | n/a | n/a | 38 | 9 | n/a |
| Orange Peel Beef | 1 | 1330 | 77 | 69 | n/a | n/a | 82 | 18 | n/a |
| Sweet and Sour Pork | 1 | 910 | 42 | 89 | n/a | n/a | 43 | 7 | n/a |
| Wok Seared Lamb | 1 | 1270 | 80 | 22 | n/a | n/a | 95 | 34 | n/a |
| **Noodles, Meins, and Rice** | | | | | | | | | |
| Brown Rice (cooked) | 1 | 350 | 7 | 73 | n/a | n/a | 3 | 0 | n/a |
| Cantonese Chow Fun Beef | 1 | 1080 | 56 | 101 | n/a | n/a | 48 | 12 | n/a |
| Chow Mein Chicken | 1 | 670 | 42 | 92 | n/a | n/a | 16 | 3 | n/a |
| Chow Mein Shrimp | 1 | 750 | 50 | 94 | n/a | n/a | 20 | 3 | n/a |
| Dan Dan Noodles | 1 | 1070 | 65 | 128 | n/a | n/a | 30 | 5 | n/a |
| Double Pan-Fried Noodles, Beef | 1 | 1240 | 57 | 111 | n/a | n/a | 61 | 13 | n/a |
| Double Pan-Fried Noodles, Vegetable | 1 | 980 | 30 | 114 | n/a | n/a | 44 | 7 | n/a |
| P.F. Chang's Fried Rice Combo | 1 | 1130 | 61 | 150 | n/a | n/a | 28 | 6 | n/a |
| White Rice (cooked) | 1 | 410 | 8 | 88 | n/a | n/a | 1 | 0 | n/a |
| **Desserts** | | | | | | | | | |
| Banana Spring Rolls | 1 | 1860 | 26 | 235 | n/a | n/a | 97 | 43 | n/a |
| New York–Style Cheesecake | 1 | 870 | 15 | 72 | n/a | n/a | 58 | 34 | n/a |
| The Great Wall of Chocolate | 1 | 1883 | 18 | 325 | n/a | n/a | 71 | 17 | n/a |

Note: Nutritional information is listed in grams and pertains to the entire dish. Because dishes are freshly prepared, nutritional values may vary slightly.
Sauces—The ingredients used to make all of our sauces is proprietary information. Should you have dietary concerns and need specific information regarding these sauces, please ask to speak with a manager or chef on your next visit to P.F. Chang's.

| FOOD ITEM | SERVING SIZE | CALORIES | PRO (g) | CARB (g) | FIBER (g) | SUGAR (g) | FAT (g) | SAT FAT (g) | SOD (mg) |
|---|---|---|---|---|---|---|---|---|---|
| **Pizza Hut** | | | | | | | | | |
| **12-Inch Medium Pizza** | | | | | | | | | |
| Chicken with Jalapeños and Mushrooms | 1 slice | 170 | 10 | 22 | 2 | 5 | 5 | 2 | 690 |
| Chicken with Onions and Green Peppers | 1 slice | 170 | 10 | 23 | 2 | 6 | 4.5 | 2 | 460 |
| Ham with Onions and Mushrooms | 1 slice | 160 | 8 | 22 | 2 | 6 | 4.5 | 2 | 470 |
| Ham with Pineapple and Tomatoes | 1 slice | 160 | 8 | 24 | 2 | 7 | 4 | 2 | 470 |
| Veggie with Green Peppers, Onions, and Tomatoes | 1 slice | 150 | 6 | 24 | 2 | 6 | 4 | 1.5 | 360 |
| Veggie with Tomatoes, Mushrooms, and Jalapeños | 1 slice | 150 | 6 | 22 | 2 | 5 | 4 | 2 | 590 |
| **14-Inch Large** | | | | | | | | | |
| Chicken with Jalapeños and Mushrooms | 1 slice | 160 | 9 | 20 | 2 | 5 | 4.5 | 2 | 630 |
| Chicken with Onions and Green Peppers | 1 slice | 160 | 9 | 22 | 2 | 6 | 4 | 2 | 420 |
| Ham with Onions and Mushrooms | 1 slice | 150 | 8 | 21 | 2 | 6 | 4 | 2 | 440 |
| Ham with Pineapple and Tomatoes | 1 slice | 150 | 7 | 22 | 1 | 7 | 4 | 2 | 440 |
| Veggie with Green Peppers, Onions, and Tomatoes | 1 slice | 140 | 6 | 22 | 2 | 6 | 3.5 | 1.5 | 330 |
| Veggie with Tomatoes, Mushrooms, and Jalapeños | 1 slice | 140 | 6 | 21 | 2 | 5 | 4 | 1.5 | 540 |
| **Quiznos** | | | | | | | | | |
| Honey Bourbon Chicken Sandwich | 1 small sandwich | 359 | 24 | 45 | 3 | n/a | 6 | 1 | 1494 |
| Sierra Smoked Turkey Sandwich | 1 small sandwich | 350 | 23 | 53 | 3 | n/a | 6 | n/a | 1140 |
| Turkey Lite Sandwich | 1 small sandwich | 334 | 17 | 52 | 3 | n/a | 6 | 1 | 1909 |
| **Red Lobster** | | | | | | | | | |
| Atlantic Salmon | 1 | 258 | n/a | 0 | 0 | n/a | 12 | n/a | n/a |
| Broiled Flounder | 1 | 240 | n/a | 0 | 0 | n/a | 5 | n/a | n/a |
| Garden Salad | 1 | 52 | n/a | 9 | 2 | n/a | 2 | n/a | n/a |
| Grilled Chicken | 1 | 314 | n/a | 0 | 0 | n/a | 8 | n/a | n/a |
| Jumbo Shrimp Cocktail | 1 appetizer | 138 | n/a | 1 | 0 | n/a | 2 | n/a | n/a |

| FOOD ITEM | SERVING SIZE | CALORIES | PRO (g) | CARB (g) | FIBER (g) | SUGAR (g) | FAT (g) | SAT FAT (g) | SOD (mg) |
|---|---|---|---|---|---|---|---|---|---|
| **Red Lobster (cont.)** | | | | | | | | | |
| Jumbo Shrimp Cocktail | 1 dinner | 228 | n/a | 2 | 0 | n/a | 4 | n/a | n/a |
| King Crab Legs | 1 | 163 | n/a | 0 | 0 | n/a | 3 | n/a | n/a |
| Live Maine Lobster | 1 | 145 | n/a | 2 | 0 | n/a | 1 | n/a | n/a |
| Petite Shrimp Topping | 1 | 30 | n/a | 1 | 0 | n/a | 1 | n/a | n/a |
| Rainbow Trout | 1 | 273 | n/a | 2 | 0 | n/a | 2 | n/a | n/a |
| Rock Lobster Tail | 1 | 258 | n/a | 0 | 0 | n/a | 3 | n/a | n/a |
| Snow Crab Legs | 1 | 262 | n/a | 0 | 0 | n/a | 5 | n/a | n/a |
| Tilapia | 1 lunch | 186 | n/a | 0 | 0 | n/a | 6 | n/a | n/a |
| Tilapia | 1 dinner | 346 | n/a | 0 | 0 | n/a | 10 | n/a | n/a |
| **Sides** | | | | | | | | | |
| Baked Potato with Pico de Gallo | 1 | 185 | n/a | 37 | 5 | n/a | 2 | n/a | n/a |
| Baked Potato without topping | 1 | 179 | n/a | 36 | 4 | n/a | 2 | n/a | n/a |
| Seasonal Vegetables with Butter | 1 | 143 | n/a | 9 | 3 | n/a | 11 | n/a | n/a |
| Seasoned Fresh Broccoli | 1 | 56 | n/a | 10 | 4 | n/a | 0 | n/a | n/a |
| **Schlotzsky's®** | | | | | | | | | |
| **Small Sandwiches** | | | | | | | | | |
| Angus Roast Beef & Cheese | 1 | 528 | 33 | 42 | n/a | 2 | 22 | n/a | 1973 |
| Chicken Breast | 1 | 330 | 26 | 50 | n/a | 2 | 4 | n/a | 1370 |
| Fresh Veggie | 1 | 330 | 14 | 50 | n/a | 4 | 9 | n/a | 839 |
| Ham & Cheese The Original™-Style | 1 | 428 | 31 | 54 | n/a | 3 | 19 | n/a | 2328 |
| Smoked Turkey Breast | 1 | 336 | 23 | 51 | n/a | 2 | 5 | n/a | 1430 |
| The Original™ | 1 | 536 | 27 | 53 | n/a | 3 | 24 | n/a | 1973 |
| Turkey Bacon Club | 1 | 454 | 41 | 54 | n/a | 3 | 31 | n/a | 1973 |
| Turkey The Original™-Style | 1 | 574 | 36 | 54 | n/a | 3 | 24 | n/a | 2179 |
| **Pizzas** | | | | | | | | | |
| BBQ Chicken & Jalapeño | 1 | 647 | 39 | 92 | n/a | 3 | 15 | n/a | 2473 |
| Combination Special | 1 | 619 | 24 | 76 | n/a | 4 | 24 | n/a | 1907 |

| FOOD ITEM | SERVING SIZE | CALORIES | PRO (g) | CARB (g) | FIBER (g) | SUGAR (g) | FAT (g) | SAT FAT (g) | SOD (mg) |
|---|---|---|---|---|---|---|---|---|---|
| Pepperoni & Double Cheese | 1 | 744 | 33 | 77 | n/a | 4 | 33 | n/a | 2244 |
| Vegetarian Special | 1 | 544 | 22 | 73 | n/a | 4 | 18 | n/a | 1715 |
| **Salads** | | | | | | | | | |
| Caesar | 1 | 101 | 5 | 9 | n/a | 2 | 5 | n/a | 345 |
| Garden | 1 | 57 | 3 | 8 | n/a | 3 | 1 | n/a | 479 |
| Grilled Chicken Caesar | 1 | 186 | 25 | 7 | n/a | 3 | 9 | n/a | 842 |
| Turkey Chef | 1 | 263 | 26 | 13 | n/a | 4 | 13 | n/a | 1466 |

Note: Salad nutrition refers to undressed salads only and does not include dressing, available in separate packets labeled with nutrition, or croutons (except for the Caesar and Grilled Chicken Caesar salads, which include croutons), also available in separate packets labeled with nutrition, and does not apply to Pick Any Two size salads.

| FOOD ITEM | SERVING SIZE | CALORIES | PRO (g) | CARB (g) | FIBER (g) | SUGAR (g) | FAT (g) | SAT FAT (g) | SOD (mg) |
|---|---|---|---|---|---|---|---|---|---|
| **Wraps** | | | | | | | | | |
| Asian Chicken | 1 | 303 | 20 | 56 | n/a | 4 | 9 | n/a | 1789 |
| Parmesan Chicken Caesar | 1 | 432 | 28 | 34 | n/a | 5 | 25 | n/a | 1380 |
| **Kids' Meals** | | | | | | | | | |
| Cheese Pizza | 1 | 475 | 18 | 72 | n/a | 3 | 13 | n/a | 1368 |
| Cheese Sandwich | 1 | 387 | 17 | 48 | n/a | 2 | 14 | n/a | 983 |
| Ham & Cheese Sandwich | 1 | 418 | 21 | 49 | n/a | 2 | 15 | n/a | 1357 |
| Pepperoni Pizza | 1 | 524 | 20 | 72 | n/a | 3 | 17 | n/a | 1554 |
| Turkey Sandwich | 1 | 291 | 15 | 48 | n/a | 2 | 4 | n/a | 1031 |
| **Schlotzsky's® Chips** | | | | | | | | | |
| Barbeque | 1 (1.5 oz) | 220 | 3 | 25 | n/a | 1 | 12 | n/a | 270 |
| Cracked Pepper | 1 (1.5 oz) | 210 | 3 | 25 | n/a | 1 | 11 | n/a | 310 |
| Jalapeño | 1 (1.5 oz) | 220 | 3 | 25 | n/a | 1 | 12 | n/a | 220 |
| Regular (Plain) | 1 (1.5 oz) | 220 | 3 | 25 | n/a | 1 | 12 | n/a | 190 |
| Salt & Vinegar | 1 (1.5 oz) | 220 | 3 | 25 | n/a | 1 | 12 | n/a | 310 |
| Sour Cream & Onion | 1 (1.5 oz) | 220 | 3 | 25 | n/a | 1 | 12 | n/a | 220 |
| **Desserts** | | | | | | | | | |
| Brownie | 1 | 220 | 3 | 25 | n/a | 1 | 12 | n/a | 270 |
| Cheesecake | 1 | 310 | 7 | 31 | n/a | 0 | 18 | n/a | 230 |
| Chocolate Chip Cookie | 1 | 162 | 2 | 23 | n/a | 1 | 7 | n/a | 54 |

| FOOD ITEM | SERVING SIZE | CALORIES | PRO (g) | CARB (g) | FIBER (g) | SUGAR (g) | FAT (g) | SAT FAT (g) | SOD (mg) |
|---|---|---|---|---|---|---|---|---|---|
| **Schlotzsky's® (cont.)** | | | | | | | | | |
| **Desserts (cont.)** | | | | | | | | | |
| Fudge Chocolate Chip Cookie | 1 | 164 | 2 | 22 | n/a | 1 | 8 | n/a | 64 |
| Oatmeal Raisin Cookie | 1 | 148 | 2 | 24 | n/a | 1 | 5 | n/a | 54 |
| Sugar Cookie | 1 | 154 | 2 | 22 | n/a | 1 | 7 | n/a | 27 |
| White Chocolate Macadamia | 1 | 169 | 2 | 22 | n/a | 1 | 8 | n/a | 56 |
| **Small Buns/Tortillas** | | | | | | | | | |
| Dark Rye | 1 | 230 | 7 | 47 | n/a | 2 | 1 | n/a | 570 |
| Jalapeño Cheese | 1 | 230 | 8 | 44 | n/a | 2 | 3 | n/a | 630 |
| Sourdough | 1 | 230 | 7 | 46 | n/a | 2 | 2 | n/a | 590 |
| Wheat | 1 | 230 | 8 | 46 | n/a | 3 | 2 | n/a | 600 |
| Wheat Tortilla, low-fat | 1 | 116 | 4 | 24 | n/a | 2 | 1 | n/a | 339 |

Note: This nutritional information is based on standard specifications and recipes, using product ingredients approved for use in the Schlotzsky's restaurant system. Variations may occur depending on the local restaurant, the season of the year, use of an alternate supplier, and/or small differences in product assembly. Some menu items may not be available in all Schlotzsky's restaurants. Schlotzsky's attempts to provide nutrition and ingredient information regarding its products that is as complete as possible. Menu items are prepared in our kitchens where dairy products, wheat, soy, peanuts and other nuts are present. If you wish further information or have special sensitivities or dietary concerns regarding specific ingredients in specific menu items, please call us at (800) 846-BUNS.

| FOOD ITEM | SERVING SIZE | CALORIES | PRO (g) | CARB (g) | FIBER (g) | SUGAR (g) | FAT (g) | SAT FAT (g) | SOD (mg) |
|---|---|---|---|---|---|---|---|---|---|
| **Café Sandwiches** | | | | | | | | | |
| Chicken Salad | 1 | 497 | 31 | 64 | 2 | | 15 | | 1,383 |
| Chicken Parmesano | 1 | 543 | 33 | 52 | 3 | | 25 | | 2,032 |
| **Souplantation/Sweet Tomatoes** | | | | | | | | | |
| **Signature Prepared Salads** | | | | | | | | | |
| Aunt Doris' Red Pepper Slaw, fat-free, vegetarian | ½ cup | 70 | 1 | 18 | 3 | 13 | 0 | 0 | 480 |
| Baja Bean & Cilantro, low-fat, vegetarian | ½ cup | 180 | 9 | 29 | 5 | 2 | 3 | 0 | 190 |
| Carrot Raisin, low-fat, vegetarian | ½ cup | 90 | 1 | 17 | 2 | 15 | 3 | 0 | 80 |
| Mandarin Noodles with Broccoli, low-fat, vegetarian | ½ cup | 120 | 3 | 19 | 2 | 5 | 3 | 0 | 380 |
| Mandarin Shells with Almonds, low-fat, vegetarian | ½ cup | 120 | 3 | 19 | 2 | 4 | 3 | 0 | 360 |
| Marinated Summer Vegetables, fat-free, vegetarian | ½ cup | 80 | 1 | 19 | 4 | 14 | 0 | 0 | 210 |
| Oriental Ginger Slaw with Krab, low-fat | ½ cup | 70 | 2 | 8 | 4 | 3 | 3 | 0 | 80 |

| FOOD ITEM | SERVING SIZE | CALORIES | PRO (g) | CARB (g) | FIBER (g) | SUGAR (g) | FAT (g) | SAT FAT (g) | SOD (mg) |
|---|---|---|---|---|---|---|---|---|---|
| Penne Pasta with Chicken in a Citrus Vinaigrette, low-fat | ½ cup | 130 | 5 | 20 | 2 | 5 | 3 | 0 | 380 |
| Southern Dill Potato, low-fat, vegetarian | ½ cup | 120 | 4 | 20 | 2 | 2 | 3 | 2 | 300 |
| Southwestern Rice & Beans, low-fat, vegetarian | ½ cup | 90 | 1 | 15 | 3 | 2 | 3 | 0 | 480 |
| Spicy Southwestern Pasta, low-fat, vegetarian | ½ cup | 130 | 5 | 21 | 4 | 3 | 3 | 0 | 350 |
| Summer Barley with Black Beans, low-fat | ½ cup | 110 | 4 | 19 | 4 | 1 | 3 | 0 | 280 |
| **Desserts and Yogurt Bar Toppings** | | | | | | | | | |
| Apple Medley (fat-free) | ½ cup | 70 | 1 | 18 | 1 | 12 | 0 | 0 | 5 |
| Banana Royale (fat-free) | ½ cup | 80 | 1 | 20 | 1 | 12 | 0 | 0 | 5 |
| Butterscotch Pudding (low-fat) | ½ cup | 140 | 4 | 24 | 0 | 24 | 3 | 0 | 160 |
| Candy Sprinkles (low-fat) | 1 tbsp | 70 | 0 | 11 | 0 | 11 | 2 | 0 | 0 |
| Chocolate Frozen Yogurt (fat-free) | ½ cup | 95 | 3 | 21 | 0 | 15 | 0 | 0 | 80 |
| Chocolate Pudding (low-fat) | ½ cup | 140 | 4 | 23 | 0 | 23 | 3 | 0 | 220 |
| Chocolate Pudding (low-fat, no sugar added) | ½ cup | 90 | 4 | 21 | <1 | 6 | 1.5 | 1 | 430 |
| Chocolate Syrup (fat-free) | 2 tbsp | 70 | 0 | 18 | 0 | 17 | 0 | 0 | 15 |
| Cranberry Crush Lemonade | ½ cup | 90 | 0 | 21 | 0 | 19 | 0 | 0 | 10 |
| Jell-O (fat-free) | ½ cup | 80 | 1 | 20 | 0 | 19 | 0 | 0 | 40 |
| Jell-O (sugar-Free, fat-free) | ½ cup | 10 | 1 | 0 | 0 | 0 | 0 | 0 | 10 |
| Nutty Waldorf Salad (low-fat) | ½ cup | 80 | 1 | 12 | 3 | 5 | 3 | 0 | 80 |
| Rice Pudding (low-fat) | ½ cup | 110 | 3 | 20 | 1 | 12 | 2 | 1 | 50 |
| Strawberry Lemonade | 1 cup | 100 | 0 | 27 | 0 | 27 | 0 | 0 | 10 |
| Tapioca Pudding (low-fat) | ½ cup | 140 | 4 | 24 | 0 | 24 | 3 | 0 | 160 |
| Vanilla Soft Serve (reduced-fat) | ½ cup | 140 | 3 | 22 | 0 | 19 | 4 | 3 | 70 |
| **Salad Dressings** | | | | | | | | | |
| Cucumber Dressing (reduced-calorie) | 2 tbsp | 80 | 0 | 4 | 0 | 3 | 7 | 1 | 290 |
| Honey Mustard Dressing (fat-free) | 2 tbsp | 45 | 0 | 10 | 0 | 9 | 0 | 0 | 160 |

| FOOD ITEM | SERVING SIZE | CALORIES | PRO (g) | CARB (g) | FIBER (g) | SUGAR (g) | FAT (g) | SAT FAT (g) | SOD (mg) |
|---|---|---|---|---|---|---|---|---|---|
| **Souplantation/Sweet Tomatoes (cont.)** | | | | | | | | | |
| **Salad Dressings (cont.)** | | | | | | | | | |
| Italian Dressing (fat-free) | 2 tbsp | 20 | 0 | 5 | 0 | 4 | 0 | 0 | 340 |
| Ranch Dressing (fat-free) | 2 tbsp | 50 | 1 | 2 | 0 | 1 | 0 | 0 | 180 |
| **Hot Pasta** | | | | | | | | | |
| Oriental Green Bean & Noodle (low-fat) | 1 cup | 240 | 7 | 45 | 2 | 4 | 3 | 0 | 780 |
| **Fresh Baked Muffins and Breads** | | | | | | | | | |
| Apple Cinnamon Bran Muffin (96% fat free) | 1 | 80 | 2 | 17 | 1 | 13 | 0.5 | 0 | 110 |
| Buttermilk Cornbread (low-fat) | 1 | 140 | 3 | 27 | 2 | 4 | 2 | 0 | 270 |
| Chile Corn Muffin (low-fat) | 1 | 140 | 3 | 27 | 2 | 5 | 3 | 1 | 320 |
| Cranberry Orange Bran Muffin (96% fat-free) | 1 | 80 | 2 | 17 | 1 | 15 | 0.5 | 0 | 110 |
| Fruit Medley Bran Muffin (96% fat-free) | 1 | 80 | 2 | 17 | 1 | 15 | 0.5 | 0 | 110 |
| Indian Grain Bread (low-fat) | 1 piece | 200 | 11 | 35 | 0 | 5 | 1.5 | 0 | 260 |
| Sourdough Bread (low-fat) | 1 piece | 150 | 9 | 27 | 0 | 0 | 0.5 | 0 | 240 |
| **Soups and Chilis** | | | | | | | | | |
| Autumn Root Vegetable with Wild Rice (fat-free, vegetarian) | 1 cup | 80 | 1 | 18 | 2 | 3 | 0 | 0 | 970 |
| Big Chunk Chicken Noodle (low-fat) | 1 cup | 160 | 15 | 17 | 2 | 3 | 3 | 2 | 480 |
| Chicken Tortilla with Jalapeño Chiles & Tomatoes (low-fat) | 1 cup | 100 | 12 | 5 | 1 | 2 | 3 | 1 | 990 |
| Classical Minestrone (low-fat, vegetarian) | 1 cup | 120 | 4 | 20 | 3 | 4 | 2 | 0 | 510 |
| Deep Kettle House Chili (low-fat) | 1 cup | 230 | 15 | 26 | 7 | 4 | 3 | 2 | 560 |
| Garden Fresh Vegetable (low-fat, vegetarian) | 1 cup | 110 | 4 | 22 | 4 | 4 | 1 | 0 | 890 |
| Garden of Eatin' (low-fat, vegetarian) | 1 cup | 150 | 5 | 25 | 6 | 6 | 3 | 0 | 770 |
| Hungarian Vegetable (low-fat, vegetarian) | 1 cup | 120 | 2 | 20 | 2 | 5 | 2 | 0 | 520 |

| FOOD ITEM | SERVING SIZE | CALORIES | PRO (g) | CARB (g) | FIBER (g) | SUGAR (g) | FAT (g) | SAT FAT (g) | SOD (mg) |
|---|---|---|---|---|---|---|---|---|---|
| Old Fashion Vegetable (low-fat, vegetarian, cholesterol-free) | 1 cup | 100 | 2 | 18 | 5 | 5 | 2 | 0 | 590 |
| Ratatouille Provencale (fat-free, vegetarian) | 1 cup | 110 | 2 | 25 | 2 | 3 | 0 | 0 | 600 |
| Rustic Tuscan Stew (low-fat) | 1 cup | 140 | 6 | 25 | 4 | 3 | 2 | 0 | 620 |
| Santa Fe Black Bean Chili (low-fat, vegetarian) | 1 cup | 190 | 9 | 26 | 8 | 2 | 3 | 0 | 580 |
| Sweet Tomato Onion (low-fat, vegetarian) | 1 cup | 90 | 2 | 11 | 2 | 5 | 3 | 0.5 | 620 |
| Three-Bean Turkey Chili (low-fat) | 1 cup | 170 | 13 | 24 | 7 | 6 | 3 | 1 | 710 |
| Tomato Parmesan & Vegetables (low-fat, vegetarian) | 1 cup | 120 | 4 | 18 | 3 | 3 | 3 | 1 | 460 |
| Vegetable Medley (low-fat, vegetarian) | 1 cup | 90 | 2 | 14 | 3 | 2 | 1 | 0 | 520 |

**Southern Tsunami Sushi**

**Salads**

| FOOD ITEM | SERVING SIZE | CALORIES | PRO (g) | CARB (g) | FIBER (g) | SUGAR (g) | FAT (g) | SAT FAT (g) | SOD (mg) |
|---|---|---|---|---|---|---|---|---|---|
| Calamari Salad | 1 container (113 g) | 148 | 8 | 22 | 1 | 6 | 3 | 0 | 1023 |
| Edamame (Soybeans) | ½ cup (75 g) | 90 | 9 | 3 | 8 | 2 | 5 | 1 | 0 |
| Edamame Salad | 1 pack (113 g) | 124 | 7 | 9 | 1 | 7 | 7 | 1 | 350 |
| Harusame Salad | 1 container (142 g) | 148 | 2 | 33 | 0 | 8 | 2 | 0 | 1401 |
| Seabreeze Salad | 1 container (113 g) | 113 | 0 | 23 | 0 | 23 | 3 | 1 | 1617 |

**Sushi**

| FOOD ITEM | SERVING SIZE | CALORIES | PRO (g) | CARB (g) | FIBER (g) | SUGAR (g) | FAT (g) | SAT FAT (g) | SOD (mg) |
|---|---|---|---|---|---|---|---|---|---|
| California Roll | 6 pieces (140 g) | 187 | 5 | 33 | 2 | 4 | 4 | 1 | 319 |
| California Roll and Inari | 4.5 pieces (155 g) | 252 | 7 | 43 | 1 | 4 | 5 | 1 | 369 |
| California Roll Plus | 4 pieces (186 g) | 247 | 7 | 44 | 3 | 5 | 5 | 1 | 424 |
| Cream Cheese Roll with Salmon | 6 pieces (140 g) | 258 | 12 | 30 | 1 | 4 | 10 | 5 | 144 |
| Crunchy Shrimp Roll | 6 pieces (147 g) | 254 | 10 | 32 | 3 | 5 | 10 | 1 | 384 |
| Dragon Roll | 6 pieces (144 g) | 254 | 9 | 33 | 2 | 6 | 9 | 2 | 206 |

## Southern Tsunami Sushi (cont.)

### Sushi (cont.)

| FOOD ITEM | SERVING SIZE | CALORIES | PRO (g) | CARB (g) | FIBER (g) | SUGAR (g) | FAT (g) | SAT FAT (g) | SOD (mg) |
|---|---|---|---|---|---|---|---|---|---|
| Eel Roll (Freshwater Eel) | 6 pieces (140 g) | 246 | 10 | 32 | 1 | 7 | 8 | 2 | 220 |
| Eel Roll (Sea Eel) | 6 pieces (140 g) | 218 | 7 | 33 | 1 | 6 | 6 | 1 | 345 |
| Fullmoon Combo | 6 pieces (140 g) | 211 | 7 | 32 | 2 | 4 | 6 | 1 | 362 |
| Futomaki | 3 pieces (158 g) | 254 | 5 | 48 | 1 | 17 | 3 | 1 | 408 |
| Inari | 2 pieces (113 g) | 210 | 5 | 36 | 0 | 3 | 4 | 0 | 248 |
| Maki & Inari | 3 pieces (162 g) | 281 | 7 | 51 | 1 | 10 | 5 | 1 | 373 |
| Marina Plate | 3 pieces (108 g) | 189 | 11 | 26 | 0 | 3 | 4 | 1 | 107 |
| Meteor Special | 7 pieces (133 g) | 192 | 8 | 34 | 1 | 4 | 2 | 0 | 153 |
| M&M Roll (Tuna & Cucumber) | 8 pieces (108 g) | 153 | 7 | 28 | 1 | 3 | 1 | 0 | 78 |
| M&M Roll (Shrimp & Avocado) | 8 pieces (108 g) | 164 | 6 | 29 | 2 | 3 | 3 | 0 | 141 |
| Ocean Crab Roll | 6 pieces (140 g) | 195 | 12 | 30 | 2 | 3 | 3 | 0 | 432 |
| Orange Roll | 6 pieces (147 g) | 191 | 10 | 33 | 1 | 4 | 3 | 0 | 664 |
| Rainbow Roll | 6 pieces (176 g) | 244 | 16 | 33 | 2 | 4 | 4 | 1 | 344 |
| Seaside Combo (Tuna & Salmon) | 8 pieces (108 g) | 180 | 10 | 29 | 1 | 3 | 2 | 0 | 87 |
| Seaside Combo (Tuna, Salmon, Shrimp, Eel) | 8 pieces (109 g) | 177 | 8 | 30 | 1 | 3 | 2 | 0 | 154 |
| Shoreline Combo | 6 pieces (165 g) | 241 | 11 | 39 | 1 | 4 | 4 | 1 | 252 |
| Snack Pack (Cucumber) | 8 pieces (108 g) | 132 | 3 | 29 | 1 | 3 | 0 | 0 | 71 |
| Snack Pack (Imitation Crab & Cucumber) | 8 pieces (108 g) | 144 | 4 | 30 | 1 | 3 | 0 | 0 | 221 |
| Spicy Roll (Salmon) | 6 pieces (140 g) | 243 | 12 | 30 | 1 | 3 | 8 | 2 | 140 |
| Spicy Roll (Shrimp) | 6 pieces (140 g) | 199 | 9 | 29 | 1 | 3 | 5 | 1 | 288 |
| Spicy Roll (Tuna) | 6 pieces (140 g) | 225 | 12 | 29 | 1 | 3 | 6 | 1 | 138 |

| FOOD ITEM | SERVING SIZE | CALORIES | PRO (g) | CARB (g) | FIBER (g) | SUGAR (g) | FAT (g) | SAT FAT (g) | SOD (mg) |
|---|---|---|---|---|---|---|---|---|---|
| Stardust Combo | 7 pieces (176 g) | 270 | 7 | 47 | 1 | 5 | 6 | 1 | 296 |
| Tempura Roll | 6 pieces (158 g) | 266 | 12 | 41 | 1 | 5 | 6 | 0 | 576 |
| Tofu Roll | 6 pieces (140 g) | 161 | 5 | 31 | 2 | 5 | 1 | 0 | 100 |
| Tsunami Roll (Imitation Crab & Fish Roe) | 6 pieces (133 g) | 234 | 10 | 35 | 2 | 6 | 7 | 1 | 630 |
| Vegetable Combo (12 pieces) | 6 pieces (140 g) | 175 | 3 | 32 | 3 | 4 | 4 | 1 | 87 |
| Vegetable Combo (24 pieces) | 12 pieces (165 g) | 223 | 4 | 46 | 2 | 6 | 2 | 0 | 120 |
| **Nigiri Sushi** | | | | | | | | | |
| Nigiri (Cuttlefish) | 1 piece (30 g) | 42 | 2 | 9 | 0 | 1 | 0 | 1 | 42 |
| Nigiri (Egg Cake) | 1 piece (39 g) | 73 | 2 | 13 | 0 | 5 | 1 | 0 | 49 |
| Nigiri (Fish Roe) | 1 piece (39 g) | 61 | 6 | 9 | 0 | 1 | 1 | 0 | 367 |
| Nigiri (Fresh Salmon) | 1 piece (38 g) | 68 | 5 | 9 | 0 | 1 | 1 | 0 | 29 |
| Nigiri (Freshwater Eel) | 1 piece (45 g) | 108 | 5 | 11 | 0 | 2 | 5 | 1 | 82 |
| Nigiri (Octopus) | 1 piece (30 g) | 57 | 2 | 9 | 0 | 1 | 1 | 0 | 50 |
| Nigiri (Sea Eel) | 1 piece (45 g) | 90 | 4 | 11 | 0 | 2 | 3 | 1 | 157 |
| Nigiri (Shrimp) | 1 piece (30 g) | 44 | 2 | 8 | 0 | 1 | 0 | 1 | 28 |
| Nigiri (Smoked Salmon) | 1 piece (38 g) | 68 | 5 | 9 | 0 | 1 | 1 | 0 | 29 |
| Nigiri (Tilapia) | 1 piece (33 g) | 49 | 2 | 8 | 0 | 1 | 1 | 0 | 26 |
| Nigiri (Tuna) | 1 piece (38 g) | 60 | 4 | 8 | 0 | 1 | 0 | 0 | 28 |
| Nigiri (Yellowtail) | 1 piece (35 g) | 54 | 3 | 8 | 0 | 1 | 1 | 0 | 25 |
| **Brown Rice Sushi** | | | | | | | | | |
| California Roll (Brown Rice) | 6 pieces (140 g) | 152 | 5 | 26 | 2 | 3 | 3 | 1 | 295 |
| Eel Roll, freshwater eel (Brown Rice) | 6 pieces (140 g) | 218 | 10 | 25 | 2 | 6 | 9 | 2 | 196 |
| Eel Roll, sea eel (Brown Rice) | 6 pieces (140 g) | 189 | 7 | 26 | 2 | 5 | 6 | 1 | 322 |

| FOOD ITEM | SERVING SIZE | CALORIES | PRO (g) | CARB (g) | FIBER (g) | SUGAR (g) | FAT (g) | SAT FAT (g) | SOD (mg) |
|---|---|---|---|---|---|---|---|---|---|
| **Southern Tsunami Sushi (cont.)** | | | | | | | | | |
| **Brown Rice Sushi (cont.)** | | | | | | | | | |
| Shoreline Combo (Brown Rice) | 6 pieces (165 g) | 205 | 10 | 30 | 3 | 3 | 5 | 1 | 222 |
| Vegetable Combo (Brown Rice) | 6 pieces (139 g) | 139 | 3 | 25 | 3 | 3 | 3 | 1 | 64 |
| **Miscellaneous** | | | | | | | | | |
| Green Horseradish | 4 g | 7 | 0 | 1 | 0 | 0 | 0 | 0 | 0 |
| Pickled Ginger | 13 g | 9 | 0 | 2 | 0 | 1 | 0 | 0 | 160 |
| Soy Sauce | 1 packet (7 g) | 16 | 2 | 2 | 0 | 0 | 0 | 0 | 660 |

Note: Southern Tsunami Sushi A Trademark of Advanced Fresh Concepts Corp. Found in better supermarkets throughout the United States and Canada. For more information, visit www.afcsushi.com.

The nutritional information listed above represents standard product formulations. AFC sushi is prepared fresh daily at each location and therefore actual product sizes may vary.

| FOOD ITEM | SERVING SIZE | CALORIES | PRO (g) | CARB (g) | FIBER (g) | SUGAR (g) | FAT (g) | SAT FAT (g) | SOD (mg) |
|---|---|---|---|---|---|---|---|---|---|
| **Starbucks** | | | | | | | | | |
| **Beverages** | | | | | | | | | |
| Café Latte, with soy milk | grande (16 fl oz) | 210 | 1 | 28 | 2 | 21 | 6 | 1 | 160 |
| Café Misto/Café au Lait, with fat-free milk | tall (12 fl oz) | 66 | n/a | n/a | n/a | n/a | n/a | n/a | n/a |
| Café Misto/Café au Lait, with soy milk | grande (16 fl oz) | 110 | 6 | 15 | <1 | 12 | 3 | 0 | 90 |
| Café Mocha, with fat-free milk, without whipped cream | tall (12 fl oz) | 174 | n/a | n/a | n/a | n/a | n/a | n/a | n/a |
| Café Mocha, with soy milk, without whipped cream | grande (16 fl oz) | 260 | 10 | 46 | 3 | 33 | 6 | 1 | 120 |
| Cappuccino, with soy milk | grande (16 fl oz) | 120 | 6 | 17 | <1 | 12 | 3 | 0 | 90 |
| Caramel Apple Cider, without whip cream | tall (12 fl oz) | 228 | n/a | n/a | n/a | n/a | n/a | n/a | n/a |
| Caramel Macchiato, with fat-free milk | tall (12 fl oz) | 168 | n/a | n/a | n/a | n/a | n/a | n/a | n/a |
| Caramel Macchiato, with soy milk | grande (16 fl oz) | 270 | 9 | 44 | 1 | 37 | 6 | 1.5 | 140 |
| Chantico Drinking Chocolate | 6 fl oz | 390 | n/a | n/a | n/a | n/a | n/a | n/a | n/a |
| Chocolate milk, soy | grande (16 fl oz) | 290 | 12 | 49 | 3 | 37 | 8 | 1 | 150 |
| Cinnamon Spice Mocha, with soy milk, without whipped cream | grande (16 fl oz) | 390 | 10 | 53 | 2 | 42 | 15 | 7 | 140 |

| FOOD ITEM | SERVING SIZE | CALORIES | PRO (g) | CARB (g) | FIBER (g) | SUGAR (g) | FAT (g) | SAT FAT (g) | SOD (mg) |
|---|---|---|---|---|---|---|---|---|---|
| Gingerbread Latté, with fat-free milk, without whipped cream | tall (12 fl oz) | 180 | n/a | n/a | n/a | n/a | n/a | n/a | n/a |
| Iced Shaken Coffee | tall (12 fl oz) | 60 | n/a | n/a | n/a | n/a | n/a | n/a | n/a |
| Iced Vanilla Latte, with fat-free milk | tall (12 fl oz) | 120 | n/a | n/a | n/a | n/a | n/a | n/a | n/a |
| Tazo Chai Iced Tea Latté, with soy milk | tall (12 fl oz) | 175 | n/a | n/a | n/a | n/a | n/a | n/a | n/a |
| Tazo Green Tea Lemonade | tall (12 fl oz) | 85 | n/a | n/a | n/a | n/a | n/a | n/a | n/a |
| Vanilla Frappuccino®, without whipped cream | 12 fl oz | 225 | n/a | n/a | n/a | n/a | n/a | n/a | n/a |
| **Baked Goods** | | | | | | | | | |
| bagel | 1 | 430 | n/a | n/a | n/a | n/a | n/a | n/a | n/a |
| blueberry muffin | 1 | 380 | n/a | n/a | n/a | n/a | n/a | n/a | n/a |
| caramel apple bar | 1 | 310 | n/a | n/a | n/a | n/a | n/a | n/a | n/a |
| cinnamon roll | 1 | 620 | n/a | n/a | n/a | n/a | n/a | n/a | n/a |
| dark chocolate graham | 1 | 140 | n/a | n/a | n/a | n/a | n/a | n/a | n/a |
| morning sunrise muffin | 1 | 330 | n/a | n/a | n/a | n/a | n/a | n/a | n/a |
| sesame bagel | 1 | 440 | n/a | n/a | n/a | n/a | n/a | n/a | n/a |
| **Subway** | | | | | | | | | |
| **Salads** | | | | | | | | | |
| BMT® | 396 g | 290 | 17 | 15 | 4 | 7 | 19 | 8 | 1360 |
| Cold Cut Combo | 405 g | 250 | 15 | 14 | 4 | 6 | 15 | 6 | 1140 |
| **Salads, 6 g fat or less** | | | | | | | | | |
| Grilled Chicken Breast & Baby Spinach | 300 g | 140 | 20 | 11 | 4 | 4 | 3 | 1 | 450 |
| Grilled Chicken Breast Strips | 392 g | 140 | 19 | 12 | 4 | 5 | 3 | 0.5 | 400 |
| Ham | 378 g | 120 | 12 | 15 | 4 | 6 | 3 | 1 | 850 |
| Roast Beef | 378 g | 130 | 13 | 13 | 4 | 6 | 3.5 | 1.5 | 490 |
| Subway Club® | 411 g | 160 | 18 | 15 | 4 | 7 | 4 | 1.5 | 880 |
| Turkey Breast | 378 g | 120 | 12 | 14 | 4 | 6 | 2.5 | 0.5 | 590 |

| FOOD ITEM | SERVING SIZE | CALORIES | PRO (g) | CARB (g) | FIBER (g) | SUGAR (g) | FAT (g) | SAT FAT (g) | SOD (mg) |
|---|---|---|---|---|---|---|---|---|---|
| **Subway (cont.)** | | | | | | | | | |
| **Salads, 6 g fat or less (cont.)** | | | | | | | | | |
| Turkey Breast & Ham | 388 g | 130 | 14 | 15 | 4 | 6 | 3 | 1 | 800 |
| Veggie Delite® | 322 g | 60 | 3 | 12 | 4 | 5 | 1 | 0 | 85 |
| **Salad Dressings** | | | | | | | | | |
| Fat-Free Italian | 2 oz (57g) | 35 | 1 | 7 | 0 | 4 | 0 | 0 | 720 |
| Ranch | 2 oz (57g) | 200 | 1 | 1 | 1 | 0 | 22 | 3.5 | 550 |
| **Sandwiches, 6 g fat or less** | | | | | | | | | |
| 6" Ham | 223 g | 290 | 18 | 47 | 4 | 8 | 5 | 1.5 | 1280 |
| 6" Oven Roasted Chicken Breast | 237 g | 330 | 24 | 47 | 4 | 9 | 5 | 1.5 | 1020 |
| 6" Roast Beef | 223 g | 290 | 19 | 45 | 4 | 8 | 5 | 2 | 920 |
| 6" Subway Club® | 256 g | 320 | 24 | 47 | 4 | 8 | 6 | 2 | 1310 |
| 6" Sweet Onion Chicken Teriyaki | 279 g | 370 | 26 | 59 | 4 | 19 | 5 | 1.5 | 1220 |
| 6" Turkey Breast | 223 g | 280 | 18 | 46 | 4 | 7 | 4.5 | 1.5 | 1020 |
| 6" Turkey Breast & Ham | 233 g | 290 | 20 | 47 | 4 | 8 | 5 | 1.5 | 1230 |
| 6" Veggie Delite® | 167 g | 230 | 9 | 44 | 4 | 7 | 3 | 1 | 520 |
| **Sandwiches, breakfast** | | | | | | | | | |
| Cheese & Egg on Deli Roll | 135 g | 270 | 16 | 35 | 3 | 2 | 9 | 4 | 670 |
| Honey Mustard Ham & Egg on Deli Roll | 170 g | 270 | 18 | 43 | 3 | 9 | 5 | 1.5 | 1080 |
| Western with Cheese on Deli Roll | 189 g | 360 | 25 | 38 | 3 | 3 | 14 | 7 | 1140 |
| **Sandwiches, cold** | | | | | | | | | |
| 6" Cold Cut Combo | 250 g | 410 | 21 | 47 | 4 | 8 | 17 | 7 | 1550 |
| 6" Tuna | 250 g | 530 | 22 | 45 | 4 | 7 | 31 | 7 | 1030 |
| **Sandwiches, deli** | | | | | | | | | |
| Ham Deli | 142 g | 210 | 11 | 36 | 3 | 4 | 4 | 1.5 | 770 |
| Roast Beef Deli | 151 g | 220 | 13 | 35 | 3 | 4 | 4.5 | 2 | 660 |
| Tuna Deli | 160 g | 350 | 14 | 35 | 3 | 3 | 18 | 5 | 750 |
| Turkey Breast Deli | 151 g | 210 | 13 | 36 | 3 | 4 | 3.5 | 1.5 | 730 |

| FOOD ITEM | SERVING SIZE | CALORIES | PRO (g) | CARB (g) | FIBER (g) | SUGAR (g) | FAT (g) | SAT FAT (g) | SOD (mg) |
|---|---|---|---|---|---|---|---|---|---|
| **Sandwiches, toasted** | | | | | | | | | |
| 6" Cheese Steak | 250 g | 360 | 24 | 47 | 5 | 9 | 10 | 4.5 | 1100 |
| 6" Spicy Italian | 226 g | 480 | 21 | 46 | 4 | 8 | 25 | 9 | 1670 |
| 6" Subway Melt® | 254 g | 380 | 25 | 48 | 4 | 8 | 12 | 5 | 1610 |
| **Soup** | | | | | | | | | |
| Brown and Wild Rice with Chicken | 1 cup (240 g) | 190 | 6 | 17 | 2 | 3 | 11 | 4.5 | 990 |
| Cheese with Ham and Bacon | 1 cup (240 g) | 240 | 8 | 17 | 1 | 5 | 15 | 6 | 1160 |
| Chicken and Dumpling | 1 cup (240 g) | 130 | 7 | 16 | 1 | 2 | 4.5 | 2.5 | 1030 |
| Chili Con Carne | 1 cup (240 g) | 240 | 15 | 23 | 8 | 14 | 10 | 5 | 860 |
| Cream of Broccoli | 1 cup (240 g) | 130 | 5 | 15 | 2 | 0 | 6 | 0 | 860 |
| Cream of Potato with Bacon | 1 cup (240 g) | 200 | 4 | 21 | 2 | 3 | 11 | 4 | 840 |
| Golden Broccoli & Cheese | 1 cup (240 g) | 180 | 5 | 16 | 2 | 3 | 11 | 4 | 1120 |
| Minestrone | 1 cup (240 g) | 90 | 7 | 7 | 1 | 1 | 4 | 1 | 1180 |
| New England Style Clam Chowder | 1 cup (240 g) | 110 | 5 | 16 | 1 | 1 | 3.5 | 0.5 | 990 |
| Roasted Chicken Noodle | 1 cup (240 g) | 60 | 6 | 7 | 1 | 1 | 1.5 | 0.5 | 940 |
| Spanish Style Chicken with Rice | 1 cup (240 g) | 90 | 5 | 13 | 1 | 1 | 2 | 0.5 | 800 |
| Tomato Garden Vegetable with Rotini | 1 cup (240 g) | 100 | 3 | 20 | 2 | 7 | 0.5 | 0 | 900 |
| Vegetable Beef | 1 cup (240 g) | 90 | 5 | 15 | 3 | 3 | 1 | 0.5 | 1050 |
| **Cookies** | | | | | | | | | |
| Chocolate Chip | 1 (45 g) | 210 | 2 | 30 | 1 | 18 | 10 | 4 | 160 |
| Chocolate Chunk | 1 (45 g) | 220 | 2 | 30 | 1 | 17 | 10 | 3.5 | 105 |
| Double Chocolate | 1 (45 g) | 210 | 2 | 30 | 1 | 20 | 10 | 4 | 170 |
| M & M | 1 (45 g) | 210 | 2 | 30 | 1 | 17 | 10 | 3.5 | 105 |
| Oatmeal Raisin | 1 (45 g) | 200 | 3 | 30 | 2 | 16 | 8 | 2.5 | 170 |
| Peanut Butter | 1 (45 g) | 220 | 4 | 26 | 1 | 16 | 12 | 4 | 200 |
| Sugar | 1 (45 g) | 230 | 2 | 28 | 0 | 14 | 12 | 3.5 | 135 |
| White Macadamia Nut | 1 (45 g) | 220 | 2 | 28 | 1 | 17 | 11 | 3.5 | 160 |

| FOOD ITEM | SERVING SIZE | CALORIES | PRO (g) | CARB (g) | FIBER (g) | SUGAR (g) | FAT (g) | SAT FAT (g) | SOD (mg) |
|---|---|---|---|---|---|---|---|---|---|
| **Subway (cont.)** | | | | | | | | | |
| **Fruizle Express** | | | | | | | | | |
| Berry Lishus | small (369 g) | 110 | 1 | 28 | 1 | 27 | 0 | 0 | 30 |
| Berry Lishus, with Banana | small (396 g) | 140 | 1 | 35 | 2 | 27 | 0 | 0 | 30 |
| Peach Pizazz | small (341 g) | 100 | 0 | 26 | 0 | 26 | 0 | 0 | 25 |
| Pineapple Delight | small (369 g) | 130 | 1 | 33 | 1 | 33 | 0 | 0 | 25 |
| Pineapple Delight, with Banana | small (396 g) | 160 | 1 | 40 | 2 | 33 | 0 | 0 | 25 |
| Sunrise Refresher | small (341 g) | 120 | 1 | 29 | 1 | 28 | 0 | 0 | 20 |

Note: Subs with 6 grams of fat or less include Italian or wheat bread, lettuce, tomatoes, pickles, onions, green peppers, and olives. All other sandwich values include cheese unless otherwise noted.
Salads contain meat/poultry, standard vegetables and do not include salad-dressing or croutons.
Addition of other condiments and fixings will alter nutrition values.

| FOOD ITEM | SERVING SIZE | CALORIES | PRO (g) | CARB (g) | FIBER (g) | SUGAR (g) | FAT (g) | SAT FAT (g) | SOD (mg) |
|---|---|---|---|---|---|---|---|---|---|
| **Taco Bell** | | | | | | | | | |
| Bean Burrito | 213 g | 350 | 13 | 56 | 9 | 4 | 8 | 2 | 1220 |
| Burrito Supreme, Chicken | 241 g | 350 | 19 | 50 | 6 | 5 | 8 | 2 | 1270 |
| Burrito Supreme, Steak | 241 g | 350 | 17 | 50 | 6 | 5 | 9 | 2.5 | 1260 |
| Enchirito, Beef | 206 g | 270 | 12 | 35 | 5 | 3 | 9 | 3 | 1300 |
| Enchirito, Chicken | 206 g | 250 | 16 | 34 | 5 | 3 | 5 | 1.5 | 1230 |
| Enchirito, Steak | 206 g | 250 | 14 | 34 | 6 | 3 | 7 | 2 | 1220 |
| Fiesta Burrito, Chicken | 198 g | 340 | 16 | 50 | 3 | 4 | 8 | 2 | 1160 |
| Gordita Baja, Chicken | 153 g | 230 | 15 | 29 | 2 | 7 | 6 | 1 | 570 |
| Gordita Baja, Steak | 153 g | 230 | 13 | 29 | 3 | 7 | 7 | 1.5 | 570 |
| Grilled Steak Soft Taco | 128 g | 170 | 11 | 21 | 2 | 3 | 5 | 1.5 | 560 |
| Ranchero Chicken Soft Taco | 135 g | 170 | 12 | 22 | 2 | 3 | 4 | 1 | 710 |
| Tostada | 177 g | 200 | 8 | 30 | 8 | 2 | 6 | 1 | 670 |
| **TCBY** | | | | | | | | | |
| 96% Fat-Free Frozen Yogurt | ½ cup | 140 | | | | | | | |
| Nonfat Frozen Yogurt No Sugar Added | ½ cup | 90 | | | | | | | |
| Nonfat Frozen Yogurt | ½ cup | 110 | | | | | | | |
| Cappucino Chiller | 16 fl oz | 481 | | | | | | | |

| FOOD ITEM | SERVING SIZE | CALORIES | PRO (g) | CARB (g) | FIBER (g) | SUGAR (g) | FAT (g) | SAT FAT (g) | SOD (mg) |
|---|---|---|---|---|---|---|---|---|---|
| Oreo Shake | 16 fl oz | 738 | | | | | | | |
| Rocky Road Shiver | 16 fl oz | 864 | | | | | | | |
| Sorbet Nonfat Nondairy | ½ cup | 100 | | | | | | | |
| Strawberry Shortcake | 1 | 450 | | | | | | | |
| Turtle Sundae | 1 | 1000 | | | | | | | |
| **Wendy's** | | | | | | | | | |
| **Sandwiches and Chicken** | | | | | | | | | |
| Black Forest Ham Frescata | 1 | 400 | 21 | 50 | 4 | 8 | 13 | 2 | 1390 |
| Jr. Cheeseburger | 1 | 320 | 17 | 34 | 2 | 7 | 13 | 6 | 820 |
| Jr. Hamburger | 1 | 280 | 15 | 34 | 2 | 7 | 9 | 3.5 | 600 |
| Kids' Meal Crispy Chicken Nuggets | 4 pieces | 180 | 8 | 10 | 0 | 0 | 11 | 2.5 | 390 |
| Roasted Turkey and Basil Pesto Frescata | 1 | 420 | 21 | 50 | 4 | 4 | 16 | 3 | 1530 |
| Roasted Turkey and Swiss Frescata | 1 | 490 | 26 | 52 | 4 | 5 | 21 | 7 | 1530 |
| Ultimate Chicken Grill | 1 | 330 | 31 | 41 | 2 | 8 | 5 | 1 | 990 |
| Ultimate Grilled Grill, chicken only, no roll, vegetables, or condiments | 1 | 120 | 23 | 2 | 0 | 0 | 2.5 | 0.5 | 630 |
| **Salads** | | | | | | | | | |
| Caesar Chicken Salad | 1 | 180 | 27 | 9 | 4 | 4 | 5 | 2.5 | 550 |
| Caesar Side Salad | 1 | 70 | 5 | 3 | 2 | 1 | 4.5 | 2 | 135 |
| Mandarin Chicken Salad | 1 | 170 | 23 | 18 | 3 | 13 | 2 | 0.5 | 480 |
| Side Salad | 1 | 35 | 1 | 8 | 2 | 4 | 0 | 0 | 25 |
| Southwest Taco Salad | 1 | 440 | 30 | 32 | 9 | 10 | 22 | 12 | 1100 |
| **Side Dishes** | | | | | | | | | |
| Baked Lay's potato chips | 1 bag | 130 | 2 | 26 | 2 | 2 | 2 | 0 | 200 |
| Baked Potato, plain | 10 oz | 270 | 7 | 61 | 7 | 3 | 0 | 0 | 25 |
| Baked Potato, sour cream and chives | 1 | 320 | 8 | 63 | 7 | 4 | 4 | 2.5 | 50 |
| Chili | small (8 oz) | 220 | 17 | 23 | 5 | 6 | 6 | 2.5 | 780 |
| Mandarin Orange Cup | 5 oz | 80 | 1 | 19 | 1 | 17 | 0 | 0 | 15 |
| Strawberry-Flavored Yogurt, low-fat | 1 | 140 | 6 | 27 | 0 | 11 | 1.5 | 1 | 85 |

| FOOD ITEM | SERVING SIZE | CALORIES | PRO (g) | CARB (g) | FIBER (g) | SUGAR (g) | FAT (g) | SAT FAT (g) | SOD (mg) |
|---|---|---|---|---|---|---|---|---|---|
| **Wendy's (cont.)** | | | | | | | | | |
| **Dressings and Sauces** | | | | | | | | | |
| BBQ Nugget Sauce | 1 packet | 45 | 1 | 10 | 0 | 8 | 0 | 0 | 170 |
| Caesar Dressing salad dressing | 1 packet | 120 | 1 | 1 | 0 | 0 | 13 | 2.5 | 220 |
| Creamy Ranch salad dressing, reduced-fat | 1 packet | 100 | 1 | 6 | 1 | 3 | 8 | 1.5 | 450 |
| French salad dressing, fat-free | 1 packet | 80 | 0 | 19 | 0 | 16 | 0 | 0 | 210 |
| Honey Mustard salad dressing, low-fat | 1 packet | 110 | 0 | 21 | 0 | 16 | 3 | 0 | 340 |
| Sour Cream, reduced-fat, acidified | 1 packet | 45 | 1 | 2 | 0 | 1 | 3.5 | 2.5 | 30 |
| Sweet and Sour Nugget Sauce | 1 packet | 50 | 0 | 13 | 0 | 11 | 0 | 0 | 120 |
| Sweet and Spicy Hawaiian Dipping Sauce | 1 packet | 70 | 0 | 17 | 0 | 13 | 0 | 0 | 350 |
| **Beverages** | | | | | | | | | |
| Milk, 2% reduced-fat | 1 | 120 | 8 | 13 | 0 | 12 | 4.5 | 3 | 135 |
| Diet Coke | medium (20 fl oz) | 0 | 0 | 0 | 0 | 0 | 0 | 0 | 15 |
| Minute Maid Light Lemonade | medium (20 fl oz) | 5 | 0 | 0 | 0 | 0 | 0 | 0 | 0 |
| Dasani bottled water | 1 | 0 | 0 | 0 | 0 | 0 | 0 | 0 | 0 |
| Junior Frosty | 1 | 160 | 4 | 28 | 0 | 21 | 4 | 2.5 | 75 |

Note: The information contained on this list is effective as of March 1, 2006. Wendy's International, Inc., its subsidiaries, affiliates, franchisees, and employees do not assume responsibility for a particular sensitivity or allergy to any food product provided in our restaurants. We encourage anyone with food sensitivities, allergies, or special dietary needs to check on a regular basis with Wendy's Consumer Relations Department to obtain the most up-to-date information.